'Dr Norbert Goldfield is a "Renaissance Physician." His interests and experience range from local to global. He is both an idealist and realist whose hopes and thoughts lead to action. This highly readable book does not merely recount his experience with the COVID-19 pandemic in practice and at the health care organizational level but leads to important thoughts about how pandemics might be managed better in the future.'

Stephen C. Schoenbaum, MD, MPH, *formerly, special advisor to the President, Josiah Macy Jr. Foundation and Executive Vice President for Programs, The Commonwealth Fund*

'For decades, Dr. Norbert Goldfield has provided a beacon for what health care and public health should be. Dedicated clinician, important health services researcher, peace activist, and policy analyst, Dr. Goldfield has a unique combination of insights about the changes we need. In this book, drawing on both his own personal stories and science, he brings all of that expertise and wisdom to a focus through the lens of the COVID pandemic, and he offers prescriptions for the future that no one who cares about American health care can afford to ignore.'

Donald M. Berwick, MD, *President Emeritus and Senior Fellow, Institute for Healthcare Improvement*

'In his compelling new book, Dr. Norbert Goldfield puts the COVID-19 pandemic in the context of badly dysfunctional US health care and political systems. How should ethical health professionals respond, not just to the pandemic, but to the broader politico-economic disruptions wrought by the Donald Trump era? Drawing on his careers in medicine, public health, health policy, as well as organizing and activism, he offers clear advice, strategies, and actions for our dangerous times.'

Prof. John E. McDonough, DrPH, MPA, *Professor of Practice, Department of Health Policy & Management, Director, Executive & Continuing Professional Education (ECPE), Harvard T. H. Chan School of Public Health*

'Dr. Goldfield has put together a very readable and meaningful first-hand account of what it means to be a compassionate physician during a global pandemic when the conduct of our public officials frequently influenced patients to ignore science and any notion of community and public health. And recognizing the potential power of organized health professionals to do public good, he acknowledges his disappointment with organized medicine and licensing boards of all health professionals in not stepping up and protecting the reputation of science and the health of the public. This is a must read for all health professionals and office holders who take an oath to protect the public good.'

Gordon H. Smith, J.D., *former Executive Vice President, Maine Medical Association*

'I've known Dr. Goldfield for well over a decade and first met him while I was serving as the Texas Medicaid Director and Deputy Health and Human Services Executive Commissioner. He is as much a visionary now as he was when we first met in 2010.' Dr. Goldfield was instrumental in re-engineering how Medicaid programs pay for services – moving away from volume and towards a model based on value. To put it simply he is passionate about improving health. This ambitious book takes the tragedy of COVID and answers the question – what next. This book will be of interest to all – health professionals and the lay public – who want a better response to this and future pandemics. His book is a hopeful, practical, and doable set of specific ideas that we can debate, learn from, and then put into action!'

Billy R. Millwee, MHA, *President/CEO, Millwee & Associates, LLC*

'This book offers a portrait of America in the throes of the COVID-19 pandemic – sharing insights of a practicing physician who is also a visionary scholar and activist. The book spans the arc of the pandemic, taking the reader from the early days to the way forward – looking not just at how individuals were impacted but also at the challenges the pandemic poses to U.S. health care and public health systems. Dr. Goldfield closes the book with a "Call to Action" to our health care community and society overall, proposing a community-centered approach to care, strengthening our capacity to reach all community members in times of substantial health challenge that we will inevitably face again in the years to come.'

E. Lee Rosenthal, PhD, MS, MPH, *Community Health Worker Core Consensus (C3) Project Director/PI, FSOM Society, Community, and the Individual Course Director, Foster School of Medicine, Texas Tech University Health Sciences Center, El Paso*

'Dr. Norbert Goldfield is a powerful champion for community-based solutions to the pressing health care challenges our country faces. I urge everyone to read his prescription for how each of us has a role to play in improving outcomes by restoring confidence in America's public health system and rebuilding trust between health professionals and the communities they serve.'

Congressman Jim McGovern, *House of Representatives*

Public Health, Public Trust, and American Fragility in a Pandemic Era

This book explores how professionals and policymakers in mental and physical health care can use lessons from the COVID pandemic to better inform future public policy and treatment.

Using the United States as a test case, Norbert Goldfield draws on his professional experience in healthcare and policy-making to explore how some societies have emerged from the pandemic with increasing internal conflicts. The author uses excerpts from his own COVID diary to revisit key stages in response to the COVID pandemic to highlight where division has entered the public health discourse, and to set out an alternative vision of how mental and physical health can be framed professionally and publicly. In addition to this account, Dr Goldfield details how our political system should change with respect to pandemics and how health professionals, together with the lay public, can help. Specifically, the book highlights the three critical issues confronting American pandemic fragility: increasing vaccinations, decreasing misinformation, and fostering greater linkages between our public and acute health systems.

This book will be invaluable for all types of health care professionals, both in mental and physical health arenas, lay people interested in the pandemic, and for policymakers.

Norbert Goldfield is CEO of the bipartisan Ask Nurses and Doctors (www. asknursesdoctors.com) that organizes health professionals in support of political candidates favoring health reform. His previous book, also published with Routledge, *Peace Building through Women's Health* (2021), builds on his peace through health work with Israelis and Palestinians (www.healingdivides.org).

Public Health, Public Trust, and American Fragility in a Pandemic Era

The Critical Role of Health Care Professionals

Norbert Goldfield

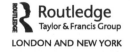

LONDON AND NEW YORK

Cover image by © Getty Image

First published 2024
by Routledge
4 Park Square, Milton Park, Abingdon, Oxon OX14 4RN

and by Routledge
605 Third Avenue, New York, NY 10158

Routledge is an imprint of the Taylor & Francis Group, an informa business

© 2024 Norbert Goldfield

British Library Cataloguing-in-Publication Data
A catalogue record for this book is available from the British Library

ISBN: 978-1-032-54705-3 (hbk)
ISBN: 978-1-032-54706-0 (pbk)
ISBN: 978-1-003-42625-7 (ebk)

DOI: 10.4324/9781003426257

Typeset in Adobe Garamond Pro
by KnowledgeWorks Global Ltd.

To health professionals everywhere in the world but especially
to those and their families who have suffered from this
pandemic and to those who have paid the ultimate price

Contents

Preface xi
COVID Timeline xv
List of Abbreviations xix

**PART I BACKGROUND PERSPECTIVES, THE COVID
"DIARY," AND AMERICAN FRAGILITY** 1

1 Introduction 3

2 Peace through Health and American Fragility: Evidence
for Peace through Health Impact 11

3 The COVID "Notes" 39

4 American Fragility during and after the COVID Pandemic:
The Role to Date of Health Professionals and Health
Professional Associations 125

**PART II INCREASING PUBLIC TRUST IN THE
UNITED STATES; THE CRITICAL ROLE OF HEALTH
PROFESSIONALS IN REBUILDING THE PUBLIC
HEALTH SYSTEM AND DECREASING FRAGILITY** 139

5 COVID-19 and the Mental Health and Substance Abuse Crisis:
Tragedy, Positive Changes, and Resilience 141

6 COVID-19 Crisis Creates Opportunities for Community Health
Resilience Plan: Community Health Workers at the Center 159

7 Fitting Community Health Resilience Plan (CHRP) into the
Existing Healthcare Delivery Patchwork: The Politics of CHRP 169

8 Building Trust in Public Health: Coordinating Our Public Health and Acute Care Systems... 181

9 Reform of Our National and International Organizations: Leadership, Trust, Power—and Money 197

10 What Can Health Professionals Do to Better Address This and Future Pandemics? 213

11 Health Professionals Can Have an Even Greater Impact on This and Future Pandemics: Final Arguments and a Call to Action 225

Index 247

Preface

How to Use This Book and Acknowledgments

March 2020 was the start of the saddest and yet one of the most personally intimate of times in my life. At that point, I had been married for 40 years, with two children in their thirties. I live in Northampton, a small town in western Massachusetts, about one and a half hours west of Boston in the northeast part of the United States. It is a rural area close to small cities, including Springfield, population of 150,000, where I practice as an internist.

For more than 45 years, I worked at a community health center as an adult medicine physician. I also founded an organization, Healing Across the Divides, that funds community health initiatives in Israel and the Palestinian Territories. In addition, until 2016, I worked as a researcher on health care systems. I resigned after the 2016 presidential election and, shortly after that, started a political consulting group, Ask Nurses and Doctors, designed to organize local health care professionals in support of competitive candidates who advocate health reform. Over the past two years, the personal and every aspect of the professional intersected and led to the writing of this book.

It has been an intimate time in that with the onset of the pandemic my daughter, my son, and my son's wife decamped from New York and Boston, respectively, and moved next door, 50 feet away, into a cottage that we own next door. Yet having your children in their thirties move back home suddenly can be an awkward situation. None of them, especially my daughter, who was just about to start her long-delayed graduate school, really wanted to live with their parents or in-laws. But the alternative was worse – much worse. Hearing ambulance sirens 24/7, my daughter in March 2020 couldn't get to sleep in her New York City apartment. My son and his wife were both working remotely in Boston. With the onset of the pandemic, they were all cooped up in their apartment and living with roommates, one of whom was a "front-line" physician – meaning she had regular contact with COVID-19 patients. My son and his wife had planned on giving up their apartment in June and were beginning to think of moving to a more rural area – in preparation, as they tell it, for the effects of climate change on coastal cities. So instead of leaving in June, they came to Northampton in April.

From a family perspective, we were suddenly thrown together. The kids – well, the bottom line is that they are not only adults chronologically but behaved like adults during this very stressful time. They pitched in and we all got along. During that first year of the pandemic, we shouldn't forget that most people, including ourselves, did not interact with others unless it was absolutely necessary. We interacted only with each other. We had our "circle" or "pod." I went shopping every two weeks as soon as the supermarket opened. Very quickly, my practice shut down, and I, as an older, at-risk individual, "saw" patients only telephonically. That was it in terms of physically going out into spaces that contained a lot of people.

On one fundamental level, it was, in some paradoxical way, the happiest of times. As I write this, my daughter is finally in graduate school, having left our home next door after almost a year. Our son and his wife, having decided to stay in Northampton, bought a house fifteen minutes away. Who knows if they would have permanently moved to Northampton if it weren't for the pandemic? It is doubtful (I fervently hope) that we will ever live together again as we did that first year of the pandemic.

Yet this period proved the most depressing of my entire professional career. Especially at the beginning of the pandemic, patient after patient of mine suffered through hospitalizations, intubation, and death. I reflected on this abysmal outcome which was the result of the United States government abdicating its core function of protecting its inhabitants. I began to keep a diary that included reflections on my patients in combination with policy observations drawn from my more than 30 years as a researcher on our health care system. At the same time, at the start of the pandemic, I was also finishing a book entitled *Peace Building through Women's Health: Psychoanalytic, Sociopsychological, and Community Perspectives on the Israeli-Palestinian Conflict*. It places the work that I've been doing for the past several decades in Israel and the Palestinian Territories, via the nonprofit Healing Across the Divides I founded, into a wider context. I looked at our work in the Middle East through two research/historical lenses: the peace through health literature and the many perspectives on the Israeli-Palestinian conflict. I've taught courses at the college level on peace through health. I taught students about the different peace through health tools (see Chapter 2). One of these tools deals with how governments that are emerging from conflict look to reestablish a functioning health system. Government officials together with health care professionals do this not just as a good unto itself but in an effort to establish the government's legitimacy, to increase trust in the possibility that the government can deliver on its promise to function effectively.

As I continued to write my diary, called "COVID-19 Notes," and forward it to about a thousand individuals throughout the world, I realized that the United States was engaged in the exact opposite of the peace through health tool described above. That is, the United States is slowly, but inexorably, entering conflict – with itself. While not the only or even the principal cause, the COVID-19 pandemic has greatly exacerbated this trend into greater conflict within the United States. Hence, paradoxically, my work with Israelis and Palestinians in one of the longest-running wars in the world today is the genesis of this book that deals with increasing American fragility during our pandemic era. Such fragility emanating from the COVID-19 pandemic is not unique to the United States, but it is most evident in this country, given that we as a nation have performed worse in this pandemic on virtually every possible metric as compared with any other industrialized country.

My "COVID-19 Notes" details this tragedy both as it affected my patients and how it played out and continues to play out at a national policy level. The "COVID-19 Notes" also highlight possible peace through health engagement of the health profession. The remainder of the book expands on health policy and health care professional peace-building themes and addresses the question of the potential roles of health care professionals in dealing with American (and beyond) fragility in this new pandemic era. The introductory chapters provide the policy (chapter 1) and peace-building frameworks (chapter 2) that lead to my diary (chapter 3). The diary is in chronological order, with my first COVID note coming first and my most recent entry coming last. Chapter 4 examines in historical and theoretical terms the word "fragility" and how it applies to the United States.

From a policy perspective, chapters 5 through 8 deal with different health professional approaches and responses to the pandemic, with chapter 5 centered on COVID-19 and mental health and substance abuse (MHSA), and chapter 6 on a reimagined population health system that places community health workers at the center. Chapter 7 highlights the political forces that will be needed to marshal any health system that focuses on community health. Recognizing that comprehensive national responses to the pandemic are virtually impossible to imagine in the present political climate, chapter 8 specifies the elements of a statewide system for Massachusetts, where I live. Policymakers and activists could apply these elements to any state, and I've already spoken with people in different states about implementing the suggested approach in their state. Chapter 9 examines national (most importantly, the Centers for Disease Control and Prevention) and international (such as the World Health Organization) entities and explores how they could evolve in response to the COVID-19 pandemic.

Chapter 10 further characterizes the roles that health professionals could possibly play, together with a call to action. I delve into the following questions: What are the different *peace through health* approaches that health professionals can undertake? How should health professionals best engage with senior-level politicians whose electoral success may be predicated on opposition to community approaches to the control of this (and future) pandemics, including vaccinations and other traditional public health interventions? How can health professionals best engage with those groups most affected by the pandemic – low-income people, nonwhite people, and Republicans? And, most important, what are the prospects for success for this health professional engagement?

Chapter 11 provides concluding comments and offers responses to the following questions: Will the United States be able to better confront this and future pandemics? How does this tie into increased American fragility? How can health professionals help to better confront current and future pandemics and thus decrease American fragility? In short, I am not optimistic, but we must try, and I hope that this book will contribute to the debate.

At this point, I don't remember in my bones a time without COVID-19. In addition, I am not hopeful about our ability to reverse the trend toward ever-increasing conflict. I am also dubious that even a substantial minority of health professionals are likely to make a significant effort to reverse American fragility by working together as a profession to create comprehensive responses to this pandemic at a state and then national level. But if we are to diminish American fragility, this book, in many ways, summarizes what I think is possible. I fervently believe that without the American government demonstrating the ability to handle pandemics such as COVID-19, our fragility as a nation will only increase. However, if a small group of health professionals take a path that could lead to comprehensive pandemic solutions, adapting it as needed, we could help reverse American fragility and protect people who live in the United States. This book is dedicated to opening the way to such a path.

I have many acknowledgments to make. I would like to first give profound thanks to my immediate family. I thank them profusely for their support during my writing and, most importantly, for being the Goldfield-Matthews-Bennett "pod" during the worst of the pandemic. My wife Sandra Matthews, in addition, spent hours going over much of my manuscript. She always couched her many suggestions in kindness. Lory Frankel also spent many hours copyediting the work. She truly is an amazing copyeditor and a friend for more than 50 years! John McDonough made some very trenchant comments that I tried my best to take to heart. I thank the editors at Routledge for their support throughout this process. They are always a pleasure to deal with.

I would like to thank and offer my profound respect and appreciation to my patients – especially to those who continue to suffer or who tragically died during the pandemic. When referring to any of my patients, I completely change every aspect of their character, identity, and what occurred to them. Any resemblance that a reader might perceive is purely coincidental.

To be sure, all errors in the book are mine and mine alone.

Lastly, I wish to thank from the bottom of my heart all the health professionals throughout the world who gave of themselves, including many who gave with their lives during this pandemic. It is to them and those who are suffering from Long COVID that I owe the most thanks. As someone who has always considered it an honor to be a health professional, it is to them that this book is dedicated. I only hope that this book will lead to changes in our response to this and future pandemics. If we can do that even a little bit, we can decrease American fragility and rebuild public trust in ourselves and public services.

COVID Timeline

2020

January 9: WHO Announces Mysterious Coronavirus-Related Pneumonia in Wuhan, China

January 21: CDC Confirms First US Coronavirus Case

January 31: WHO Issues Global Health Emergency; U.S. follows shortly after

Beginning of March: Public health professionals encourage everyone to stay at home

March 17: our practice changes in 2 hours – gowns, masks, no one with cold symptoms allowed

March 17: CMS Expands Use of Telehealth

March: California Issues Statewide Stay-at-Home Order;

March 30: My First Patient Dies of COVID – all alone

April 2: All my visits become telephonic

April 15: I can now order tests for COVID;

April: Republicans Drs Scott Gottlieb and Marc McClelland propose national contact tracing and economic recovery program – goes nowhere

April 23: Trump said re bleach: "can we do something like ... injection inside... a cleaning?"

May 7: Irish Times: The world has loved, hated and envied the US. Now... we pity it.

May 15: USA Today: 50 states 50 different approaches

May 2020: Remdesivir given FDA EUA as the first scientifically proven treatment for COVID

May 22: My patient who was intubated for weeks – goes home

May 28: US COVID-19 Deaths Pass the 100,000 Mark

June: article in Science – contact tracing, social distancing, and travel restrictions work

July: Scott Atlas, who has no relevant background except his anti-science punditry on Fox News hired by the White House as COVID advisor

September 28: Global COVID-19 Deaths Surpass 1 Million

September 30: Dylan Scott says: 20 million more will lose their health insurance under Trump, 25 million will gain under Bide

October 22: FDA Approves Remdesivir as First COVID-19 Drug

November 17: The hospital I admit in NYT Magazine: "The Trump administration had achieved one of its goals: It had trained Americans not to rely on it. Everyone was on his or her own in this pandemic. That was the American way.

November 4: US Reports Unprecedented 100,000 Cases in 1 Day

November 18: Pfizer, BioNTech Vaccine Is 95% Effective; December FDA Agrees to Emergency Use Authorization (EUA) for COVID-19 Vaccine from Pfizer

December 15: I get my first COVID vaccine

2021

January 6: A mob attacks the U.S. Capitol.

February 1: Where I live, only people over 75 are "eligible" (many ineligible people I know are cutting in line).

April: According to the National Center for Health Statistics, suicides totaled fewer than 45,000 in 2020. Drug overdoses increased dramatically last year; more than 88,000 overdose deaths.

Paper: Vaccination protects the person being vaccinated but lower community infection rates.

Vaccines available for all who want it

May 2021: Senator Ron Johnson: "over 3,000 deaths … within 30 days of taking the vaccine."

June 2021: Fauci quote: more than 99% of people who die of COVID in June in the U.S. weren't vaccinated.

July: I go back to seeing patients face to face; More than 99% of the deaths and 97% of the hospitalizations are among the unvaccinated.

August 11: The country reported more than 900,000 cases in a week for the first time since February 4, while deaths surpassed 4,500 a week. Cases are rising in 46 states.

August 23 FDA announced the first approval of a COVID-19 vaccine. I had several patients who were immediately willing to get the vaccine.

August 25: Seventy-five doctors in Palm Beach Gardens staged a symbolic walkout to protest unvaccinated people who are flooding Florida hospitals.

September: Governor Ron DeSantis announces the appointment of Dr Joseph Ladapo to become Surgeon General of Florida.

A group of physicians in Atlanta recently pleaded with Georgians to get vaccinated. "Hours later, Gov. Brian Kemp announced an executive order blocking cities from forcing private businesses to enact mask rules, mandate vaccines or take other actions to mitigate the coronavirus."

September 14: one of my antivax patients tells me I got the vaccine instead of being fired;

Sturgis Motorcycle Rally in South Dakota – a mega super spreader event

September 29: Research documents that vaccine mandates work – saving many lives

October: I get my COVID booster

December: Paxlovid given emergency use authorization

Scientific article documents that: people living in counties that went 60% or higher for Trump in November 2020 had 2.7 times the death rates of those that went for Biden

Trump's White House doctor, a physician, now a congressman, claimed that Omicron is a Democratic mid-election ruse

December: Son of one of my patients secretly gives Ivermectin to his anti-vax parents who are both hospitalized with COVID pneumonia

Francis Collins, director of NIH retires. Resisted Trump's pressures to fire Fauci and to endorse unproven therapies. His one regret is a wish to better understand vaccine hesitancy and resistance

Senate Republicans vote to defund vaccine mandates

Senator Ron Johnson from Minnesota claims that gargling Listerine® kills COVID

2022

January 2022: 3 million cases and 145, 000 hospitalizations – highest ever

I hospitalize three patients – all unvaccinated

Patient after patient of mine, all vaccinated, became COVID-positive in the last 24 hours. All of them are eligible for treatment, as they have significant chronic illnesses. To avoid hospitalization, several were lucky to get outpatient medication. The rest received nothing, as we've run out of the medication in our part of the state.

January 6, 2021: *Journal of the American Medical Association* (*JAMA*) publishes articles amounting to "extraordinary, albeit polite critique" of much of President Biden's COVID policy.

January 13, 2022: The U.S. Supreme Court blocks enforcement of the Biden's COVID-19 vaccine mandate for workers at larger businesses but upholds mandate for health workers.

January 2022: President Biden announces a plan to give out 400 million free N95 masks.

February 2022: Government Accounting Office investigators "found persistent deficiencies" in how the CDC has led the response to the coronavirus pandemic and past public health emergencies dating to 2007 citing "continued problems coordinating among public health agencies, collecting infectious-disease surveillance data, and securing appropriate testing and medical supplies, among areas it said are unresolved.

Kaiser Permanente broke its own profit record in 2021

March: Two-year anniversary for COVID: As reported in the NYT: What if China had been open and honest in December 2019? What if the world had reacted as quickly and aggressively in January 2020 as Taiwan did? What if the United States had put appropriate protective measures in place in February 2020, as South Korea did?

April: Due to the COVID pandemic, life expectancy in the U.S. fell by two years in 2020 to about 77 years – a drop greater than in any other high-income country.

April 22, 2022: CDC reports that COVID third leading cause of death in the U.S. in 2021.

May 14: The US surpassed 1 million COVID-19 deaths.

May: Cruises are back. Yet 76 of 92 ships have reported cases of the coronavirus on board.

May 31: Growing vaccine hesitancy is one of the WHO's top 10 threats to global health.

June 2022: 34% of the people killed by the virus lived in nursing homes (1% of the U.S. population). Resident outcomes significantly worse at for-profit nursing homes.

August 2022: Harassing public health officials was justified rose 5.4 percentage points.

Never happened to me: 3 vaccine-resistant patients jabbed in 1 day; high-fiving all over.

September 2022: Scott Jensen, Republican candidate for Governor of Minnesota said that Democratic Gov. Tim Walz's COVID policies were comparable to Kristallnacht "the night of broken glass," that heralded the beginning of the Nazis' antisemitic mass violence.

10.5 million children were orphaned or lost a primary caregiver to COVID.

2023

January 2023: Nurses just went on strike at a number of NYC hospitals.

40,000 hospitalized patients and 750 deaths per day.

February 2023: Biden declares end of public health emergency to take effect in May.

Governor DeSantis would like to enshrine into Florida law the right of health professionals to spread misinformation about a vaccine that only 11% of Floridians have chosen to receive.

List of Abbreviations

ACA — Affordable Care Act
AMA — American Medical Association
AND — Ask Nurses and Doctors
ARP — American Rescue Plan
CDC — Centers for Disease Control and Prevention
CHRP — Community Health Resilience Plan
CMS — Center for Medicare and Medicaid Services
DCCC — Democratic Congressional Campaign Committee
DHS — Department of Homeland Security
ER — Emergency Room
FBI — Federal Bureau of Investigation
FDA — Food and Drug Administration
GAO — Government Accounting Office
HHS — Department of Health and Human Services
IRA — Inflation Reduction Act
LTE — Letter to the Editor
NIH — National Institutes of Health
NYT — *New York Times*
OPT — Occupied Palestinian Territories
PCR — Polymerase chain reaction
PtH — Peace through health
VA — Veterans Affairs
WHO — World Health Organization

BACKGROUND PERSPECTIVES, THE COVID "DIARY," AND AMERICAN FRAGILITY

I

Chapter 1

Introduction

Introduction

I should be melancholic as I write this book, but as my family and friends know, that is not my nature. I am by no means optimistic. Ever since I started thinking about the world as a teenager, I've always felt that the situation in the world has gotten worse. Between climate change and pandemics (HIV and now COVID-19), in particular, I don't expect any turnaround in my lifetime. But I am trying; I feel I have no choice but to try. I've often thought about how to best rationalize my efforts in an ever-darkening world. Italo Calvino in his book Invisible Cities says it best about how to engage with the "hell" we increasingly live in.[1]

Looking through the lens of the COVID-19 pandemic, this book highlights what we could do to change our political system in order to deal with pandemics effectively and what health professionals can do to help bring about this change.

From "COVID-19 Notes,"

> March 2020: I called one patient at work to tell him, he was positive; ten more in past two weeks. Need national policy now. You need to see this brief video advocating for people to wear masks and be Covid safe.[2] The first sentences in the video feature Dr Williams: "We are tired because the numbers are overwhelming.... we have nurses being pushed to the limits emotionally ... we are watching patients in the turmoil of dying and families being torn apart."[3]

From a 2021 *New York Times Magazine* article about the efforts of the hospital where I work (Baystate Medical Center, Springfield, Massachusetts) to procure N95 masks: "The primary wisdom that Artenstein [a Baystate employee] was providing to other health care systems asking for his advice was to not expect substantial help

DOI: 10.4324/9781003426257-2

from the federal government. In a sense, the Trump administration had achieved one of its goals: It had trained Americans not to rely on it. Everyone was on his or her own in this pandemic, Artenstein warned. That was the American way."[4]

What are the net results of this "approach" to the American way:

> More than 6 million COVID-19 deaths have been confirmed worldwide, but in many ways that number severely understates the death toll.... One estimate suggests that between 14 million and 25 million total human beings lost their lives because of the virus.[5]

> Not only have millions died; we've lost trillions in economic output, countless families have been scarred by loss, and a generation of youth has seen childhood and education interrupted. The devastatingly personal nature of this crisis, even to the wealthy and well connected, can't be overstated. And yet, there's little evidence that our current political system has adjusted to take long-term threats any more seriously.[6]

This chapter lays out the central arguments of the book within a framework of who suffers most during pandemics throughout history.

Epidemics and History

Epidemics have literally plagued every society and culture throughout history. In reading and rereading the history of epidemics and their impact on human society, several threads continuously emerge. Throughout history, people always mess up when dealing with pandemics. Second, the poor suffer the most. Third, we, as human beings, learn very few lessons from past pandemics. Finally, the idea of "God's punishment" is present in every epidemic right up to and including COVID-19. Such proclamations are almost all suffused with hate. Frank Snowden, in his magisterial *Epidemics and Society: From the Black Death to the Present*, quoted the right-wing evangelist Jerry Falwell: "AIDS is not just God's punishment of homosexuals, it is God's punishment for the society that tolerates homosexuals."[7]

Until recently, we had little in the way of scientifically validated treatment for the viral, bacterial, or other infectious causes of epidemics. The medical historian Thomas McKeown has written about the key role of sanitation in eliminating pandemics.[8] Effective treatment did not emerge until the twentieth century, with the dramatic development of vaccines, initially targeting polio, and antivirals, starting with HIV. What is remarkable and sad at the same time is the rapidity with which scientists developed treatment and vaccines in the case of COVID-19. It is sad in that, as we will see, it is the unwillingness of organized health professional organizations and politicians, especially some Republicans, to act in the public interest that limited the impact that the path-breaking scientific miracle of vaccines could have made on the course of the pandemic.

The Poor, Pandemics, and Individual Responsibility

Over and above pandemics, it is clear that the poor, in general, have always suffered more than the well-off, a truth reinforced throughout history. In the nineteenth century, the debate on the causes and solutions of this problem was between advocates of social medicine, such as Rudolf Virchow, and those, such as Sir Edwin Chadwick in England, who focused on the idea that filth caused poverty.[9] In Chadwick's worldview, it is the poor themselves who are to blame. In contrast, Virchow argued that social forces lead to or at least contribute to poverty. The latter impact falls under the category of "the social determinants of health." Despite all the evidence staring him in the face, Chadwick opined that it was up to the poor to pull themselves up by their bootstraps.

To this day, in the United States we have not resolved, at either a cultural or a policy level, the debate between Chadwick and Virchow. In contrast, all European countries acknowledge via government programs and legislation the impact of social determinants on the health of the poor and disadvantaged. These European countries have enacted, albeit at different levels of support, universal health coverage, paid family leave, and other benefits that recognize the impact that socioeconomic disparities have on disease. As we will see in Chapter 4, in particular, some branches of the Republican Party, together with elements of the Democratic Party, have completely denied, despite ample data, the veracity of the effect of socioeconomic disparities on health.

The Politics of Socioeconomic Disparities

Since the United States has never acted to address socioeconomic disparities in health in a systematic manner, it has, on many metrics during this pandemic, performed worse than any other industrialized country, especially on COVID-19 deaths adjusted for population.[10] We in the United States continue to perpetuate the nineteenth-century approach of concentrating solely on individual responsibility for disease. For example, an examination of the America First policy platform, which is closely allied with especially the Trump wing of the Republican Party, advocates the repeal of vaccine mandates as a primary health objective; in fact, the military vaccine mandate was repealed in late 2022 on the insistence of Republicans.[11] Tragically, the Republican Party's approach to the pandemic has led to the following outcomes for members of their own party:

> Male and female residents of Democratic counties experienced both lower mortality rates and twice the relative decrease in mortality rates than did those in Republican counties. Black Americans experienced largely similar improvement in age adjusted mortality rates in both Democratic and Republican counties. However, the mortality difference between white residents in Democratic versus Republican counties increased fourfold. Rural Republican counties experienced the highest mortality rates and the least improvement.[12]

In the naked pursuit of power, Trump and his acolytes in the form of Ron DeSantis, Josh Hawley, Greg Abbott among others go much further:

> The chilling amalgam of Christian nationalism, white replacement theory and conspiratorial zeal—from QAnon to the "stolen" 2020 election—has attracted a substantial constituency in the United States, thanks in large part to the efforts of Donald Trump and his advisers. By some estimates, adherents of these overlapping movements make up as much as a quarter or even a third of the electorate.[13]

In addition, for many Republican politicians, an almost exclusive focus on individual responsibility for disease together with the amalgam of opinions described above is complemented with, simply put, lies.[14] Reacting to the arrest of Dr. Simone Gold, Representative Louie Gohmert (R-TX) told *Newsmax*,

> "If you're a Republican, you can't even lie to Congress or lie to an FBI agent or they're coming after you." He claimed that the grand jury acquitted lawyer Michael Sussman of lying to the FBI about his contact with Hillary Clinton's 2016 campaign with the argument that "[o]f course you're gonna lie. Everybody lies!"[15]

What are the political consequences of this approach that combines complete disregard for science and outright lies? One might think that, in response, citizens would not vote for people who lie in virtually every sentence. Yet, as researchers have documented, "In sharply polarized electorates, even voters who value democracy will be willing to sacrifice fair democratic competition for the sake of electing politicians who champion their interests. When punishing a leader's authoritarian tendencies requires voting for a platform, party, or person that his supporters detest, many will find this too high a price to pay."[16]

Fragility, How Changing Our Health System Can Impact This Trend, and the Important Role of Health Care Professionals

In short, the United States is an increasingly fragile country. What does that term mean? Fragility, as used in the peace through health field, describes countries that are emerging from conflict. The United States, in contrast, is increasingly going into conflict.[17] The United States, assessed in 2018 to be the country most able to deal with a disaster,[18] has tragically performed the worst of any industrialized country. There are two components to this fragility: the political polarization around the COVID-19 pandemic and the dramatic disproportional impact of the pandemic on the lower socioeconomic strata. These two factors continue and, in fact, have become exacerbated, despite many American strengths. We are, as a country, increasingly going into conflict—both physically (exemplified by constant mass shootings[19]) and politically (from the polarization described above).

Health care is a significant economic driver in the United States. Without the active leadership of a bipartisan group of senior elected officials to lead this and future pandemic responses, economic interests that underlie our health care system will continue to struggle with each other, resulting in a lackluster or failed public health response. Grants from the government or foundations are not sufficient. They are time-limited and do not represent a national commitment to resolving an existential challenge—in this case, an appropriate permanent response to this and future pandemics. What should the "goal" or model be? Given our political polarization, a national program is not possible. However, the United States has a long tradition of state-led efforts that occasionally become the foundation for national programs. The Affordable Care Act is just one of the many examples. As discussed in Chapter 8, we need a statewide public health system led by elected officials in a bipartisan manner that places community health workers (CHWs) at the center of the network. Such a model provides ample opportunity for variation in implementation. Numerous CHW-led models exist (see Chapters 6 and 8 for more details):

The central arguments for a statewide public health initiative are:

a. *We will continue to face ongoing pandemics and endemics.*
b. *Effective public health is one ingredient in improved public trust in an increasingly "fragile" United States.*
c. *An effort to implement a national, federally directed public health response to the COVID-19 pandemic is not politically feasible at the present time.*
d. *States have historically taken the lead on important national issues. We can implement a statewide public health initiative that links acute and public health that builds on existing strengths.*
e. *A linked public-acute health initiative needs to place community health workers (CHWs) at the center for at least low- and middle-income counties in the state.*
f. *This initiative can function effectively in our fragmented health care system only if bipartisan, senior statewide elected political officials play an active leadership role.*

This book also addresses the question, how should we, as health professionals, respond? In broad terms, health professionals have a unique role to play. As trusted validators, health professionals can take the perspective of Virchow and emphasize the social determinants of health. It could make a dramatic difference if we as health professionals work with and, in fact, encourage elected, preferably bipartisan, politicians to act in the public interest using science as our basis for action.

The seeking of power is another crucial element in health care organizations. Who seeks it? What do people do with power when they have it? To what extent are they truly motivated by the interest of the public? While health professionals like Joseph Ladapo, the surgeon general of Florida, who believes in neither science nor the social determinants of health, are a minority, they cause incalculable suffering and death.[20] Such health professionals assist politicians like Ron DeSantis, the governor of Florida, who dissociate science from their decision making. In our time, we are in a position of witnessing health professionals who assist politicians in causing more death (though this is not unique to our time). What can or should health professionals do about this? What about health professionals working in the private sector? How have they behaved with respect to the public interest both historically and recently? More important, what should these health professionals be doing today?

Of critical concern, how have health professional organizations tried to mitigate the COVID-19 pandemic? Health professional organizations are the licensing body for all health professionals. Have these licensing health professional boards suspended the licenses of health professionals who contribute to the death of individuals with vaccine misinformation or outright lies? If not, should they?

This book considers the health professional roles that could lead to needed changes in our health system through the lens of the COVID-19 pandemic—a defining issue in both my personal and professional life. The pandemic has been and continues to be a life-and-death issue for millions throughout the world. In order to determine the possible roles that health professionals could play, it will be necessary to examine the tools that health professionals have at their disposal. These tools are best summarized under the rubric of peace through health—the focus of the next chapter.

Notes

1 Paraphrased in Calvino, I. (1972) *The Invisible Cities* from *Empty Square Journal* https://www.theemptysquare.org/stories/that-which-is-not-hell; Accessed: December 24, 2022.
2 BSA Health System. (2022) Help your hospitals. Wear a mask. *BSA Health System* Available at https://www.youtube.com/watch?v=pD-i-zDTZq4; Accessed: November 19, 2022.
3 Ibid.
4 Clark, DB. (2020) Inside the chaotic cuthroat gray market for N95 masks. *The New York Times Magazine*. Available at: https://www.nytimes.com/2020/11/17/magazine/n95-masks-market-covid.html; Accessed: August 31, 2022.
5 Giattino, C., Ritchie, H., Roser, M. et al. (2022) Excess mortality during the coronavirus pandemic. *Our World in Data*. Available at: https://ourworldindata.org/excess-mortality-covid?country=IND~USA~GBR~CAN~DEU~FRA&utm_source=newsletter&utm_medium=email&utm_campaign=atlantic-daily-newsletter&utm_content=20220725&utm_term=The%20Atlantic%20Daily Accessed: November 19, 2022.
6 Congressional Research Service. (2021) *Global Economic Effects of Covid-19*. Available at: https://sgp.fas.org/crs/row/R46270.pdf?utm_source=newsletter&utm_medium=email&utm_campaign=atlantic-daily-newsletter&utm_content=20220725&utm_term=The%20Atlantic%20Daily. Accessed: November 19, 2022.

7 Reed, C. (2007) The Rev Jerry Falwell. *Guardian* Available at: https://www.theguardian.com/media/2007/may/17/broadcasting.guardianobituaries. Accessed: November 19, 2022.

8 As discussed in Snowden, F. (2020) *Epidemics and Society: From the Black Death to the Present*. New Haven: Yale University Press, pp 184–185.

9 Ibid, pp 200–202.

10 Masters RK., Aron, LY. and Woolf, SH. (2022) Changes in life expectancy between 2019 and 2021 in the United States and 21 peer countries. *JAMA Netw Open* 5:4 e227067. doi: 10.1001/jamanetworkopen.2022.7067. PMID: 35416991; PMCID: PMC9008499. Available at: https://www.ncbi.nlm.nih.gov/pmc/articles/PMC9008499/. Accessed: January 14, 2023

11 America First Policy Institute. *Health Care*. Available at: https://americafirstpolicy.com/priorities/healthcare. Accessed: November 19, 2022. O'Brien, C. (2022) Biden signs defense bill repealing military mandate. *Politico*. Available at: https://www.politico.com/news/2022/12/23/biden-defense-bill-military-vaccine-mandate-00075437. Accessed: December 26, 2022.

12 Warraich, HJ., Kumar, P., Nasir, K. et al. (2022) Political environment and mortality rates in the United States, 2001–19: population based cross sectional analysis. *The British Medical Journal*. Available at: https://www.bmj.com/content/377/bmj-2021-069308. Accessed: November 19, 2022.

13 Edsall, T. (2022) The MAGA formula is getting darker and darker. *The New York Times* Available at: https://www.nytimes.com/2022/05/18/opinion/christian-nationalism-great-replacement.html. Accessed: November 19, 2022.

14 Kessler, G., Rizzo, S., Kelly, M. (2022) Trumps false or misleading claims total 30,573 over four years. *Washington Post*. Available at: https://www.washingtonpost.com/politics/2021/01/24/trumps-false-or-misleading-claims-total-30573-over-four-years/. Accessed January 6, 2023. It should be made clear that the Republican party doesn't own the phenomenon of lying. It is bipartisan but it is my assessment that there is a qualitative difference between the two parties. See Kaplan, T. (2019) Elizabeth Warren apologizes at Native American Forum: 'I have listened and I have learned'. *New York Times*. Available at: https://www.nytimes.com/2019/08/19/us/politics/elizabeth-warren-native-american.html. Accessed January 6, 2023.

15 Vakil, C. (2022) Gohmert: 'If you're a Republican, you can't even lie to Congress or lie to an FBI agent or they're coming after you'. *The Hill*. Available at: https://thehill.com/homenews/house/3511477-gohmert-if-youre-a-republican-you-cant-even-lie-to-congress-or-lie-to-an-fbi-agent-or-theyre-coming-after-you/. Accessed: November 19, 2022.

16 Edsall, T. (2022) Trump poses a test democracy is failing. *The New York Times*. Available at: https://www.nytimes.com/2022/04/13/opinion/trump-democracy-decline-fall.html. Accessed: November 19, 2022.

17 https://www.foreignaffairs.com/articles/united-states/trump-americas-coming-age-instability

18 Center for Health Security, Johns Hopkins University and NTI Building a Safer World (2019) *Global Health Security Index* Available at: https://www.ghsindex.org/wp-content/uploads/2019/10/2019-Global-Health-Security-Index.pdf. Accessed: November 19, 2022.

19 Ledur, J. and Rabinowitz, K. (2022) There have been almost 600 mass shootings so far in 2022. *Washington Post*. Available at: https://www.washingtonpost.com/nation/2022/06/02/mass-shootings-in-2022/ Accessed: November 19, 2022.

20 Bump, P. (2022) Florida's Surgeon General makes the conspiracy theory podcast rounds. *Washington Post* Available at: https://www.washingtonpost.com/politics/2022/10/21/florida-covid-vaccines-desantis-surgeon-general/. Accessed: November 19, 2022.

Chapter 2

Peace through Health and American Fragility

Evidence for Peace through Health Impact

Introduction

The COVID-19 pandemic has exacerbated American fragility. As a country, as graphically shown in a recent cover of the *Economist* in which the legs of a Statue of Liberty are splayed apart, the United States is entering into increasing conflict.[1] By rallying for the public interest utilizing science, health professionals can mitigate this state of affairs. We have several techniques at our disposal to decrease fragility and encourage greater peace. These techniques or tools fall into the general rubric of peace through health (hereafter abbreviated as PtH).

This chapter will provide a research and political summary of a remarkable, relatively recent effort on the part of health care organizations and health professionals to fuse a connection between PtH. These PtH tools form the basis of the types of activities that health professionals can undertake, and to a modest extent are already undertaking, to address increasing fragility in the United States. I will introduce the concept of fragility as it is understood in much of the research and policy literature. I argue in this book that fragility in the United States, a country that is increasingly descending into conflict, is similar in many ways to the fragility of countries that are emerging out of conflict or outright war.

DOI: 10.4324/9781003426257-3

In this chapter, I will

■ Provide a background section

  ■ Presenting sociological theories that underlie PtH.
  ■ Highlighting the impact of conflict on health (in its various dimensions) and the impact of health interventions on peace and conflict dynamics.
  ■ Briefly defining PtH and PtH Tools.

■ Review of the evidence for PtH.

Background

Sociological Underpinnings of PtH

This background section consists of a short introduction to sociological theories that underlie PtH and a very brief historical introduction to the term PtH. I then continue with definitions of the different mechanisms that PtH practitioners and organizations utilize. I introduce the separate category of Peace to Health; I conclude with a very brief summary of the impact of conflict on health. In Chapter 4, I explore the concept of fragility particularly as it pertains to the United States.

Health professionals typically utilize an individually based biological model and translate that biological outlook into actions that impact the entire society, failing to recognize that an individual health professional's biological model worldview is shaped by surrounding societal forces.[2] There are biological facts surrounding COVID-19 that are absolutely true. Vaccines work to decrease death. Medication exists that decreases hospitalization. Masks work to decrease the transmission of the disease. Today, the bigger challenge for health professionals is to convince people that these biological facts are not only true but should be acted on. How can health professionals work with social and political forces that see it in their political interest to fight against these facts? If health professionals are to engage in society, we must grapple with the many social forces that seek to deny scientific facts, the social forces that seek to promote social chaos for their own political purposes.

Weber defined sociology as "a science which attempts the interpretive understanding of social action in order thereby to arrive at a causal explanation of its course and effects."[3] The term "science" conjures up empirically verifiable facts, such as those that health professionals learn in the biological model in the health sciences—for example, penicillin is an established treatment for streptococcal infection of the throat. Sociological researchers such as Peter Berger and Thomas Luckmann highlight "the social construction of reality."[4] They emphasize how most people share a conception of the world that eventually "passes for knowledge in a society, regardless of the ultimate validity or invalidity (by whatever criteria) of such knowledge." In any activity such as PtH, socio-psychological theory posits that an individual's thoughts, emotions, and resultant actions are impacted by social factors or society.[5] A societal culture of conflict serves to increase an individual's socio-psychological barriers to resolution of any conflict. Health professionals committed to PtH who live either inside or outside a conflict zone seek to identify ways of engaging with and, hopefully, interrupting this culture of conflict.

Individuals operate as members of society. Max Weber, in particular, together with many others, pointed to the human need for leadership, especially charismatic leadership.[6] Leadership and bureaucratic use of knowledge and resultant power can be wielded to promote economic development, or its implementation may result in social suffering. Arthur Kleinman and Veena Das theorized that "social suffering results from what political, economic, and institutional power does to people and, reciprocally, from how these forms of power themselves influence responses to social problems."[7]

Social suffering might be considered analogous to Johan Galtung's concept of structural violence.[8] Violence, according to Galtung, can be defined as avoidable insults to basic human needs (survival, identity, well-being, and freedom) that reduce the human potential. Direct violence describes visible acts (physical, psychological, emotional, spiritual) where we usually know the perpetrator and certainly see the effect on a known victim. Structural violence characterizes more hidden processes resulting in inequalities or violation of needs, where the perpetrator, working through structures or institutions, may not be so obvious but the effects on individuals are equally strong. Finally, cultural violence emerges from "isms," the belief systems that allow for direct and structural violence to occur. Galtung also developed the concept of negative (absence of violence) and positive peace, encompassing acts, structures, and belief systems promoting human potential, in which sense peace, adapted from Galtung, might be "a state of integrated, respectful, positive, cooperative, nurturing, relationships."[9] As we will discuss in further detail in Chapter 4, increasing fragility as is occurring in the United States involves both direct and structural violence and diminishing positive peace. Thinking about PtH, any increase in any form of violence or diminished positive peace might lead to more macro-level direct violence. In many respects, with the regular occurrence of mass shootings, the United States has already entered an era of macro-level direct violence.

The physician and sociologist Paul Farmer stated that different forms of power are often a type of structural violence.[10] This structural violence can occur at a national level in many manifestations, including cultural, gender, or race-based forms. Farmer asserts that this form of social suffering "is structured by historically given (and often economically driven) processes and forces that conspire—whether through routine, ritual or, as is more commonly the case, the hard surfaces of life—to constrain agency. For many including most of my patients, choices both large and small are limited by racism, sexism, political violence, and grinding poverty."[11] Health professionals are confronted daily by both structural violence and the direct violence of conflict. By impacting both direct and structural violence, health professionals may integrate peace and health to try and alleviate social suffering.

The Constitution of the World Health Organization (WHO) defines health as "not merely the absence of disease or infirmity," but more holistically as a "state of complete physical, mental and social well-being."[12] Health professionals try to improve the health of their patients by attending to their diseases and, possibly even more important, addressing both direct (from all types of conflict) and structural violence. A determinants-of-health model includes much that might be related to structural violence; the Ottawa Charter for Health Promotion explicitly lists peace (presumably as the absence of direct violence) as the first determinant of health.[13]

"The role of physicians and other health workers in the preservation and promotion of peace is the most significant factor for the attainment of health for all."[14] This brings us full circle from the opposite direction, in the field that integrates peace and health, much as Galtung used health and well-being as his basis for defining peace and its components.

The Impact of Conflict on Health

Conflicts have changed over the last 50 years. They have become more protracted and complex, involving, for example, nonstate actors, and resulting in more fragile or shock-prone countries. A state that is fragile has several attributes, and such fragility may manifest itself in various ways. As will be seen, several of these attributes are apparent in the United States. Some of the most common attributes of state fragility[15] may include:

■ Either the loss of physical control of its territory or a monopoly on the legitimate use of force. Today in the United States, some members of the Republican Party advocate political violence against opponents.[16]
■ The erosion of legitimate authority to make collective decisions.
■ An inability to provide reasonable public services. As discussed extensively here, the United States has performed by far the worst of any comparable country in its efforts to address the COVID-19 pandemic.
■ The inability to interact with other states as a full member of the international community.

An estimated 1.8 billion people live in fragile states, most of which have weak health care systems.[17] The outcome of these weak health care systems can be seen in a life expectancy of 62 in South Sudan, a country still in active conflict, as opposed to 84 in Japan, with a strong health system and no conflict at present. One manifestation of the increased fragility of the United States is the dramatic drop in life expectancy (the most dramatic drop in 100 years), which has occurred as a direct consequence of the country's dismal performance on the COVID-19 pandemic.[18]

Overall life expectancy is also impacted by the many deaths from mass conflict, genocide, pandemics, and mass murder—an estimated 191 million people in the twentieth century, more than half of whom were civilians. War has changed in many ways over the past century, the most dramatic change being the negative impact on civilians. Of all civilians, children and women are particularly vulnerable.

Aside from death, conflict has many other effects on individuals. Appendix 1 contains two examples that anticipate the ultimate emergence of mental health challenges as a consequence of conflict. These examples are taken from one of the oldest protracted conflicts in the world today, the Israeli-Palestinian conflict.

Conflict carries both short- and long-term mental health consequences. For example, a recent study of survivors of the Rwanda genocide documents that the prevalence rate for current post-traumatic stress disorder (PTSD) was 25% in the survivor group.[19]

The impact of conflict on physical health includes significant physical disability, with attendant health system needs. These impacts can last for decades. Children are at particular risk during a conflict, suffering traumas ranging from malnutrition to forced labor or becoming a child soldier or sexual slave. Weak health systems in partially resilient states often lead to lower immunization rates.[20] Invisible "wounds" of violent or non-violent conflict are not simply psychological. Conflict results in often permanent disability for many,[21] severely impacts job opportunities,[22] and negatively impacts the environment.[23] Increasing conflict has also led to the worst refugee crisis since records have been kept.[24]

Both ongoing/protracted conflict (conflicts that have gone on for decades) and immediately postconflict often have dramatic impacts on health systems. Combatants try to destroy the opposing side's health care system in an effort to undermine support for that side. Appendix 2 provides a brief case example.

Lastly, and in some ways most tragically for the purposes of this examination, conflict has evolved in a particularly negative way on health professionals and facilities both during and after a conflict. Health professionals and facilities are increasingly considered part of the opposing side and killed or targeted if treatment is provided to any civilians/military from the opposing side. Physical attacks on health professionals clearly contravene the Geneva Conventions. Nonetheless, health professionals and institutions taking care of patients, notably hospitals, have been attacked by opposing sides since time immemorial. However, this tragedy has rapidly accelerated in scope and extent since 2000. As stated in a December 2019 article in the *New York Times* sadly entitled "Where Doctors Are Criminals":

> The Syrian government considers some health workers enemies of the state…. There was the medical student who volunteered in eastern Aleppo even after his classmates were tortured and killed as a warning…. Each took enormous risks to provide medical care to areas in Syria aligned against President Bashar al-Assad. Some were imprisoned and tortured, evidence of how the nearly 9-year-old conflict in Syria has normalized the criminalization of medical care. Physicians for Human Rights, which has documented the collapse of Syria's health care system, said in a recently released study that Mr. al-Assad has successfully made medical assistance given to his enemies a terrorist act.[25]

Briefly Define PtH and PtH Tools

PtH was defined in 1995 by the WHO as follows: "When there is an underlying genuine thrust towards peace and reconciliation, Health can play a role as catalyst in the peace process."[26] Such initiatives were described in a United States Institute of Peace paper of 2010: "They are premised on the idea that cooperation among health professionals and health interventions in conflict zones can contribute not only to improved outcomes for populations who suffer from the impact of war, but also to building a lasting peace."[27] While not developed as a concept until the past 30 years, the idea of "peace through health" has already been realized through numerous efforts, starting with the Pan American Health Organization (PAHO) program Health: A Bridge for Peace, initiated in the early 1980s, which included a vaccination initiative. The perceived impact of PtH is reflected in the awards of the Nobel Peace Prize to International Physicians for the Prevention of Nuclear War in 1985 and several other health-focused entities, such as the International Committee of the Red Cross (ICRC, three times), the International Campaign to Ban Land-mines, and Médecins sans Frontières/Doctors without Borders.

If we are to evaluate the evidence supporting PtH, it is necessary to define and specify the different PtH mechanisms that health professionals have used over the past 30 years. These are the different health mechanisms that can contribute to peace, which have been adapted from the McMaster model.[28] Moving from peace to health is a separate category (no. 8) and is described immediately below the seven mechanisms. Each mechanism or category is defined immediately below. The following section of this chapter provides the evidence for each PtH tool.

1. Health diplomacy: Mediation and conflict transformation; Construction of goals in common; Superordinate goals

    Superordinate goals, such as health professional-mediated humanitarian ceasefires, are those goals that appeal to both parties of a conflict but are attainable only if both sides cooperate. Mediation for conflict transformation must happen in order to make these superordinate goals a reality.
2. Limiting the destructiveness of war

    Health professionals have tried to limit the destructiveness of war and by implication redefine a conflict situation by documenting the gruesome impact of some war technologies, such as chemical weapons, including chlorine gas or phosphorus, or nuclear weapons.
3. Communication of knowledge

    Health professionals communicate knowledge when they report on the impact of deaths on a conflict to the outside world. They may also communicate knowledge to an opposing side of a conflict or across the divides for the purpose of increasing capacity on one or both sides of a conflict.
4. Evocation and extension of altruism

    Impartially caring for individuals needing care on both sides of a conflict when the possibility exists that the health professional may be harmed in conflict is the ultimate form of altruism.
5. Personalizing the enemy

    Health professionals may attempt to place an individual "human face" on an enemy in an attempt to change public opinion in a conflict.

6. Solidarity and support; Noncooperation and dissent

    When there is a clear imbalance between opposing sides in a conflict, health care professionals/organizations on the stronger side may elect to provide support to the weaker side. Health care professionals and/or organizations may also refuse to cooperate or dissent from policies of their own government.

7. Social healing; Strengthening resilience; Increasing Trust

    Health professionals can improve health care outcomes and strengthen resilience in protracted conflict, thus leading to peace building.

8. Peace to health, or public health to public trust; Rebuilding the fabric of society/Strengthening of communities; Building trust between citizens and state through people-centered health systems

    Public health to public trust is a critical PtH tool that can be used to address American fragility—as is true for many of the above tools. See Chapters 3 through 9 for an in-depth examination of the many ways in which a pandemic can diminish peace within a country and how enactment of a strengthened public health system could reduce American fragility. In addition, each of the other tools listed have relevance for health professionals as we seek to address American fragility.

Integrating Peace and Health—A Review of the Evidence

I examined the literature on PtH in the following ways:

a. A search strategy was developed and reviewed by a health science librarian. For scientific literature, we searched for articles on PtH with MEDLINE, Scopus, and APA PsycInfo from the inception of these databases to March 15, 2021, using a combination of indexed terms, free text words, and MeSH (Medical Subject) headings. There were no date or language restrictions. I searched for any studies that met our inclusion criteria of PtH. In addition, I examined Google Scholar and did Google searches in particular for "gray literature." I consulted PtH experts to identify any additional studies I may have missed. A bibliography is available directly from the author.

    For the purposes of this bibliography, I largely restricted myself, with the exception of some review articles, to publications that move from health to peace. Of the thousands of articles in the peace to health field, I included only a few review articles and key reports. Thus, for example, a recently published review of peace to improved mental health outcomes had 146 references representing only a small portion of the field.

b. A number of PtH documents not published in the peer-reviewed literature will be found in this bibliography available from the author (for example, documents from the WHO). Many of them were collected by the author over the past 30 years.

The vast majority of the documents that I reviewed are descriptive, calls to action, and general descriptions of PtH and/or summaries of results of PtH interventions.

Evidence is presented by each PtH mechanism, though some of the evidence of the impact interventions apply to more than one PtH mechanism. This review determined that most articles in support of PtH are case studies that describe an event or a happening that could be classified as PtH, with minimal follow-up. A general category consisting of overview articles, critiques, supportive articles, teaching material, and monographs precedes a discussion of each PtH mechanism.

After the review of all the PtH mechanisms is completed, I address the last PtH category, focused on the obverse goal: health through peace. Next, I make general observations on the overlap between peace, health outcomes, and fragility.

General PtH Articles and/or Monographs

The vast majority of the articles in the bibliography describe either general principles of PtH or provide short-term tracking of results. Long-term follow-up of PtH interventions is rare. In addition, most of the articles highlight, often within an analytic framework, the author's either personal or, if representing a group, collective perception of the impact of a PtH program. Because of the large number of articles that fall into the general article or monograph category, this chapter briefly summarizes four articles/monographs.

For this general section, in the first article to be discussed, Randi Garber summarizes years of PtH pertaining to the Israeli-Palestinian conflict in her article "Health as a Bridge for Peace: Theory, Practice and Prognosis Reflections of a Practitioner."[29] She highlights outcomes achieved (which are summarized in Appendix 3). She does not report on any long-lasting impact of these initiatives. More importantly, the downward spiral of the political process between Israelis and Palestinians culminating in the second intifada (beginning in 2000) not surprisingly dominated and eliminated to this day most interorganizational PtH engagement between Israelis and Palestinians.

A second article, the monograph entitled *How Can Health Serve as a Bridge to Peace?* by Rosalía Rodriguez-García and colleagues, summarized years of PtH experience.[30] After a literature search, the authors identified the impact of five interventions, including those in El Salvador, Haiti, and Angola.

> Though outcomes varied among the cases studied, a common thread was found emphasizing that joint action and common points of interest can engender a gradual renewal of trust and sense of mutuality among former combatants, which can lead to local reconciliation and successful peace building…. It is too early to say whether the positive short-term outcomes of initiatives will make real contributions to the peace process or the improvement of health status and services in the long term. These long-term outcomes should be the subject of future research and evaluation activities.[31]

This detailed monograph concluded with recommendations. Among these, interestingly, is the development of much more in-depth evaluation of PtH programs.

> There seems to be an overwhelming need for further evaluative research
> of HBP initiatives to date. Methodologies should be developed and
> tested in the course of new and ongoing activities, leading to overarching
> guidance in the form of general protocols and lessons learned. As part
> of these efforts, the theory behind Health as a Bridge for Peace should
> continue to be built and developed.[32]

What are the boundaries of peace and health activities? This was addressed in the early 2000s.[33] Abuelaish and colleagues published in December 2020 an article in the peer-reviewed literature that fits well in this first general category. Entitled "Interdependence between Health and Peace: A Call for a New Paradigm," it encourages us to be aspirational and consider that:

> Health promotion and peace promotion are intrinsically interrelated:
> health promotion and peace promotion share the goal of creating social
> harmony and cooperation, leading to just societies and communities....
> To be at peace and to be healthy, individuals and communities need to be
> resilient, tolerant, and adaptable to life-circumstances, especially under
> conditions that result in, or foster, personal or community fragility. The
> relationship between health and peace is evident in the mutual roles
> played by resilience and adaptation in restoring healthy functionality, and
> restoring positive peace when challenged by disease and other life-issues.[34]

Finally, Abuelaish and Arya ask us to push the boundaries of health and peace and include hatred as a public health problem.[35] The authors do not highlight a specific path forward for such a program, and thus far, few have taken up the cause of hatred as a public health issue.

A Review of Evidence for Each PtH Tool

1. Health diplomacy: Mediation and conflict transformation; Construction of goals in common; Superordinate goals

PtH advocates have written extensively about two famous initiatives that fall under health diplomacy and superordinate goals: immunization ceasefires and the prevention of nuclear war.

Ian Maddocks and many others have discussed how a very young organization, the International Physicians for the Prevention of Nuclear War (IPPNW), rapidly gained more than 100,000 members.[36] IPPNW activism against the health effects of nuclear war resulted in a 1987 meeting with the then leader of the Soviet Union, Mikhail Gorbachev. IPPNW leaders may very well have influenced him to pursue an end to the production, testing, and deployment of nuclear weapons. The IPPNW received the Nobel Peace Prize in 1985. Maddocks summarized the rationale behind the award: "The Norwegian Nobel Committee cited IPPNW for having performed a considerable service to mankind by spreading authoritative information, contributing to an increase in public opposition to atomic weapons, and giving arms limitation negotiations a new perspective and seriousness. In addition, great importance was attached to the fact that IPPNW was founded as a joint initiative by Soviet and American physicians."[37]

Two-thirds of unimmunized children live in conflict-affected countries.[38] Vaccination campaigns on both sides of a conflict could represent a superordinate goal and a form of mediation between two sides of a conflict. A classic example is offered by El Salvador in 1985. UNICEF (United Nations Children's Fund), led by James Grant, identified the issue of children dying of preventable diseases. Infant mortality was far higher in El Salvador, Nicaragua, and the Honduras than in neighboring countries at peace. UNICEF and PAHO approached the Salvadoran government and the Roman Catholic church interceded with the FMLN (Farabundo Martí National Liberation Front) rebels. They found each side could view the future of their children as a superordinate goal. Beginning with a humanitarian ceasefire in El Salvador, Rodriguez-Garcia documented that UNICEF, the Roman Catholic Church, and other organizations negotiated ceasefires resulting in the immunization of hundreds of thousands of children. Dramatically, these efforts reduced the incidence of polio to zero.[39]

Operation Life Sudan was another effort that provided medical aid to both sides in a conflict, in this case, the Sudanese civil war. Simon Taylor-Robinson summarized the challenges of humanitarian aid and the benefits of an even-handed approach:

> In any humanitarian disaster caused by war, medical aid workers should be aware that their presence, however well intentioned, can prolong political conflicts, either because the negotiations that allow NGOs to operate can legitimise warring factions, or more nefariously, because aid money can become misappropriated into non-civilian channels. An evenhanded approach to aid distribution to all sides in a civil war is warranted, both in terms of emergency response and with respect to longer term aid.[40]

As Taylor-Robinson's and other articles emphasize, the relation, if any, between peace and these ceasefires promulgated for immunization programs is open to debate.[41]

2. Limiting the Destructiveness of War

Health professionals have been at the forefront of efforts to ban particular weapons because of their destructiveness. IPPNW, for example, inverted what was perceived as a political or military issue into a medical or health issue. The reasons for this were twofold: first, in the case of a nuclear attack, health professionals would be killed in extraordinary numbers, and second, because of this, there could be no meaningful medical response to even a limited nuclear war.

Since the St. Petersburg Declaration in 1868 and the Hague Declaration of 1899 banning dumdum (expanding) bullets, health professionals and, in particular, the International Committee of the Red Cross (ICRC) have advocated against numerous other instruments of war that cause "superfluous injury or unnecessary suffering"[42] from a PtH perspective, including napalm, poison gas, landmines, and blinding lasers. It is unclear to what extent, if any, these attempts to ban weapons limit the destructiveness of war, let alone lead to peace.

3. Communication of Knowledge; Health Professional Practice across the Divides

Communication of knowledge between both sides constitutes the most common PtH mechanism. There are several different types of communication of knowledge, including training and providing direct services. In addition, health professionals have been engaged both in war zones and in neutral territory. The following summarizes a PtH communication of knowledge initiative described in detail in *Healing under Fire: The Case of Southern Thailand*, by Virasakdi Chongsuvivatwong, Louisa Chan-Boegli, and Supat Hasuwannakit:

> The initiatives involved negotiating sustained access to populations residing in "red zones" which were off limits to governmental health workers; mental health services targeting children who had witnessed violence with a view to preventing cycles of violence; active participation in the peace process representing civil society and community interests; and, integration of health and peace topics into the medical curriculum of the Prince of Songkla Medical Faculty. Almost one year following the joint workshop, implementation of the initiatives were still in place, and plans were made to conduct health and peace conferences to further disseminate the concept amongst health workers in the region.... The most acceptable practice amongst peacebuilding activities was building relationships and mutual understanding with counterparts from the "opposing" side. A small minority saw their own potential in engaging directly in a peace process. Three years on, even with the official peace process stalled, participants in the original workshop are continuing some kind of activity related to their peacebuilding skills.[43]

International Physicians for the Prevention of Nuclear War (IPPNW) got its start with American and Soviet physicians working together across the Iron Curtain. This work began by relying on evidence gathered in the 1960s on the projected impact of a nuclear attack on the city of Boston, and with the friendship between two eminent cardiologists, both renowned authorities on sudden cardiac death, Bernard Lown and Evgeny Chazov.

Much of Pan American Health Organization's Health as a Bridge to Peace work in the 1980s involved collaboration and the sharing of knowledge among the health ministries of governments across the political spectrum in Central America.

As another example, Physicians for Human Rights-Israel (PHR-Israel) provides training and direct services in the Gaza Strip and has been doing so for many years.

The communication of knowledge is often one-sided, reflecting a lack of equivalence in strength between the two sides of a conflict. In this situation, the weaker side desiring the knowledge often prefers to have an outside party provide the training. Unfortunately, this results in neither side of the conflict engaging with each other. There is no literature specifically exploring the relation, if any, between the communication of knowledge programs and peace. At the same time, in the above-quoted southern Thailand example, a number of health professionals who participated in the communication of knowledge pursued peace building, even though as individuals rather than as members of their health organization.

4. Evocation and Extension of Altruism

In contrast to extending solidarity and support (see below), health workers have an ethical obligation to provide care to both sides of a conflict. Médecins sans Frontières, the ICRC, and the Red Crescent all adhere to this goal. Similarly, the WHO is involved in health care issues pertaining to postwar reconstruction on both sides. While such an activity can expose both sides in a conflict to health professionals, this may not function as a PtH mechanism unless the health professionals take this work to the next level in the form of health diplomacy, as discussed above. This is especially important in light of a recent study that concluded "on the aggregate, aid in conflict zones is more likely to exacerbate violence than to dampen violence."[44]

Buhmann, Santa Barbara, Arya, and Melf, in part, addressed the issues raised primarily in this mechanism in an article focused on the roles of health professionals before, during, and after an active conflict.[45] Buhmann and colleagues, for example, highlight the insider versus outsider health professionals who are engaged, pointing out the advantages and disadvantages of each. The insider has more intimate knowledge of the conflict, while the outsider often has access to greater resources. Setting aside the obvious military role that health professionals play in treating soldiers, the humanitarian role they take on is most akin to the PtH mechanism of altruism. By its nature, the WHO works with governments; the ICRC aims, within the framework of the Geneva Conventions, to provide health care to the suffering of all sides in a conflict; Médecins sans Frontières/Doctors without Borders will act as a witness to denounce violations of international humanitarian law. None go as far as Dr. Che Guevara or others willing to fight hostile powers in the name of justice.[46]

5. Personalizing the Enemy

Physicians for Human Rights-Israel (PHR-Israel), Physicians for Human Rights-USA (PHR-USA), Healing Across the Divides (HATD), and many other organizations have endeavored to put a human face on suffering that takes a toll on both sides of the conflict. HATD has sponsored speaking tours in the United States of, for example, directors of HATD-funded initiatives aiming to improve diabetes care among Palestinians living in the Occupied Palestinian Territory (OPT), early detection of breast cancer among Orthodox Jewish women in Jerusalem, and health improvement among Arab or Palestinian women living in extremely impoverished conditions in the northern part of Israel. One of the many challenges for organizations such as PHR-Israel, PHR-USA, and HATD is that they play a marginal role in the national discourse on the conflict disrupting societies. Desensitization to the violence[47] due to the ubiquity of social media may also play a role in diminishing the relevance of "personalizing the enemy" for peace-building efforts.

I would like to emphasize that two opposing sides "breaking bread" together does not personalize the enemy. Simply having contact does not personalize the enemy, especially in the case of a protracted conflict. Establishing "communication of knowledge" calls for an organizational engagement on the part of the party with the superior power balance between the two sides. Otherwise, the communication of knowledge serves only to protract the conflict to the benefit of the occupier and deepens the challenges facing the occupied.

6. Solidarity and Support; Noncooperation and Dissent

As highlighted above under superordinate goals, many health professionals attempt to work on bringing the two sides together by identifying goals in common. In some situations, the power imbalance between the two sides in a conflict is so significant that a few health care organizations decide to support the opposing side. In an effort to provide "solidarity and support," Physicians for Human Rights-Israel has since its inception critiqued the Israeli occupation of Palestinian Territories. Quoting from one of its many statements,

> The report, "The Casualties of Conflict: Medical Care and Human Rights in the West Bank and Gaza Strip," found that thousands of Palestinians suffered from both physical abuse and mental illness resulting from unprovoked violence. This included systematic but indiscriminate beatings in Palestinian homes and communities who were not engaged in demonstrations or provocations at the time of the beating, as well as the inappropriate use of tear gas indoors. PHR was unable to see Israeli military hospitals or clinics where military casualties might have been treated, nor Israeli civilian hospitals where civilian casualties might have

been treated. A review of published unofficial sources yielded a total of two serious Israeli civilian injuries, one Israeli soldier shot and killed, and 186 minor injuries to Israeli soldiers and police.[48]

While offering solidarity and support is likely to have minimal impact on opportunities for peace in a conflict such as that between Israelis and Palestinians, many Palestinians, health professionals, and the public alike, nonetheless frequently express appreciation. PHR-Israel has moved

> beyond the provision of immediate health services, to identifying, uncovering, and addressing the root causes of these health inequities. PHR's political activism, representing Palestinians before the Israeli Supreme Court, writing petitions, writing reports (in English, Arabic, and Hebrew), organizing demonstrations, even maintaining contact with the almost completely cut-off Gaza to try and advocate for their rights, is what allows the organization to gain credibility to work closely with Palestinian partners. As the President and Founder, Ruchama Marton, states: "I think that everyone, including doctors, needs to be politicized. Otherwise, it is a kind of mild, blind, non-affective activity. Even though a person can come home at night and tell himself how wonderful he was today, it is not very helpful to the dynamics of the whole thing. The organization and each and every one in the organization must be outside the consensus, which is not an easy place to be.[49]

Expressions of solidarity might be found to have a measurable impact; it might, for example, increase Palestinian resilience. However, there is no published data on this possibility.

7. *Social Healing; Strengthening Resilience; Increasing Trust*

Strengthening resilience, a critical PtH mechanism, calls for more than a simple definition. In examining resilience and its individual impact, I first specify the antecedents to resilience, such as readiness of change and confidence.

■ The Stages of Change Model developed by James Prochaska and Carlo DiClemente[50] specifies the levels of readiness of change for an individual who, for example, has diabetes and ideally should modify her diet. The stages are precontemplation (i.e., not ready); contemplation; preparation; action (i.e., ready to make change and take charge). Social disparities in health resulting in food insecurity or the presence of a conflict may impact, delay, or freeze any of the stages of change necessary to reach the goal.

■ Interventions to increase a person's confidence can be adapted from interventions drawn from the scientific literature or from the beliefs of those implementing the intervention. The Chronic Disease Self-Management Program (CDSMP) represents one intervention from the scientific literature that researchers have implemented among participants from many countries and across wide socioeconomic disparities.[51] The fact that it is well validated and lay-led makes it very attractive for immediate postconflict situations or even in the setting of protracted conflict.

■ People with a chronic illness who develop confidence via an intervention such as the CDSMP are able to manage all aspects of their life and desire to do so.

■ Resilience represents "a balance of biological, psychological, and social interactive effects for developing an adaptive trade-off between tolerance and sensitivity to stress."[52] If one is confident, one must be resilient; if one is resilient, one is likely to be confident, but not necessarily so.

The human need for resilience unfortunately emerges from the consequences of conflict. Put differently, the need for resilience emerges from humiliation. According to a Somali proverb, "Humiliation is worse than death; in times of war words of humiliation hurt more than bullets."[53]

> Perhaps the primary psychological effect of war on victims generally is through their witnessing the destruction of a social world embodying their history, identity, values and roles of everyday life. Such suffering has largely to be resolved collectively, in this same social world, albeit one which has been intentionally weakened. Thus, as the World Health Organization and other authorities confirm, the major thrust of humanitarian interventions must be towards the depleted social fabric and its institutions, for herein lie the sources of resilience and capacity for recovery for all. Beyond that, history has shown that social or political reform is the best medicine, and for victims of oppressive violence this means acknowledgement and justice.[54]

A blunt view of resilience holds that most people don't want to be resilient; they just want to have their needs met. "All too often, Palestinian 'resilience' is over-rated and sometimes used as a means of avoiding acknowledging and addressing the issue of injustice to Palestinians with humanitarian and international support divorced from the calls for justice, as happens elsewhere."[55] In contrast, Jeyda Hammad and Rachel Tribe recently reviewed Palestinian "culturally informed resilience," or *sumud*, and found a shift in the expression of resilience from a suspension of activities such as celebrations in the immediate aftermath of the 1948 war to efforts at affirming life as the Israeli-Palestinian conflict has continued.[56]

However, the reality is that there are many ongoing conflicts throughout the world today, with countries involved either paying no attention or making the conflicts worse. In addition, we are now witnessing the worst refugee crisis since

World War II. This explains the emergence and importance of resilience as a human response in the effort to simply survive.

Local community groups in the OPTs, funded, in combination with technical training, by Healing Across the Divides (HATD), have implemented several initiatives aimed at increasing resilience covering several thousand individuals in both Gaza and the West Bank. The local groups tracked intermediate outcomes through biological markers of diabetes and measures of confidence translated and culturally validated in Arabic. While not specifically measured, the thousands of individuals participating in these initiatives, having derived a direct benefit from the service, have developed trust in the ability of the community groups to deliver the service.[57] This does not automatically translate into trust in the health care system, since the nominally independent Palestinian health care system in the OPT is under aspects of military law.[58]

Next, I discuss what we consider to be a separate category, moving from public health to public trust. Moving from peace to health entails strengthening resilience that is explicitly linked to the macro level, such as the rebuilding of a health system after a conflict recedes. This section has special relevance for the increasing fragility perceived in the United States.

8. Peace to Health, or Peace to Public Health and Public Trust

Peace may have several impacts on health:

- Peace may lead to efforts to rebuild the health care system.
- Peace may also lead to efforts to reconcile parties to a conflict in a manner that specifically focuses on the sources of a conflict. Truth and reconciliation efforts represent one notable example of such efforts. These efforts can impact the health of the population.
- Finally, peace may lead to informal efforts to strengthen community cohesion.
- In relation to the connection between peace and health system improvement, peace may result in the strengthening of the health care system if political leaders make that a clear objective. When peace comes to a conflict-ridden zone, one of the first tasks of the local government is to "erect" or rebuild the health care system. As documented by many, better evidence linking peace and health system improvement is called for.

A nongovernmental organization (NGO), Rebuild Consortium, "examines health system resilience in fragile settings experiencing violence, conflict, pandemics and other shocks."[59] According to Rebuild Consortium,

> resilient health systems have been characterized in one framework as having five key features: knowledge of available resources and emerging challenges; versatility to take action against a broad range of challenges;

ability to contain health crises and avoid damaging reverberations in other parts of the health system; capacity to form a multi-sectoral response that integrates a range of actors and institutions; and flexible processes that allow for adaptation during crises.[60]

Rebuild Consortium, for example, linked the successful peace to health response to Ebola virus disease in Uganda in 2001 to "local, national and international contextual factors that included trust between service users and a key non-governmental (faith-based) provider, a supportive environment for health workers and a quicker, coordinated response by donors."[61] In another example, reporting on a case study consisting of interviews conducted in Zimbabwe, health professionals under difficult economic circumstances tried to encourage, for example, patients to report incidents of domestic violence to the police, a measure of health professional trust in the governmental entity, in this case, the police.[62]

If a conflict terminates, people's desire for better health may lead to efforts to influence, in a positive feedback loop, the health care system under "construction." However,

> Post-conflict states usually have very low capacity to improve service delivery even if they have the will. Investments in health in these contexts normally aim to bring the privatised provision of healthcare by NGOs and others under a government umbrella with calls for increased equity and inclusion of underserved populations. During the last decade, the provision of a basic package of health services, free of charge, to all citizens, as a core policy element has become a commonly promoted approach. Part of this approach may be contracting third parties, often NGOs, to provide the services on behalf of the government. One concern with this approach may be low visibility for the government and hence fewer legitimacy gains. This concern may be off-set by co-branding and by providing comprehensive services of higher quality ... that in principle are much more accountable than the government's service delivery mechanisms, and have the potential for a wider impact on both health outcomes as well as on socio-economic determinants of health.[63]

If at least part of the population is confident and/or resilient, as described in the previous section, citizens are more likely to want and be able to provide feedback on ways to improve a health system under development. Improved health outcomes that occur as a consequence of an increasingly functional government may engender measurably increased social trust. This resultant increased social trust may in turn strengthen a peace still new and frangible.

Rebuilding a health system can further resilience and improve citizens' health and well-being. However, it should be kept in mind that health systems are extremely labor-intensive and, as such, furnish significant opportunities for patronage, nepotism, and, in fact, corruption, especially for a partially resilient new government.

In addition, the need to spend an ever-increasing amount of a health system's budget on certain elements, such as pharmaceuticals, increases incentives for corruption.

Researchers, particularly from Rebuild Consortium, have demonstrated both positive and negative results on the relation between states recently emerging from a conflict and health system reconstruction:

> Effective provision of health services during crises can promote state-building, while inadequate provision undermines the process. In Nigeria and Mozambique, privately contracted health services that were more accessible and of better perceived quality were associated with better perceptions of the state by the public, and failures in health service provision by private contractors were blamed on the state.[64] Evidence therefore indicates that state-building can be supported by effective public and private provision, however there is also evidence that extensive private contracting for health service management and provision during crises can undermine legitimacy of the state, as reported in Afghanistan.[65]

Peace may also lead to efforts to reconcile parties to a conflict in a manner that specifically focuses on the sources of a conflict. In this regard, researchers have explored the health effects of "truth and reconciliation efforts." One such study examining the impact of this process on health found that:

> reconciliation had both positive and negative consequences. It led to greater forgiveness of perpetrators and strengthened social capital: Social networks were larger, and people contributed more to public goods in treated villages. However, these benefits came at a substantial cost: The reconciliation treatment also worsened psychological health, increasing depression, anxiety, and posttraumatic stress disorder in these same villages. For a subset of villages, we measured outcomes both 9 months and 31 months after the intervention. These results show that the effects, both positive and negative, persisted into the longer time horizon.[66]

With respect to the impact of peace on social cohesion, it is certain that for the vast majority of people, peace will result in a stronger sense of well-being. Countries just emerging from conflict and rebuilding their health system can further increase well-being by involving citizens in decision-making processes and deliberately addressing social, physical, and economic barriers to health system engagement. Emperatriz Crespin, an interviewee for this brief, provided an excellent example of an initiative on youth gang violence:

> Over the past five years, the increasing number of youth groups involved in violence has become a major public concern in many areas in Central America. The youth gang problem is linked to and made even worse by

the legacies of unresolved dynamics going back to former conflicts, the onset of democratic governments, and the confluence of illegal migration and the drug trade. This problem is proving a constant threat to the security and stability of local populations.[67]

In another study on a different conflict, acknowledging that there was no long-term follow-up and that the study was done at only one health center, Cathryn Christensen and Anbrasi Edwards interviewed individuals in the aftermath of a still-simmering conflict. They analyzed data in a structured manner, a positive feature that distinguishes this article from many others. One quote from an informant stands out. It goes to the heart of the connection between health, peace, and fragility—the themes of this book

> When there is no health in the household first, there won't be peace, everybody will be stressed out and worried, you won't be able to work, you won't be able to eat, and then that will create tension....
>
> In the community it is the same thing: if a neighbor is sick all the time, people can say their neighbor poisoned them and there can be jealousies and blame....
>
> It is the same thing for the country: if there is no health, there is no production, and there is stress between people.... It is just what I see every day. If you see that someone is sick ... how can you know that there is peace? How can there be peace in your country if you do not feel peaceful yourself ... if you see that no one cares about you.[68]

Conclusions

As discussed in detail above, the literature on the young field of PtH consists of many papers, of which 246 from all over the world were systematically collected and analyzed for this chapter. While most of the interventions described in these papers did not benefit from follow-up, many of the initiatives point to at least positive short-term outcomes. We also discussed the challenges and opportunities of the peace to health category.

Tragically, to my mind, all the interventions discussed in this chapter are the same ones that form the critical underpinnings of the work that health professionals must engage in if we are to address the increased—not decreasing, as is typically researched—fragility in the United States. This increased fragility and what health professionals can do to address it constitute the subject of the remainder of this book. But it is important to first provide an in-depth sense of American fragility. My "COVID-19 Notes," a diary I kept during the pandemic, provides this direct sensibility of the challenges that confront us and that we continue to face.

Notes

1 See graphic available at: https://www.economist.com/weeklyedition/2022-09-03. Accessed: December 24, 2022.
2 Though beyond the scope of this chapter, in the past 20 years there have been dramatic strides on research into the impact of social deprivation on the physical/mental health of individuals In addition, remarkable recent research has demonstrated not only a relationship between stress, in general, chronic illness, and poverty but also how these negative experiences of stress, especially if they occur in childhood, can impact the genes of children in their lives as well as those of their offspring. In more technical terminology: "chronic psychosocial stressors and related emotional states lead to dysfunctional mitochondria, which in turn contribute to stress pathophysiology via multiple mechanisms including changes in gene expression and the epigenome, alterations of brain structure and functions, abnormal stress reactivity, inflammation, and by promoting cellular aging." Picard, M. and McEwan, B. (2018) Psychological stress and mitochondria: a conceptual framework. *Psychosom Med.* 80:2. 126–40. Available at: https://www.ncbi.nlm.nih.gov/pmc/articles/PMC5901651/ Accessed: December 24, 2022. See in general the research of Bruce McEwan.
3 Weber, M. (1978) The Nature of Social Action in *Max Weber: Selections in Translation*, ed. Runciman, WG., trans Matthews, E. Cambridge: Cambridge University Press as quoted in Hanna, B. and Kleinman, A. Unpacking Global Health: Theory and Critique in Farber P., Kim JY., Kleinman, A., Basilico, M. (2013) *Reimagining Global Health*. Berkeley: University of California Press, p. 16.
4 Berger, PL. and Luckmann, T. (1996) *The Social Construction of Reality: A Treatise in the Sociology of Knowledge*. New York: Irvington Publishers, p. 3.
5 Bar-Tal, D., Halperin, E., and Pliskin, R. (2015) Why Is It So Difficult to Resolve Intractable Conflicts Peacefully? A Sociopsychological Explanation. In M. Galluccio (Ed.), *Handbook of International Negotiation: Interpersonal, Intercultural, and Diplomatic Perspectives*. Switzerland: Springer. See also Bar-Tal, D. (2013) *Intractable conflicts: Socio-psychological foundations and dynamics*. Cambridge: Cambridge University Press.
6 Weber, M. (1947) *The Theory of Social and Economic Organization*, trans AM Henderson and Talcott Parson. New York: Free Press.
7 Kleinman, A., Das, V., Lock, M. eds. (1997) *Social Suffering*. Berkeley: University of California Press, p. ix.
8 Galtung J. (1969) Violence, Peace, and Peace Research. *Journal of Peace Research*. 6:3. 167–91. Available at: http://www2.kobe-u.ac.jp/~alexroni/IPD%202015%20readings/IPD%202015_7/Galtung_Violence,%20Peace,%20and%20Peace%20Research.pdf. Accessed: December 24, 2022. See also Galtung, J. (1996) *Peace by Peaceful Means: Peace and Conflict, Development and Civilization*. London: Prio/Sage.
9 Arya, N. (2004). Peace through Health I: Development and use of a working model. *Medicine, Conflict, and Survival*. 20: 242–57. 10.1080/1362369042000 248839.
10 Farmer, P. (2003) *Pathologies of Power: Health, Human Rights and the New War on the Poor* Berkeley: University of California Press.
11 Ibid p. 40.
12 Constitution of the World Health Organization. Originally published 1946. https://www.who.int/about/governance/constitution; Accessed January 16, 2023.

13 Ottawa Charter for Health Promotion. Available at: https://www.euro.who.int/__ data/assets/pdf_file/0004/129532/Ottawa_Charter.pdf?ua=1. Accessed December 24, 2022.

14 World Health Assembly. (1981) Resolution WHA34.38. The role of physicians and other health workers in the preservation and promotion of peace as the most significant factor for the attainment of health for all. *Thirty-fourth World Health Assembly*, Geneva: World Health Organization Available at: https://apps.who.int/iris/handle/10665/155679. Accessed April 11, 2020–February 20, 2023.

15 Fragile States Index. (2022) Available at: https://fragilestatesindex.org/frequently-asked-questions/. Accessed November 19, 2022.

16 Frum, D. (2022) Only the GOP celebrates political violence *The Atlantic*. Available at: https://www.theatlantic.com/ideas/archive/2022/10/pelosi-republicans-partisan-political-violence/671934/. Accessed December 24, 2022.

17 For more on information given in this sentence and the following sentences, see various chapters in Levy, B., and Sidel, V. (2008) *War and Public Health*. New York: Oxford University Press.

18 Shmerling, RH. (2022) Why life expectancy in the U.S. is falling. *Harvard Health Publishing* Available at: https://www.health.harvard.edu/blog/why-life-expectancy-in-the-us-is-falling-202210202835. Accessed November 19, 2022.

19 Musanabaganwa, C., Jansen, S., Fatumo, S. et al. (2020) Burden of post-traumatic stress disorder in postgenocide Rwandan population following exposure to 1994 genocide against the Tutsi: A meta-analysis *Journal of Affective Disorders*. 275:10. 7–13.

20 Nnadi, C., Etsano, A., Uba, B., Ohuabunwo, C., et al. (2017) Approaches to vaccination among populations in areas of conflict. *Journal of Infectious Disease*. 216(suppl_1): 7: S368–72.

21 See Levy, B. and Sidel, V. op cit.

22 Ibid.

23 Ibid.

24 UNHCR (2015) Worldwide displacement hits all-time high as war and persecution increase *UNHCR*. Available at: https://www.unhcr.org/558193896.htmll. Accessed March 28, 2021.

25 Ewing, J., Shoumali, J. (2019) Where doctors are criminals *The New York Times*. Available at: https://www.nytimes.com/2019/12/20/world/middleeast/syria-medical-criminalization.html. Accessed January 15, 2023.

26 WHO (2022) Health as a Potential Contribution to Peace. 'Realities from the field: what has WHO learned in the 1990s' *WHO* Available at: https://www.who.int/initiatives/who-health-and-peace-initiative. Accessed December 24, 2022.

27 Rubenstein, L. (2010) Peace Building Through Health Among Israelis and Palestinians. *United States Institute for Peace*, Available at: https://www.usip.org/sites/default/files/resources/PB7%20Health.pdf. Accessed December 24, 2022.

28 MacQueen, G. and Santa Barbara, J. (2000) Peace Building through Health Initiatives. *BMJ* 321: 293. doi:10.1136/bmj.321.7256.293. Available at: https://www.ncbi.nlm.nih.gov/pmc/articles/PMC1118283/pdf/293.pdf. Accessed December 24, 2022.

   MacQueen, G., McCutcheon, R. and Santa-Barbara, J. (1997) The Use of Health Initiatives as Peace Initiatives." *Peace and Change 22: 175–197.10.1111/pech. 1997.22.issue-2 in Arya, Neil. (2004).* Peace through Health I: Development and Use of a Working Model. *Medicine, conflict, and survival.* 20:3. 242–57. 10.1080/1362369042000248839.

29 Garber, R. (2001) Health as a Bridge for Peace: Theory, Practice and Prognosis Reflections of a Practitioner *Journal of Peacebuilding and Development*, 1:1. 69–84.

30 Rodriguez-Garcia, R.; Macinko, J., Solorzano, FX., Schlesser, M. (2001) How Can Health Serve as a Bridge for Peace? *CERTI Crisis and Transition Tool Kit*. Retrieved from http://hsrc.himmelfarb.gwu.edu/sphhs_global_facpubs/228. Accessed December 24, 2022.

31 Ibid. 66–67.

32 Ibid. 81.

33 Arya, N. (2004) Peace Through Health I: Development and Use of a Working Model *Medicine, Conflict and Survival* 20:3. 242–57. 10.1080/1362369042000248839. Available at: https://www.researchgate.net/publication/8208122_Peace_through_Health_I_Development_and_Use_of_a_Working_Model. Accessed December 24, 2022 and Abuelaish, I., Fazal, N., Doubleday, N., Arya, N. et al (2013). The mutual determinants of individual, community, and societal health and peace. *International Journal of Peace and Development Studies*. 4:1. 10.5897/IJPDS12.008. Available at: https://www.researchgate.net/publication/261874402_The_mutual_determinants_of_individual_community_and_societal_health_and_peace. Accessed December 24, 2022.

34 Abuelaish, I., Goodstadt, MS., and Mouhaffel, R. (2020) Interdependence between health and peace: a call for a new paradigm. *Health Promot Int*. 35: 6: 1590–600. 10.1093/heapro/daaa023. PMID: 32219393.

35 Izzeldin A. and Neil, A. (2017) Hatred-A public health issue, *Medicine, Conflict and Survival*, 33: 2: 1–6. 10.1080/13623699.2017.1326215.

36 Maddocks, I. (1996) Evolution of the physicians' peace movement: a historical perspective. *Health Hum Rights*. 2: 1: 89–109.

37 Maddocks, I. (1996) Evolution of the physicians' peace movement: a historical perspective. *Health Hum Rights* 2: 1: 98.

38 UNICEF (2016) Two-thirds of unimmunized children live in conflict-affected countries *UNICEF*. Available at: https://www.unicef.org/png/press-releases/two-thirds-unimmunized-children-live-conflict-affected-countries-unicef. Accessed December 24, 2022 and Nnadi, C., Etsano, A., Uba, B., Ohuabunwo, C. et al. (2017) Approaches to vaccination among populations in areas of conflict. *Journal of Infectious Disease*. 216: Suppl 1: S368–372.

39 Rodriguez-Garcia, R., Macinko, J., Solorzano, FX., and Schlesser, M. (2001) *How can health serve as a bridge for peace?* Washington, DC: George Washington Center for International Health. Available at: https://hsrc.himmelfarb.gwu.edu/sphhs_global_facpubs/228/. Accessed December 24, 2022.

40 Taylor-Robinson, SD. (2002) Operation Lifeline Sudan. *J Med Ethics*. 28: 1: 51.

41 Ibid.

42 Arya, N. and Santa Barbara, J. eds. (2008) *Peace through Health: How Health Professionals Can Work for a Less Violent World*. Sterling, VA: Kumarian Press, p. 43 and Coupland, R. The Effect of Weapons: Defining Superfluous Injury and Unnecessary Suffering *International Physicians for the Prevention of Nuclear War*. Available at: http://ippnw.org/pdf/mgs/3-coupland.pdf https://ihl-databases.icrc.org/customary-ihl/eng/docs/v1_rul_rule70. Accessed November 19, 2022.

43 Chongsuvivatwong, V., Louisa, CB., and Supat, H., eds. (2015) *Healing under Fire: The Case of Southern Thailand*. Available at: https://peaceresourcecollaborative.org/en/deep-south/overview-analysis/healing-under-fire-the-case-of-southern-thailand-2#.

Accessed March 14, 2021. Appendix 4 provides greater detail on this specific intervention, together with results.

44 Zürcher, C. (2017) What Do We (Not) Know About Development Aid and Violence? A Systematic Review, *World Development,* 98:C. 508. Available at: https://ideas.repec.org/a/eee/wdevel/v98y2017icp506-522.html. Accessed December 24, 2022.

45 Buhmann, C., Barbara, JS., Arya, N., and Melf, K. (2010) The roles of the health sector and health workers before, during and after violent conflict. *Medicine, Conflict and Survival.* 26: 1: 4–23.

46 Whittall, J. (2019) Medical humanitarian needs in a changing political and aid environment *Medicins Sans Frontieres.* Available at: https://msf-analysis.org/medical-humanitarian-needs-changing-political-aid-environment/. Accessed December 24, 2022.

47 Stevis-Gridneff, M. (2020) Child Dies at Sea as Greece Cracks Down on Migrants From Turkey. *New York Times.* Available at: https://www.nytimes.com/2020/03/02/world/europe/migrant-death-greece.html. Accessed December 24, 2022.

48 Physician for Human Rights - Israel Available at: https://phr.org/countries/israel/#:~:text=In%201988%2C%20PHR%20physicians%20visited%20Jerusalem%2C%20the%20Gaza,abuse%20and%20mental%20illness%20resulting%20from%20unprovoked%20violence. Accessed December 24, 2022.

49 Ibid.

50 Prochaska, JO. and DiClemente, CC. (1992) Stages of change in the modification of problem behaviors. *Progress in Behavior Modification.* 28: 183–218.

51 Lorig, KR., Sobel, DS., and Stewart, A. (1999) Evidence suggesting that a chronic disease self-management program can improve health status while reducing utilization and costs: A randomized trial. *Medical Care.* 37: 1: 5–14.

52 Davydov, DM., Stewart, R., Ritchie, K., and Chaudieu, I. (2010) Resilience and mental health. *Clin Psychological Review.* 30: 5: 479. 10.1016/j.cpr.2010.03.003. Epub 2010 Mar 25. PMID: 20395025

53 as quoted in Barber, BK., McNeely, C., Olsen, JA., Belli, RF. et al. (2016) Long-term exposure to political violence: The particular injury of persistent humiliation. *Social Science & Medicine.* 156: 154–66.

54 Giacaman, R. (2020) Reflections on the meaning of 'resilience' in the Palestinian context. *Journal of Public Health* (Oxford). 42:3: e369–400.

55 Ibid. 370.

56 Hammad, J and Tribe, R. (2021) Culturally informed resilience in conflict settings: a literature review of Sumud in the occupied Palestinian territories, *International Review of Psychi*atry. 33: 1–2: 132–39.

57 See for example chapter 3 of Goldfield, N (ed) (2021) *Peace Building through Women's Health.* New York: Routledge.

58 Barnea, T. and Husseini, R. (2002) *Separate and Cooperate, Cooperate and Separate: The Disengagement of the Palestinian Health Care System from Israel and its Emergence as an Independent System.* New York: Praeger.

59 See https://www.rebuildconsortium.com/

60 Witter, S. and Hunter, B. (2017) Resilience of health system during and after crises – what does it mean and how can it be enhanced *Rebuild Consortium.* Available at: https://rebuildconsortium.com/media/1535/rebuild_briefing_1_june_17_resilience.pdf. Accessed: November 19, 2022.

61 Ibid https://rebuildconsortium.com/media/1535/rebuild_briefing_1_june_17_ resilience.pdf

62 Evans, S. and Maheshvari, N. (2020) Mapping the role of health professionals in peace promotion within an urban complex emergency: the case of Chegutu, Zimbabwe, *Medicine, Conflict and Survival.* 36: 4: 314.

63 Ndaruhutse, S. (2011) State-Building, Peace-Building and Service Delivery in Fragile and Conflict-Affected States: Literature Review *Department for International Development (DFID)* Available at: http://www.gsdrc.org/docs/open/sd34.pdf. Accessed December 24, 2022.

64 Eldon, J. and Waddington, C. (2008) Health systems reconstruction: Can it contribute to state building. *Health and Fragile States Network* London: HLSP Institute http://bit.ly/2qqiOeN and Witter, S., Falisse JB., Bertone, M.P., Alonso-Garbayo, A, et al. (2015) State-building and human resources for health in fragile and conflict affected states: exploring the linkages. *Human Resources for Health* 13: 33. Available at: http://bit.ly/2qLLYYv. Accessed November 19, 2022.

65 Palmer, N., Strong, L., Wali, A., and Sondorp, E. (2006) Contracting out health services in fragile states. *BMJ* (Clinical Research ed), 332 (7543) http://bit.ly/ 2raMmjm. Both this and the previous two references are drawn from. Witter Sophie and Hunter Benjamin. (2017) Do health systems contribute to reduced fragility and state-building during and after crises? *Rebuild Consortium Briefing* #6. Available at: https://www.rebuildconsortium.com/resources/do-health-systems-contribute-to-reduced-fragility-and-state-building-during-and-after-crises/. Accessed November 19, 2022.

66 Cilliers, J., Dube, O., and Siddiqi, B. (2016) Reconciliation after civil conflict increases social capital but decreases individual well-being. *Science*, 352: 6287: 787–94.

67 SICA signs MoU with Interpeace to strengthen capacities of member states to confront youth violence (2009) Available at: https://www.interpeace.org/fr/2009/06/ sica-signs-mou-with-interpeace-to-strengthen-capacities-of-member-states-to-confront-youth-violence/ Accessed November 19, 2022.

68 Cathryn, C. and Anbrasi, E. (2015) Peace-building and reconciliation dividends of integrated health services delivery in post-conflict Burundi: qualitative assessments of providers and community members, *Medicine, Conflict and Survival*, 31: 1: 39.

69 Transcribed testimony of Yerachmiel Kahanovich. Sivan E. (2012) Towards a Common Archive – Video Testimonies of Zionist Fighters in 1948. Available at: https:// www.youtube.com/watch?v=lDEiUY8mW0Y. Accessed December 24, 2022 as quoted In Ross A. (2019). *Stone Men: The Palestinians who Built Israel.* New York: Vero, pp. 13–14.

70 Mann-Shalvi, H. (2016) *From Ultrasound to Army: The Unconscious Trajectories of Masculinity in Israel.* London: Karnac pp: 140–41.

71 Levy, B. and Sidel, V. (2000) *War and Public Health.* Washington DC: American Public Health Association, p. 247.

72 Garber, R. (2002) Health as a Bridge for Peace: Theory, Practice and Prognosis Reflections of a Practitioner. *Journal of Peacebuilding and Development*, 1: 1: 81.

73 Arcadu, G. Louisa, CB., Urs, B., Virasakdi, C. et al. (2022) *Healing Under Fire – The Case of Southern Thailand.* See specifically chapter 9. Available at: https:// sites.google.com/site/thaibookproject/chapter-9-capacity-building-for-health-and-peace-work-a-collaborative-effort-in-southern-thailand. Accessed December 24, 2022.

Appendix 1: Two case examples that presage the development of the mental, physical, and invisible consequences of war

Operation Broom. Interview with Palmach (part of the pre-Israel Jewish army) machine gunner Yerachmiel Kahanovich (YK) by filmmaker E. Sivan:

INTERVIEWER (I): Operation Broom, what is it? You simply stood in line and just....

YK: Yes, you march up to a village, you expel it, you gather round and have a bite to eat, and go on to the next village....

I: But how?

YK: You mean by shooting?

I: How do you mean?

YK: We shot, we threw a grenade here and there. Just listen—there is one thing you have to understand: at first, once they heard shots, they took off with the intention of returning later.

I: But wait a sec, that was before May 15 (declaration of Israeli independence), that was before the Arab armies came.... Operation Broom then. How does it happen? Do you receive any information? Is it an organized campaign? ...

YK: Yigal Allon (at the time commander of the Palmach; eventually a general and acting Israeli Prime Minister) himself planned it. We moved from one place to the next.

I: What places? Can you tell me?

YK: We passed by Tiberias and moved from one village to the other, from one to the next.

I: So, you had orders to expel and clean up the villages?

YK: And then go home.[69]

A historical vignette highlighting one terrorist attack on Israeli Jews, Interview with Naftali Lau Levi, a child survivor of the Holocaust, by psychoanalyst Hanni Mann-Shalvi:

> Among other incidents, Naftali talks of how in April 1974, he found himself in the coast town of Maalot in Northern Israel, as terrorists took control of the local school.... "When the firing stopped, I ran ... to the building. Tens of boys and girls and several adults lay dead or injured on the floor, and several sat leaning against the wall screaming for help. The horrific scene sent me back thirty years to scenes I hadn't found release from since Auschwitz and Buchenwald. I stood there, helpless, feeling my legs collapsing beneath me. I hurried outside and sat on a curbstone...."

The Israeli warrior, who can protect his own life and that of his family, is pitched against Naftali's father or grandfather, who couldn't do a thing. Unlike the Holocaust, the Israeli soldier is an answer to the helplessness of the school children and of Naftali, who once again faces the Holocaust. When Naftali read my interpretation of his emotions, he admitted wholeheartedly that I had hit the nail on the head.[70]

Appendix 2: Example of the impact of conflict on health systems from the Nicaraguan "Contra" war, which began soon after the Nicaraguan Sandinistas came to power

Health workers were often targeted. Interrupting services was intended to help erode popular support for the government. Malaria control programs, immunization programs, and health posts had to be closed down in many rural zones. By the late 1980s, malaria re-emerged in some zones along with epidemics of measles and other vaccine-preventable illnesses that had diminished markedly by the mid-1980s. A new rural hospital was closed. Medicines and medical supplies were destroyed, most dramatically in the 1983 bombing of the port of Corinto.[71]

Appendix 3: Extract of Randi Garber, "Health as a Bridge for Peace: Theory, Practice and Prognosis Reflections of a Practitioner"

Outcomes (a) Health—Positive outcomes were found in two areas: professional development, and health services improvement. The main benefits of professional development found were increased professional knowledge and skills, gaining cross-cultural knowledge, and professional networking. Concerning health services improvement, over three-fourths of the project directors said that the health-related goals of their project were achieved. Specific examples of health-related outcomes were noted for nine projects. These include:

- Training of health personnel—specialist training of 23 Palestinian physicians; accredited training in family medicine for four Palestinian physicians; training of 380 teachers as health educators.
- Development of infrastructure—contributing to the establishment of the Health Promotion and Education Directorate in the Palestinian Ministry of Health; establishment of a state-of-the-art laboratory at a Palestinian university.
- Direct provision of service to over 20,000 Palestinians in rural areas and 80,000 students in elementary schools.
- Generation of data—to assist policy planning and development of intervention programs in both the Palestinian Authority and Israel in the fields of adolescent health behaviors, leishmaniasis, and beta-thalassemia.

b) Conflict—Outcomes measured related to the conflict include:

■ Opportunities to meet and learn about each other—Israeli respondents said they were able to learn firsthand about Palestinian people, their needs, and their culture (as opposed to secondhand reports in the media), and Palestinian respondents said they learned about Israeli professionalism.
■ Changing attitudes—the work on a cooperative project showed the participants that cooperation is possible, enhanced the desire to live in co-existence and moderated views on the conflict.
■ Spreading the word—ninety percent of health professionals involved in cooperative activities shared their experiences with colleagues or friends.

The projects presented here show that HBP projects exist even in difficult political circumstances and have positive impacts in the health field, on the conflict at individual and local levels, but are very much at the whim of the political processes surrounding them. While writing this article, a new cycle of violence erupted between Israelis and Palestinians.[72]

Appendix 4: Extract of Article on the Impact of the South Thailand Intervention, One-year follow-up

Of the four initiatives developed during the workshop, two had concrete follow-up activities.

1. **Curriculum development**

    The proposal of the health and peace course inserted into the core curriculum of the medical school was under deliberation by the Board of Directors of the Faculty of Medicine of the Yale University. It has been decided, however, to include topics relevant to health and peace in the extracurricular courses and seminars. As part of the extracurricular program, the lectures given by tRI and DSRR evaluation team were well received by both faculty staff and medical students. Further, the translation of Medical Peace Work online material in Thai has started.

2. **Healthy Mosques**

    This is an ongoing program in one of the conflict-affected districts in Narathiwat province, with ten of 34 mosques now designated as "Healthy." These Healthy Mosques offer primary health care to restricted groups of families. After participation in the workshop, the director of the district hospital negotiated access to the Healthy Mosques for everybody, including the communities in areas where health workers have no access. In some cases, these Healthy Mosques are used to conduct outreach services for the off-limits villages.

One new initiative—not planned but inspired by the workshop—is the "twinning of red and green villages" (red villages are insurgent controlled and green villages are Government controlled). The initiative focuses on reaching out through health promotion to selected "green areas" located in the proximity of "red villages." Through these outreach activities, contacts between the red and green communities may be increased. In time, confidence in health services would also grow and eventually allow access to villages that at present are off-limits to Government personnel.

In addition, a process was discreetly started to request that wise and influential elders visit and engage communities, teaching the Islamic way to reduce violence and to foster non-violent ways of resolving disputes.

The evaluation found that not all the participants at the workshop were ready to engage in peace work. The culture of the Thai society generally involves non-interference, particularly in political affairs. Any kind of peace work is considered political. Other dimensions are fear of reprisals, loss of credibility and access to communities in need. In this light, the success of the workshop can be attributed to the fact that the knowledge and skills offered through the workshop are not only part of the peace workers' toolkit but are also powerful tools to enhance the capacity of health professionals to cope and deliver health care in complex and difficult situations.[73]

Chapter 3

The COVID "Notes"

Preface

At the beginning of March 2020, I had no idea that my life, personal and professional, would change forever. By the middle of March 2020, life began to rapidly change, and I began to keep this largely professional diary. I would complete an entry every approximately two weeks. It is the feedback of approximately 1000 readers together with my ongoing efforts, via Ask Nurses and Doctors (AND), to improve our health system that encouraged me to write this book. The diary is at the center of this effort. As I write this preface in December 2022, I am reading a headline in the *Washington Post*: "Rejoice! Despair! The office holiday party is back in person."[1] This diary hopefully gives a sense of the road many of us, especially health professionals, have taken since March 2020. What follows is an excerpt from the diary. The entire diary with more extensive references can be found at the website for AND the organization I founded in 2018 to help elect individuals who believe in reform of our health system.

March 14, 2020. Executive Branch Is COVID Clueless; What Health Professionals Can Do

We live under an executive branch that decimated its own office created to fight pandemics.[2] To put it differently, health experts say Trump is breaking all the rules when it comes to communicating about the crisis.

Who will suffer the most? The poor, the undocumented, the homeless, (and sometimes they are one and the same), people of color.

Please see the links to a post regarding COVID from Andrew Goldstein, one of the most politically committed progressive and thoughtful health professionals

DOI: 10.4324/9781003426257-4

I know and work with: "Wrote some of my thoughts on our pandemic. While optional social distancing is helpful, it ultimately is still a path leading to many preventable deaths. To me, the public health and moral argument is clear: we need a societal halt coupled with humane isolation. Feedback, counterarguments, questions are welcome."[3] Public health professionals are encouraging this manifesto on staying at home.[4]

March 17, 2020. The Day We Changed; How We Completely Changed Our Practice

We can be thankful that the news media outpolls the executive branch when it comes to trust in the information. Despite this, 37% of Americans and 85% of Republicans still believe in what comes out of the political side of the executive branch of the U.S. government.

This issue of the *Economist* has a good article on the politics of pandemics.[5]

I and all practicing health care professionals are learning the meaning of the term "front-line." Many health professionals will have stories such as mine, and many will be more intense.

Yesterday was a day to remember. Though late in the game, the staff at our practice (I am an internist) and senior management at the hospital system (the practice is owned by a hospital system) came together and, within two hours (!!), totally changed the way our practice operated. A completely gowned person with security (we always have security guards at our office) behind her was questioning each and every person as to why they were coming in. Most of my visits were done by phone. No one with flu symptoms was allowed in the door. I had one HIV patient who had a runny nose. I took off all my clothes when I got home and put them in the wash. A day unlike any other. Too late; but better later than never. Eternally optimistic, but I deal with reality.

March 23, 2020. This Is What WWII Was Like Except That Instead of Bombs There Is Silence; AND Political Roundtables with Congressional Candidates

On Sunday, I spoke with my last surviving relative (94) of World War II. She is from Hong Kong and was in a civilian camp under Japanese occupation for much of the war. She lives in a small town in England and is restricted to home. Yes, she said, the COVID pandemic is very much like World War II (for her, I emphasize), but instead of hearing bombs falling, she said … there is just silence … I spoke with a physician colleague in Italy Sunday. Clearly exhausted from the 12-hour workdays, and home restriction. And no mail service – period. Yet, every person in Italy who is not working gets sick-leave pay – that is simply part of a humane political system (just as everyone in Italy has health insurance – a mixture of public and private).

At my practice, today I am dealing with patients who work at nursing homes and were exposed to COVID-infected patients, have symptoms, and were still told to come in to work (I told her to stay out of work); a prison guard who has flu-type symptoms and is afraid of COVID (I prescribed Tamiflu and told her to stay home); and then there is the usual – two patients with asthma out of control (Prednisone, etc.); and a diabetic patient with a gangrenous toe (antibiotic and evaluate again tomorrow) – all managed by phone – for now.

Re AND: I'm largely focused on organizing round tables in the next one to two weeks between health professionals and their member of Congress. I am also working on my contacts who know people one step removed from Republican governors. I am still hoping that Republican governors will lean on Trump to put in place the recommendation of my colleague.

According to my colleague Dr. Andrew Goldstein, we need to shelter in place. Response so far from one Republican governor: It is challenging for any politically astute governor to back a statewide shelter-in-place order. And why is that? Well, this morning's headline explains it: Trump suggests coronavirus containment measures may be too extreme as more states issue stay-at-home orders. On a more positive note: a shout-out of thanks to Don Berwick on AND's Board of Advisors for his great article in today's *NYT*, about health care workers risking their lives to treat COVID patients.[6]

March 30, 2020. Death of My First COVID Patient

Three days ago, I had no COVID-19 patients in the hospital. Two days ago, there were two in critical care. One of the two, a patient for more than twenty years, died Sunday at 3 pm. Her daughter cried to me, "She didn't deserve to die this way, all alone." She's right. My first, not my last, patient to die of COVID-19. When the daughter gave me details of who else was exposed to her mother, the need for testing of these people, I said ashamedly that I have no access to testing or tracking of exposed individuals. Another patient of mine is intubated. I believe he will survive.

Before Trump's inauguration, a warning from the Obama administration: "'The worst influenza pandemic since 1918'… officials briefed the incoming administration on this exact scenario."[7] What's Trump's planning approach? "Trump ties coronavirus decisions to personal grievances."[8] Priorities for this president: "Trump took to Twitter Sunday afternoon to tout the ratings of his news conferences, claiming without evidence that mainstream media are going 'CRAZY' because of his popularity on television."[9]

In the meantime, my physician colleague has been extubated and continues to improve but is still in the hospital. A song that my colleague Rich Averill sent me highlights the importance of "#staythefuckhome."[10]

April 2, 2020. How to Do a "Telephonic Visit"; Passover Questions for Fauci

All my patient visits are telephonic. Not the ideal way to "see" patients. There are presumed COVID (easy), maybe COVID (much harder to assess, including the patient who had clear shortness of breath with both myself and the nurse on the line, probably because of anxiety) and then, most people who are just getting sick with other problems, such as the patient likely with gout for whom I can't give the full treatment because of his diabetes, kidney disease, and heart failure.

The last few days have seen the lack of federal coordination in full display. Just three ominous examples and then what we can do about them. "Desperate lawmakers hunt for medical supplies as Trump takes hands-off approach; House members are taking it upon themselves to secure gear for the most at-risk health care workers in their districts."[11] Secondly, Trump suggests coronavirus testing is no longer a problem. Governors disagree.[12] I am just now under very difficult circumstances able to get testing. Many are already getting billed thousands of dollars for COVID care.[13] Lastly, the executive branch response to the millions about to lose health insurance: Trump said yesterday that Pence's response wasn't addressing the question of uninsured people. "It's one of the greatest answers I've ever heard... Because Mike was able to speak for five minutes and not touch your question. I mean that's what you call a great professional."[14]

What to do? Harvey Fineberg in yesterday's *New England Journal of Medicine* provides a good summary of most of the needed next steps, entitled "Ten Weeks to Crush the Curve!"[15] I and other colleagues have written a paper tentatively entitled "A Crisis Means There Are Opportunities for Community-Centered Population Health Care" (see Chapter 6 of this book).

For those of you thinking about Passover, questions you might want to ask Dr. Fauci to put a smile on your face[16]: I quote:

- How do I disinfect a Seder plate?
- Because this debate will come up (it's the nature of the beast): Would wandering in the desert be advisable at this time? That is assuming there is manna from heaven and/or Amazon Prime, enough water and shelter, and we keep six feet away from other wanderers.
- I'd love to be sure I'm coronavirus-free before asking my husband and kids to the table, but the only tests I can get my hands on are an expired ClearBlue Easy and a gently used Cologuard. Which do you think would reassure my family more?
- My Uncle Murray insists on tweeting that Manischewitz cures coronavirus. In case the president sees this, please tell him it's not true. Also that he shouldn't retweet it, no matter how tempted he is by Uncle Murray's use of all-caps.
- Can the president use the Defense Production Act to have gefilte fish factories converted to make... literally anything else?

April 10, 2020. Another Patient Died, All Alone; Telephone Appointment Suggestions

Sadly, another of my longtime patients died yesterday of COVID-19. Again, all alone. I spoke to the family – by phone. Starting at 9 am, I will start my telephonic phone visits with patients. What are these encounters like? I received an email yesterday from administrators at my medical practice that gave a suggested communication sequence for us health professionals. It may be of interest if you are on the receiving end of a telephone encounter with your health professional:

> Take a breath before you call the patient. Smile when you greet the patient (Research shows that people can tell if you're smiling by the tone of your voice). Acknowledge the elephant in the living room: ask how the patient is coping with the COVID-19 pandemic. Remember to engage the patient in agenda setting. Elicit reactions to recommendations overtly. Shorten your educational spiels. Break up your explanations into short chunks. Elicit reactions and questions regularly. Remember that the summary and teach-back are vital.

Yes, I am sad as a practicing physician for this almost completely avoidable situation, and it's not surprising consequences.[17] I channel any sadness – I don't have anger – into organizing via AND. I look to all of you for suggestions of health professionals interested in working with AND on swing states so that we can win this election in November. In addition, I am pleased to be working with the DCCC in a number of congressional districts.

Of course, family and friends are key at this time. Art is also very inspiring. This article from the *LA Times* on art at the time of the black death 600 years ago reprises a paper that I wrote as a high school student more than 50 years ago.[18]

April 15, 2020. My Third ICU COVID-19 Patient Is Not Doing Well; I Can Now Get Testing; Millions of Unemployed Will Lose Their Health Insurance

My third COVID patient ICU patient is not doing well; intubated. For the past two weeks, I speak to family members every night around 7 pm, giving them an update. Every COVID death is a tragedy; these deaths were largely avoidable. But this 27-year-old is especially painful for me, as I spoke with her the day before she was hospitalized. She called me about symptoms that were likely COVID, but she said she was feeling much better. But in a familiar COVID scenario, the next day she had trouble breathing, was hospitalized, and has been intubated ever since.

I am now able to order COVID tests. Of course, nothing is so simple, as it can give false negatives. But I do feel that I am making progress when yesterday I was able to order the COVID test for someone who had just been exposed to the virus and was coming down with symptoms.

By now, the (barest) outline of how the United States will emerge out of this totally avoidable human tragedy that is still unfolding is clear. The two main questions that remain are: Will the executive branch of the federal government be held to account (i.e., over the next four months) for its sheer incompetence, brazen mendacity, and authoritarian tendencies? Will Congress assert its authority and pass significant legislation checking the executive branch?[19] Thus far, Congress has been on the sidelines.[20] The important recommendations[21] for a strong federal response made by Scott Gottlieb and Mark McClellan, two excellent health policymakers who served under Republican presidents, will likely not come to pass. States will do their best to respond, and many will do just fine, though the political polarization will stop for some, for example, New York and Florida, from working together.[22]

Lastly, will we, as was done in the aftermath of the Great Depression, be able to take this unique once-in-a-century opportunity to address the gross inequities in our health system?

April 20, 2020. No Contact Tracing; Germany on the Mark; Federal Government MIA

In my last note, I wrote about the first COVID test that I was able to order. Friday, it came back positive. No contact tracing is available in Springfield, MA. So…my patient has exposed many new people to COVID and until they are symptomatic, we simply won't know who. I couldn't reach him Saturday. On Sunday, he didn't "sound" all that great, and I encouraged him to go the ER. He was dehydrated and he received fluids intravenously. A chest X-ray showed viral pneumonia – but his symptoms were not serious enough for him to be hospitalized. My intubated COVID patient is alive but continues to be in critical condition. I delivered a meal to my physician colleague who made it home and is ready to "take a walk around the block."

The politics are straightforward. This administration leads the fight against this virus by retweeting this kind of statement by Trump supporters: "Now, more than ever, we need the Wall With China Virus spreading across the globe, the US stands a chance if we can control of our borders President Trump is making it happen."[23] Contrast this with what is occurring in Germany, where 80% support Angela Merkel, the country's prime minister.[24]

I am always asked: When is this all going to end? We are in for a significant period of uncertainty. The approach summarized in this headline won't work: "Congress shovels trillions at virus, with no end in sight."[25]

April 25, 2020. My Patient Extubated! Birx Says Nothing About Trump's Touted Bleach Treatment; Millions of Newly Uninsured

Preliminary data shows that 88% of people on ventilators die.[26] Am happy to report that my last intubated patent is now extubated! But by no means is she out of the woods. She has large venous clots, a relatively common problem in COVID patients.[27] Examples of people avoiding care: "Telephonically saw" a new-to-me 27-year-old farmworker yesterday with abdominal pain for weeks. Her delayed diagnosis with infected gallstones for weeks diagnosed yesterday; immediately hospitalized and had her gallbladder removed.

Germany is being praised for a near-textbook response to the pandemic, thanks to a robust public health care system, but also a strategy of mass testing and trusted and effective political leadership.[28] The U.S. has *none of these three ingredients* – at present. On the scientific side in the executive branch, health professionals led by Adams, Birx, and Fauci are unwilling to confront executive malfeasance publicly or privately, especially on Trump's bleach pronouncement: "I see the disinfectant that knocks it out in a minute, one minute… And is there a way we can do something like that by injection inside, or almost a cleaning?"[29] Congress is thus far politically incapable of stepping up to the executive branch, i.e., still no forward thinking or response to the executive branch's refusal to support millions of newly uninsured or implement contact tracing/testing.

Data points: this paper discusses how the economic downturn primarily driven by the COVID pandemic could impact enrollment in Medicaid, the ACA Marketplaces, and employer-sponsored coverage, as well as the potential change in the number of uninsured individuals.[30]

Controlling this pandemic will be up to the states. Will states be able to coordinate? It will happen haphazardly, but the answers are clear (see Gottlieb, McLellan documents reported in previous COVID Notes and in the references; I and others have also written about long-term possibilities). I have no contact tracing available yet. Most important, we need a link between testing and contact tracers.[31]

April 29, 2020. Increased Anxiety (and Deaths); Consequences of Mistrust

My extubated patient continues to improve. She isn't speaking yet. Three weeks of intubation has affected her brain. It is too early to tell how much of her mental function will return but I am always hopeful and communicate that daily to her family – they are all of Italian extraction, my birthplace.

The consequences of this pandemic are easy to hear (I am still doing only telephonic visits) from a sample of yesterday's 17 patients – one is simply paralyzed by anxiety and doesn't want to return to work (Rx: counseling, medication, and more frequent visits with me); another experienced a hypertensive emergency including blurry vision/headache and didn't want to go to the ER because of COVID (Rx: frequent daily encounters managing his hypertension; he is doing much better); then a patient who wants to go back to work and who ten days ago had COVID pneumonia on his X-ray (Rx: encouraging him to check his diabetes, be aware of relapse).

Many of my medical encounters wouldn't occur if the U.S. had the three key elements: trust, a massive testing strategy, and a strong public health department. Ohioans do have trust in the governor (but little testing and little public health). This Ohio poll showed overwhelming support for the governor. Mr. DeWine's data-driven response has won the support of top Democrats in the state. Every morning at 11:30, Mr. DeWine holds a conference call with the mayors of Ohio's seven largest cities, all Democrats: "It's so refreshing – it's how governing should work."[32] In contrast, Attorney General Bill Barr directed all 93 U.S. attorneys on Monday to "be on the lookout for state and local directives" that curtail individual rights in the name of containing the novel coronavirus.[33]

May 5, 2020. My Patient Is Speaking! and "Unknown Unknowns"

Amazingly, my extubated patient continues to improve. I spoke to her yesterday for the first time by phone! She will likely be discharged to a rehabilitation hospital in the very near future. While she is starting to speak, there are mental health challenges, long road ahead.

After two COVID deaths, my other surviving COVID patients are well. I am able to order COVID tests. Our office parking lot is now a drive-thru testing operation, but only for people with symptoms. There are not enough tests to test an adult living in a group home exposed to someone hospitalized with COVID! And … no contact tracing yet. Long way to go!

In this COVID Note, I would like to step back and summarize a very good article I read in the *Times Literary Supplement* entitled "Models and Muddles." Put aside the fact that this administration will never examine issues from a scientific perspective. Let's look to the future. The author, Paul Collier, starts out by specifying the concept of radical uncertainty, which orients our thought to two fundamental questions: "how to face identifying known unknowns" and "how to face unknown unknowns," Collier continues:

> The answers to the former are to build resilience while encouraging rival teams of experts. The answers to the latter are to learn from others while investing in finding out new information… The value of using rival teams is that this method flushes out these known unknowns while discouraging exaggerated claims to knowledge.[34]

A *NYT* article summarizes many of the current COVID "known unknowns."[35]

So where does that leave us? A friend sent me this: From a lead editorial of the *Irish Times* from Dublin: **"The world has loved, hated and envied the US. Now, for the first time, we pity it."**[36] Yes, pity is the right word.

May 7, 2020. Another COVID Patient Hospitalized; Opening This Country Economically?

My patient was short of breath Friday. I am just happy she went to the ER without calling me. Hospitalized immediately. And another family: mother and son are both patients. Son tested positive on Friday. I told him he had to stay at his girlfriend's house as his mother is very at risk clinically. Mother calls me Sunday – worried about her son. He was doing reasonably well, and nothing was needed. I smiled to myself – mothers are at work every day – even Mother's Day!

While more tests are available, of course, no contact tracing – yet. This past Tuesday: The White House Council of Economic Advisers released a model that showed deaths dropping to zero[37] by the middle of May. There is continual disagreement even on the actual COVID death toll.[38]

Two days later, I've read this sentence from the *Washington Post* any number of times: "this administration is … asking Americans to accept – a devastating proposition: that a steady, daily accumulation of lonely deaths is the grim cost of reopening the nation." Accepting this proposition is not pitiable. It is simply disgusting.[39]

Although he is now tested every day with a rapid-result machine, Trump has questioned the value of extensive testing as the gap between available capacity and the amount that would be required to meet public health benchmarks has become clearer.[40]

A bipartisan group of former health officials seeks to sell a $46.5 billion coronavirus plan to the White House.[41]

May 15, 2020. Two More Patients Hospitalized with COVID; Ongoing National Confusion; Executive Branch to People: Testing Isn't Necessary – Really?

I had two more patients hospitalized this week with COVID. Both discharged. We are getting better in our care for COVID patients, and we are testing more. Still no contact tracing where I work – which is a hot spot!! My patient who was intubated for weeks is not only extubated, not only in rehab – but she is COVID-negative!! She is about to be discharged – home!! Wow. American health care at its best.

But sadly, the overall picture is dismal. What are the results of no national response to this pandemic? As the *USA Today* headline stated: "We Have 50 States and 50 Different Approaches."[42] *I've highlighted the millions of newly uninsured.* The Kaiser Family Foundation found: Between March 1 and May 2, 2020, more than 31 million people had filed for unemployment insurance.[43] So … what to do about this? But first a historical point: Just a few years ago, the Affordable Care Act passed by just a few votes in the House of Representatives. The question is, what if anything can we do to get health insurance to the unemployed? Right now, the Democrats don't have the votes and/or control of the White House.[44]

Finally, please look at these faces in the reference below. They belonged to health care professionals who fought for your, for our health ... and have died. They have died because of the sheer incompetence of this administration; the sheer maliciousness of this administration; the sheer wallowing in narcissism of all members of this executive branch. But ... let it be known that more and more of us get that, and we will win the presidency, the House, and the Senate in November and elect politicians to serve us in Washington who are in favor of science and the health of all people in the United States. That is the only way to open this economy which is on its knees. But first ... look at these faces.[45]

May 22, 2020. Domestic Abuse; My Intubated Patient Is Home!

It is now 6 am. I was up till 10:30 last night speaking to a longtime patient – a victim of domestic abuse – another by-product of the COVID era, which has seen a dramatic rise in violence against women and children. I was trying to convince her to call the police, but I could tell she wasn't willing or able emotionally. As I've known her for years, I made a clinical decision to trust her assertion that she could stay the night in the home with the perpetrator. I have already texted her this morning. The rise in domestic abuse that we've heard about is paralleled by a rise in child sex abuse and a drop in the reporting of child abuse.[46]

Meanwhile, my patient who was intubated for weeks is now home!! I've met with her twice telephonically this week. Again, she represents the best that U.S. medicine has to offer. But now comes the hard part – she is having difficulty with her memory; can barely walk; has leg pain (due to clots) that is very significant. COVID-19 is much worse than the flu.[47] She has a long road to recovery. It will cost tens of thousands of dollars – minimum. But, living in Massachusetts, we both have access to good home care services – including physical therapy, nursing services, and even in-home psychological therapy.

In an article published today in the *NYT*, gallery owner David Zwirner writes: "Art is how we justify our existence." I remember last year in southern Italy seeing a carving in stone of an animal that was 25,000 years old. It is art that makes human beings unique in the world.[48]

June 1, 2020. Extubated Patient Is Home; COVID Impact on Blacks

My patient who was intubated for weeks was extubated, discharged from the acute hospital, and sent to a rehabilitation facility. Ten days ago, she went home. She needs a cane; memory is poor; depressed but is happy to be alive. Another COVID patient was just discharged from the hospital. COVID question I addressed today: A symptomatic (fever, cough, sore throat) COVID-positive patient who managed herself at home, wants to go back to work. I checked in on her by phone 14 days later. No more fever. But a residual cough. What to do? test or no test? Answer: no test and send her back to work.

COVID continues to decimate the Black community. As reported today by Dylan Scott in his excellent column, "this weekend we saw the collision of two public health crises: police violence and the coronavirus."[49]

> Covid illustrates this nation's structural racism in two important ways. **First, police violence is a public health risk.** In almost any way you measure it, the US criminal justice system is prejudiced against black Americans, and black people are much more likely to be subjected to state-sanctioned violence in the US compared to white Americans. Black men, by far the most at-risk group, face one in 1,000 odds of being killed by the police over the course of their lives. Suicide in prison accounts for 34% of all deaths (suicide rates for prisoners is 4 times the rate of the general public)![50] **Second, people are coming out to protest police violence in the middle of a pandemic that has disproportionately impacted Black Americans:** Black people are more likely to work in jobs considered "essential," exposing them more to the virus. America's failure to build an equitable health system means its Black residents have high rates of preexisting conditions that make them more vulnerable to Covid-19. They also live in places with more air pollution and have less reliable access to clean water.

Can one protest safely? Here are the precautions one should take.[51]

Lastly, I do the food shopping; have you noticed skyrocketing food prices? They are predicted to stay high, making it more difficult for the poor to eat nutritious meals, worsening their chronic conditions.

June 10, 2020. Husband COVID-Negative, Wife COVID-Positive and Symptomatic; Masks and Social Distancing Work

From the *Washington Post*: "The scale of the coronavirus has made it hard to take in. In the period of four months, it has devastated the world," Anthony S. Fauci, director of the National Institute of Allergy and Infectious Diseases, told CNN on Tuesday.[52] "And it isn't over yet."

So, to bring it down to scale: What a week! The usual with my COVID patients – for now all discharged from the hospital – but this week I had the following twist – husband COVID-negative; wife COVID-positive and symptomatic. In the same building (but a different apartment) is the elderly mother who has asthma. All patients of mine. They are all isolating from each other. So far everyone is managing at home. The question was whether the husband should go to work. Even though the wife started feeling better, I was going to tell the husband that he needed to hold off going to work (his negative is probably a false negative and, and even if not, he has been exposed to his wife and thus needs a quarantine period). In response, he told me that the owner of the store where he works told him not to come in, as the owner's mother had just died of COVID! Yes, it is hard to take in, but this what it is like at the human level. And despite all the COVID patients in our practice, we are still struggling with contact tracing.

One of my standard questions these days is "do you have enough food on the table?" There is a great deal of food insecurity among both the poor and the newly poor middle class.[53]

People ask me all the time why it is that Blacks, and young Black people are disproportionately impacted. We know some of the reasons, which are poignantly described in this article.[54]

In the absence of any movement in Washington on health insurance for the many millions of newly uninsured (and this policy initiative must come from Washington), we will continue to get stories like these: COVID tests for $7,000 and, for those that have health insurance, policies that don't cover COVID tests.[55]

My belief is that when it is potentially lifesaving people will be willing to get the vaccine if the scientific community endorses it. It is at least my hope; it may be a challenge, considering how strong the anti-vaxxer movement has grown since its beginning in the now thoroughly debunked article linking vaccines to autism. In the meantime, we know that masks work. We also know, from a just-published article in Science, that contact tracing, social distancing, and appropriate travel restrictions work.[56]

June 24, 2020. Steady Stream of COVID-Positive Patients with Symptoms; Lives and Years Lost

Yesterday, another husband-and-wife pair were diagnosed as positive. Both with mild symptoms. The wife has significant chronic mental health issues, and she is simply distraught. The husband, my patient, has significant risk factors. Thus far, his symptoms are mild. My other husband-and-wife team diagnosed two weeks ago are fine; he is back at work. My patient who was intubated for weeks is stable on the outside (right now, the number of hospitalized patients has plummeted). My patient who was intubated is clearly disabled both physically and mentally; we meet by phone once a week; she is getting physical therapy and nursing services. In our practice, we are doing self-nasal swabs/health professional nasal swabs or drive-by testing. Just to reemphasize for mild symptoms (i.e., I can treat them), the only treatment is supportive care and services. The tricky part is when the patient is short of breath

(SOB). That is where knowing the patient makes all the difference in the world. I sent right to the ER my obese diabetic who had shortness of breath (SOB); I was in contact several times a day with my anxious obese asthmatic who had the same SOB.

This is the human context to this remarkable article published yesterday in Vox. **138,000 deaths**.[57] I still think about my patients who've died of COVID and their families. But as the byline says: "'Years of potential life lost' is the most sobering and sad Covid-19 statistic I've seen." When you break down the number by ethnic group you find: **Black Americans under the age of 65 have lost, collectively, 45,777 years of life, the researchers' analysis found. Hispanics and Latinos lost 48,204. White Americans under age 65 have lost, collectively, 33,446 years of life.**[58]

I have a number of patients who work as prison guards. In one of the prisons, one of my patients (a prison guard) said that 60% of the prisoners had COVID and more than a dozen died. This is similar to a just-published Pro Publica story.[59] Our practice provides the medical care to prisoners at one of the local jails, and I am pleased to say that there have been no deaths.

Lawyers for the executive branch are filing briefs this week with the Supreme Court with the executive branch advocating dismantling the Affordable Care Act (ACA). Before the COVID pandemic, it was estimated that 20 million would lose their health insurance if the ACA is struck down. That number is likely much higher now. What you may not know is that there are some winners: The highest-income 0.1 percent (1 in 1,000) households would receive tax cuts averaging about $198,000 per year. This group has annual incomes over $3 million.[60]

As Brian Resnick, the author of a Vox article put it regarding wearing masks and COVID deaths: "That number (138,000) does not seem to be enough to inspire all Americans to wear masks, to inspire self-sacrifice to save lives, to inspire more politicians in states to action." – Yet!

July 10, 2020: Native Americans, Rural America, and Social Distancing

We are living in a time of extreme parallel pandemic universes; of literally "normal" life vs COVID-19 fear, illness, or death; COVID-related economic privation or, for now, Wall Street results that do not compute for most Americans. At the human/clinical level, this week I negotiated with a patient who wanted to get out of quarantine after being symptomatically COVID-positive; I examined a young person with a rapidly expanding bald spot that he and I attribute to the stresses of not finding enough work in a COVID economy; and I hospitalized another patient who died of complications of Alzheimer's exacerbated by her COVID. But in a sign of the era we live in – was the COVID gone by the time that she died? If not, the family cannot view the body. That is the question I am researching as I write this COVID Note. While we are learning a great deal about COVID, there is much we do not know about, e.g., the impact of COVID on our body systems.

The next issue of the *Journal of Ambulatory Care Management* that I edit is focused on the COVID pandemic. A vignette from the Navajo Nation in the Southwest:

> Mae-Gilene Begay, the Director of the Navajo Nation Community Health Representative (CHR) Program, has just gotten back from staffing a curfew checkpoint when we get her on the phone. The CHRs have been helping the police at the roadblocks by providing COVID-19 education and information to the passersby. She recounts a story of a COVID positive patient they encountered that day. "This individual had run out of food and water and was very emotional, so the CHR stepped aside to take care of that," she said. "The traveler had been told to self-isolate but ran out of food and she needed to get something to eat and she was out of water. She had to leave her house to get supplies.[61]

From Rural Maine:

> On May, 10, 2020, the outbreak that started at Tall Pines Healthcare (nursing home) on April 8, 2020, was officially closed, sixteen days after the last patient tested COVID-19 positive. Our Tall Pines community was changed beyond the toll imparted by thirty-two patient cases, eleven staff cases, nineteen recovered cases, and thirteen deaths due to COVID-19. The wards, the remaining patients and staff, and Alana and I looked different. We are different; we weathered April ("the cruelest month") and emerged at the end of the outbreak with mixed feelings: relief tempered by apprehension; self-doubt laced with a modicum of pride for a "job well-done" (or at least for being of use); grief not ready to be comforted by fond memories of our patients and their families. The Tall Pines community shared a COVID-19 outbreak experience that is uniquely our own; we will need time and the will and courage to heal ourselves by facing each other and acknowledging the "different."[62]

Two headlines from today's *Washington Post* hammers home the parallel universes that we are living through in the U.S.: "Time to Shut Down Again?" And "Trump Sidelines Health Advisers in Rift over Coronavirus Response."

From a Letter to the Editor published today in the *Jacksonville Union* signed by members of the Florida AND group:

> Of the five-county area around Jacksonville (where a major COVID outbreak is occurring), only Duval (and some specific municipalities) now require masking in public and indoor places or in other situations where individuals cannot be socially distanced.... If there is still doubt

as to the effectiveness of face masks, next time you or a family member must have surgery, ask the surgeon and the team to not wear masks. It is a small request to wear a mask.

Signed: **Representatives of "Ask Nurses and Doctors" of Florida.**[63]

Lastly, this article shows how to put on, fit, and care for your mask.[64]

July 17, 2020. I Have Symptoms – Can I Afford to Get Tested; Impact on Health Workers; Political Vaccines

I had a patient yesterday who had very suspicious symptoms, but didn't feel very sick, and thus felt that for purely financial reasons she didn't want to get tested. If she gets tested and is positive; she is out of work. Workers in the U.S. do not have the same unemployment benefits as their compatriots in Western Europe. I encouraged her to wear a mask both in and out of the house and to be washing everything separately from other family members.

Another death from COVID. The family of this patient, whom I'd known for decades, was able to view his body – a very consequential act for anyone – especially as they were not allowed to see him in the hospital. In the past, I would have ordinarily gone to the wake but … no more.

I saw my patient who was intubated for weeks with COVID respiratory failure and also with a large blood clot in the neck. This week, I am trying to figure out with cardiology whether and for how long she should say on the anticoagulants – COVID is a new disease.

What's the current science on who should quarantine? Anyone who has been in close contact with someone who has COVID-19. This includes people who previously had COVID-19 and people who have taken a serologic (antibody) test and have antibodies to the virus. What about my daughter coming back from NYC who has tried to be careful? Should she quarantine when she comes back home? We have no data on that.

Lastly, I very much like Jeff Lerner's just-published piece in the *Philadelphia Inquirer*, for his brilliant metaphor of the need to deploy our *political vaccine*: All health care professionals can play a critical role in creating a "political vaccine" against disinformation. We need to speak out publicly for science now.[65]

August 3, 2020, Still Working with Patients with Aftereffects; Local COVID Outbreak; No National Plan

My COVID experiences this week in part revolve around helping one of my patients now permanently disabled from the aftereffects of COVID; large numbers of patients refusing needed treatment for their ongoing chronic illnesses due to extreme anxiety about COVID exposure; and patients who were COVID-positive with continued symptoms almost certainly related to anxiety.

A few days ago, a local health facility I am affiliated with identified several COVID-19-infected employees and patients on a clinical unit. The facility, being the transparent and thorough facility that it is, identified 23 COVID-positive employees and 12 COVID-positive patients. Contact tracing and testing is being conducted for any patients who test positive. It is likely that the outbreak resulted from several factors: employees who traveled to areas within the United States identified as "hot spots" and were found to be infected after return; staff convening in break rooms and removing their masks without observing proper social distancing protocols; some staff members coming to work with symptoms; and inappropriate or inconsistent mask use in common and public areas of the unit. Likely, a combination of these factors contributed to the transmission of the virus.

The best tools we currently possess to stave off any resurgence of this virus remain proven public health interventions – hand hygiene, face masking, social distancing, no communal meals, avoid travel, and don't go to work with symptoms. Sound familiar? But we have no national policy that advocates firmly for these measures and provides the financial and organizational resources to implement them. In fact, we will never have a national policy from this administration. For example, because of federal incompetence, we cannot get testing efficiently done, thus missing most cases.

Let's keep in our hearts health professionals who have lost their lives to the pandemic without any recognition.[66]

August 25, 2020, Fear of Going to the Hospital; Politics Tramples Science

AG, a long-standing patient of mine, has had children killed by random gunfire. His wife died of cancer years ago. He not unexpectedly has severe anxiety in addition to his diabetes, obesity, and asthma. This week I treated his cough and asthma with steroids. Unfortunately, one of the side effects of steroids is to increase blood sugar; his sugar went above 500 (normal is up to 100). I convinced him to go to the ER, but AG took one look at the busy ER and left – he was afraid of catching COVID. The next day I prevailed on him to go the ER, and he was hospitalized. Fear of COVID delayed his hospitalization by several days – an almost fatal delay.

We as health care professionals also need to balance appropriate concerns about COVID with sound medical advice based on our clinical judgment. Our clinical judgment needs to always include a healthy dose of skepticism whenever one is discussing a new illness such as COVID, which brings us to the scientific and political fiasco around plasma treatment.[67] I am not so concerned by the fact that plasma was approved under emergency use authorization (EUA) as by the process and the hype of its efficacy without scientific support.

A scientific outcry ensued after FDA Commissioner Stephen Hahn's misleading statement: 35 out of 100 COVID-19 patients "would have been saved because of the administration of plasma." On Monday night, Hahn acknowledged his error.[68] No such correction has come from either HHS or the executive branch. While Trump called it a "historic announcement," the treatment is unlikely to make a major difference against COVID, a virus that's killed more than 170,000 in the United States.

My suggestion, and of others as well – that the medical leadership in the executive branch consider resigning – is not going to happen;[69] in fact, the executive branch has settled on a new strategy – bring on physicians, such as Scott Atlas, who have no relevant background except their antiscience punditry on Fox News.

The race is on as to whether the Democrats or the Republicans can control the narrative about the responsibility of the executive branch for the extent of this pandemic. This 30-second video, produced by a colleague of mine, highlights the importance of controlling the narrative.[70] This could make the difference in encouraging people to vote – in favor of science. AND is also working with others creating videos and headshot screens for selected Congressional races. There is a new way to register to vote that involves health professionals.[71]

September 8, 2020, Contact Tracing; Voting 101

Political meddling with guidelines from the Centers for Disease Control (CDC) feeds fear. This past week, a febrile patient of mine tested positive for COVID. What to do? What type of contact tracing should I do? Who should I order tests on? While we have trusted the Centers for Disease Control for our entire working lives, we cannot now trust CDC guidance, as three recent examples highlight: the abrupt change in testing guidelines, the shifting school opening guidelines, and the reassignment of COVID and other health data analysis from CDC experts to HHS political appointees.

The change in testing guidelines is the most damaging of all. The executive branch essentially told the CDC to change its guidelines,[72] and the leadership of the CDC has largely folded under political pressure, adding more confusion for the public.

Since it is the weekend, I did my own contact tracing. The first positive individual was from New Jersey, who in turn transmitted to the patient's sister who was visiting Springfield Massachusetts where my patient lives and I practice. The patient's sister then returned to her home several thousand miles away! The patient is married with three children. Contact tracing is not easy! Despite the currently useless CDC guidelines, I am ordering COVID testing on everyone who has had close contact with the patient, including a repeat on one child who had tested negative a month ago.

We continue to have shortages of PPE equipment months and months after the outbreak. But the deficiencies are very solvable "if the federal government gives the Strategic National Stockpile agency greater clout, provides it with access to better information and technology, and beefs up its expertise."[73]

Worried about the surfaces in a voting booth? Various disinfectants (including ethanol at concentrations between 62 and 71%) inactivate a number of coronaviruses related to SARS-CoV-2 within one minute. That is what happens after every patient I see at the practice – all surfaces including doorknobs are wiped down.

Surgeon General under Ronald Reagan C. Everett Koop once said, "Health care is vital to all of us some of the time, but public health is vital to all of us all of the time." This crisis we are facing offers us a unique opportunity to rebuild our public health system.[74] Americans are looking for leadership on the worst crisis to impact us in a century and, in response, the U.S. has failed to protect its citizens, the most basic function of government.

September 18, 2020. COVID-19's Human Toll; New Knowledge; Challenges Ahead

I've spoken in past COVID Notes about one patient in her thirties who luckily survived weeks of intubation. While I've spoken to her almost on a weekly basis, I saw her for the first time only yesterday. Outwardly, she looks the same. Yet she is permanently scarred – both physically and emotionally. She will likely never work again.

Almost all my patients have an overarching sense of anxiety. In terms of my own behavior, I wash my hands incessantly with sanitizer; I wear a head screen over a mask whenever I am with a patient. When I come home, I undress and take a shower.

AND is totally focused on the upcoming election. We are organizing health professionals in Fl, PA, and Michigan on behalf of Biden via videos that will be circulated.

If you are celebrating the Jewish New Year (starts tonight!) – may it be as sweet as possible, while understanding that whoever wins the White House and Congress will have many challenges.[75] In the spirit of resolution, this, which my friend Isa Aron passed on to me, is mine: *Question what is; Imagine what can be; And then do it.* Let's do it together! I am lucky to know all of you.

September 30, 2020. This Week's Patient Highlights; COVID Challenges; Millions More Uninsured in 2020

On Yom Kippur, just after I reflected on the life and death of my parents – via Zoom – one of my patients called on my cell. I took the call as I know him and realized something significant must be up. He told me that he and his whole family all tested positive for COVID-19. His wife was exposed to a positive person. I know that the local health department is doing tests. But I have no way of confirming that, as there is no communication between the health department and the "traditional" health system (where I work). There is no contact tracing. And therein lies our challenge. Once this pandemic is under control, another one will appear. Several of us[76] and others[77] have made proposals on how to best link the public health and traditional doctor-patient health care system.

Despite all the chaos in school openings, some did very well. There is no secret to their success.[78] Sadly, there is not only no national COVID policy but, in fact, different executive branch health professionals are fighting with each other[79]. We've passed the grim, avoidable number of 200,000 deaths. Accompanying this unfathomable tragedy are ongoing PPE shortages,[80] ongoing challenges with the release of testing supplies to states, and many thousands at campaign rallies[81] without PPE. In contrast, Biden has been very clear on what his COVID policy would be: "a test-trace-isolate program, making mask-wearing and social distancing mandatory, and, once the science supports it, an equitably distributed vaccine."[82]

The number of uninsured increased by a million in 2019. Many estimates point to 15 million more losing their health insurance in 2020.[83] More to the point, "reducing protections for patients with greater health needs isn't a bug in the GOP plans; it's a key feature."[84] Or as Dylan Scott starkly summarized: 20 million more will lose their insurance under Trump, 25 million will gain under Biden.[85]

In our last month of electoral work, AND is focused on several congressional races; also helping Biden win in Fl, MI, PA. Most important, please vote!

October 21, 2020. COVID Pneumonia in Asthmatic Patient; White House MD: Masks Don't Work

My feelings in the last 48 hours whipsawed between caring for a patient with uncontrolled asthma and reading about how the U.S. non-national COVID policy has devolved into total chaos.[86] My patient, in her thirties, has asthma and it was out of control starting last Wednesday. I attended to her telephonically on Thursday and then again Friday early morning. Thursday, I started her on asthma meds (steroids, etc.); Friday, I added an antibiotic. She went to the ER Friday night, and they diagnosed COVID pneumonia. They discharged her as she was stable. Monday, she felt worse and started vomiting everything she ate though she said she could hold down her meds. I prescribed antinausea medication. It didn't help. She went back to the hospital Monday evening and was hospitalized. In a nutshell, this is why herd immunity will not work.[87]

We don't need leadership that believes that any human cost is acceptable.[88] We do need support for basic services such as food.[89] Last week, our practice gave out the last food vouchers for our undocumented patients; employees continue to replenish the till.

One of the health professionals I work with in Florida as part of AND was in Massachusetts briefly; he said everyone in Massachusetts was wearing masks.

He returned last week to Florida – where few were wearing masks. But what should we expect from ignorant physicians[90] in Florida who are in power and downplay the importance of masks?

In these last two weeks before the election, AND is organizing in states for Biden and congressional races such as Maine-2. In MI-3, we are helping with an event for Hillary Scholten. Be healthy; stay safe – the global sales of condoms have surged as social distancing rules have relaxed!

November 23, 2020. Post-Election COVID Notes; I Called One Patient at Work to Tell Him He Was Positive; Ten More in Past Two Weeks

We truly need a national COVID policy now. You need to see this brief video,[91] which recounts the horrors that health professionals have witnessed throughout this pandemic – people hungry for air, chest compressions for hearts that have stopped.

I've had more than ten COVID-positive patients in the past ten days. This past Friday, I called one patient at work and told him that he was positive/should go home/quarantine. Another young patient was hospitalized with COVID pneumonia but did well enough to be discharged a few days later. He still has significant fatigue and joint pains. I also had a 65-year-old female patient whom I had to convince to get a COVID test; her asthma was out of control and she was COVID-positive. I monitored her every day by phone. The vengeful upsurge is here.

The *New York Times* just featured the hospital (Baystate) I admit patients to; it provided a devastating summary of the national COVID chaos we confront.[92] The conclusion was painful for me to read:

> In a sense, the Trump administration had achieved one of its goals: It had trained Americans not to rely on it. Everyone was on his or her own in this pandemic, Artenstein warned. That was the American way.

I don't believe that is the American way. It is this federal government chief executive's way.

Most of my patients, and many health professionals, are suffering emotionally from the pandemic. Light-box therapy lamps could help with seasonal depression.[93]

School closings are a significant factor in childhood mental health difficulties. We need to consider alternatives, as it appears that schools are not spreading COVID. This new data makes the case.[94] States such as Vermont, instead of relying only on stay-at-home orders or curfews, have responded with the needs of high-risk groups in mind: state-supported housing for the homeless, hazard pay, meal deliveries, and free, pop-up testing in at-risk communities. The state's Republican governor, Phil Scott, is even proposing $1000 stipends for people who've been asked to self-isolate.[95]

Health professional staffing shortages are now becoming commonplace in many parts of the U.S.[96] 1,396 health care workers, and counting, have died COVID expert Michael Osterholm has set up a foundation to help the families of health care workers who have died. Confronting their own death, health professionals are sounding the clarion call[97] for more restrictions as the virus surges. Where I work, we are up to almost 6% community COVID case rate (up from 2% just a few weeks ago). I've stopped going into the office and starting last week all my work is again all telephonic – just as intense.

Biden shouldn't be waiting for January 20 to implement his ideas.[98] He and his COVID task force need to roll out a national policy now.[99] We cannot wait till January 20. Without a policy, thousands more will die before then.

2020 End of Year AND Notes: Misery, Mourning, and Vaccine Types

The surge has become a veritable flood.[100] At least half of my patients these days have a COVID-related symptom and/or are living with the aftereffects of this new disease.

I balance several thoughts simultaneously these days as we experience festivals of lights in several traditions, deeply appreciate family time, and face the closure of a very dark year with so much ongoing and completely avoidable[101] suffering.

Most importantly, in the coming days I will call the families of my patients who have died this year. I knew these patients for decades. Calling families reminds me of my own good fortune – at the moment both of my two adult children and daughter-in-law live next door. I also look to the future via the conversations I am already having on the vaccine, such as with the 911 dispatcher patient of mine questioning me about the advisability of getting the vaccine. I respond by calmly addressing the points that patients have raised and pointing to the fact that I received the vaccine on December 20.

I regularly check up on patients who are still suffering from long-term complications, and there are many of those. Many of these individuals are young, including a man in his twenties who gets winded whenever he walks up a flight of stairs.

As an at-risk (elderly) individual, I see all my patients telephonically with the return of the pandemic – not by video. I do see a future in which we will combine telephonic and face-to-face visits for routine primary care.

AND participated in the Georgia Senate races via this op-ed published last Friday in the *Atlanta Journal-Constitution*.[102] The bottom line: "Now is the moment for every health professional to widely distribute the 'political vaccine' against unreliable health information on the frontline because it is a duty both for ourselves and our patients."

February 1, 2021. Hospitalizations and Vaccine Supply

Many of my patients call for the vaccine. Where I live, only people over 75 are "eligible" (many ineligible people I know are cutting in line). Most of my patients do not have access to the internet and cannot get through on phone lines.

Until now, it is hospitals that have controlled much of the vaccine supply, as hospital employees needed to be understandably vaccinated first. Where I work, hospital-affiliated outpatient practices deliver most of the care for low-income patients. Our practice contacted the over-75 age patients to make them aware of the vaccine availability. As at least 25% of my hospital system's employees declined the vaccine, elsewhere, I would assume at least a similar number are declining the vaccine. This has implications for us as a country. For now, and for the foreseeable future in the U.S., the issue is supply, an issue that is purely a production and supply chain question – one that health professionals like me cannot influence.

Feb 8, 2021. Mind-Numbing Deaths. Vaccine Acceptance – Local Health Professionals Can Help

The numbers are mind-numbing. January saw the greatest number[103] of COVID-19 fatalities and the highest average number of coronavirus hospitalizations of any month. More than 120,000 people were hospitalized in the U.S. for coronavirus in January. At least 95,211 people died from COVID-19 in the U.S. in January; December previously held the grim record of over 77,000 fatalities.

We know about the underreporting of COVID-related deaths. The underreported mental health consequences of the pandemic were brought home to me at a memorial service I attended on Sunday for the son of a friend of mine who may have died of a drug overdose; COVID-related isolation is killing many, but these deaths are not reported as COVID-related. Drug overdose deaths in the U.S rose after declines in 2017–18.[104] No boundaries for this virus except in countries like Australia, where they lock down a state after one case.[105]

Scientists are trying to untangle whether people who get COVID-19 during pregnancy will pass on some natural immunity to their newborns. Recent studies have hinted that they might.[106] The Centers for Disease Control and Prevention (CDC) is studying the effectiveness of double masks; no hard data, though anecdotally some experts are recommending double masks.

Even if we had enough vaccine against COVID-19 (which we don't), many would not be vaccinated. Currently, we have refusal rates ranging up to 75%, including up to, for example, 60% of nursing home workers.[107] The reasons are fear based on

■ Past experiences that the collective (race,[108] family, culture) has suffered through

- Individual negative experiences (e.g., I got sick after getting the flu vaccine)
- Social media and immediate family pressures
- Lack of absolute scientific information on a vaccine that is very new and a disease that is almost as new.

A just-published article in *Politico* summarizes exactly what AND is trying to do.[109] "People working with skeptical or hard-to-reach groups say personal, better targeted messages will prove more effective at encouraging vaccinations." An example: "A community health clinic in Oregon has local business owners and clinical staff texting, tweeting and Snapchatting messages encouraging their contacts to get vaccinated." For the next six months, AND will work with local health professionals on vaccine acceptance. We hope to coordinate with all groups. For example, there is Shots Heard Throughout the World[110] (what a great name!!), a group that "defends & protects Vaccine Advocates from large, coordinated AV social media attacks."

February 15, 2021. Mental Health COVID Impact; Wednesday Vaccine Listening Session

I've highlighted the mental health tragedies emanating from COVID for all ages and all professions. This report from Wuhan[111] highlights the emotional toll where it all started:

> Another woman had spent days begging for an ambulance – at that time private cars were also barred from Wuhan's streets – for her father, but once it came she could not get him a hospital bed. She brought him home, where he lay on the first floor because she didn't have the strength to carry him up the stairs. "He passed away there in front of her. She was making congee for him," Xu said. "She didn't get to say good bye." To ease such trauma may take years. It is easier for many of Wuhan's residents to block memories of the darkest days. There is also a shortage of good psychologists.

For myself, I have a constant sense of dread hanging over me; this pandemic gnaws. One of my patients last week who had been hospitalized with COVID pneumonia was discharged and needed to stay under quarantine. I encouraged her, in a positive but firm tone of voice (I've known her for years) that she needed to be in quarantine for five more days. She told me she just couldn't take it mentally anymore and had already gone to the store – even though she was highly infectious. Who knows how many people she might have infected by going out? If you "have" to go out, we now know the importance of not only double masking but also how to put them on to minimize discomfort.[112]

School opening continues to be a flash point of debate despite recent CDC guidance.[113] Safe school openings need[114] federal funding for testing, protective gear, well-ventilated spaces, and other safety measures.

We need more vaccine, but we also need to reckon with skyrocketing drug prices. But for now, the U.S. is focused on increasing vaccine supplies from the same pharmaceutical companies that are charging unconscionably high prices for their other medications. It takes a long time to produce the vaccine – here's why.[115] In the meantime, for all pining for the vaccine, look at this Jimmy Kimmel Valentine Card.[116]

February 24, 2021. Pandemic Improvement; Sent a COVID Patient to the ER

The COVID headlines are definitely good: COVID deaths throughout the world fell by 20% compared to the previous week; U.S. vaccine production and supply increases after snowstorm caused delays. Yet at a patient level, I don't yet see the impact. Last night, the daughter of one of my patients texted me saying that her mom was having shortness of breath and had just been diagnosed with COVID. I called the patient back just before I went to sleep; I could hear her difficulty breathing. I immediately suggested that she consider going to the emergency room. Still not clear on the outcome. Most of my patients are eligible for the vaccine now but can't access the system.

Yet a disturbing percentage of my eligible patients yesterday did not want the vaccine. One of them heard me out and said she would think about it. I used approaches as summarized in a just-published NEJM article,[117] which I recommend to all. We will get to a point when there will be increased supplies of vaccine and our challenge will be to gently nudge as many as possible to getting the vaccine rather than other approaches, including job termination.

Last week we had upward of 60 people from throughout the U.S. attend the AND meeting on vaccine acceptance. We have a long way to go on vaccine acceptance; here at AND we plan to continue this work and appreciate any input. I was struck by the heartfelt comments and passion about acceptance or hesitancy. Two health professionals spoke movingly of their mothers who till now refused the vaccine. But they aren't giving up!

March 4, 2021. COVID "Long-Haulers"; Vaccine Access; 2000 Deaths a Day

I had a phone appointment with a patient who was intubated for weeks in the early stages of the pandemic (I've written about her extensively). She is nine months out and a "long hauler" patient who survived but continues to have symptoms. I have quite a number of these patients and we have a lot to learn on how to best treat them.[118] I had two new COVID patients Tuesday (these are all treated telephonically) – one who lives with his father, who is symptomatic, and the other who went to the ER with symptoms but did not need to be hospitalized.

Nationally, last week we had 67,000 cases per day compared to 300,000 in January. However, the data is plateauing at a time when many states are "opening up." Texas, without health professional input, is dropping the mask mandate. Texas went from 23,000 cases per day to 7,700 per day in the last few days and half as many people are in the hospital; yet test positivity is 11%, much higher than needed to keep the spread under control. Many people are still dying – 2,000 a day nationally. If we don't have enough vaccine by May, another 175,000 individuals will die. Contrast that with zero deaths in people receiving the vaccines in the clinical trials and in Israel, the country with the greatest vaccination rate; no one has died after receiving the vaccine (20% + of the population has thus far refused!).

We are reaping the failure of the previous administration's COVID policy. Two failures continue to impact us today: we didn't hire at a national level the needed contact tracers/community health workers at the beginning of this pandemic as advocated by both Republican and Democratic health policy experts, and we didn't commit to purchasing enough vaccine supply for the entire country.[119]

In response to the need to encourage vaccination, groups such as the Ad Council are organizing campaigns.[120]

April 8, 2021. Still Have COVID Patients; Vaccines and Hesitancy Are Here

I have no COVID patients in the hospital, but I still have COVID patients. Thus far, most COVID patients of mine have lucked out. From a mental health point of view, suicides have gone down but drug overdoses have significantly increased. According to the National Center for Health Statistics,[121] suicides totaled fewer than 45,000 in 2020, down from about 47,500 in 2019 and more than 48,000 in 2018. This appears to be true globally. In contrast, drug overdoses increased dramatically last year;[122] more than 88,000 overdose deaths up from nearly 70,000 in the same time period of 2019.

Vaccination, together with well-established public health practices, such as mask wearing and social distancing, is key to defeating the COVID-19 pandemic. Should health care workers be required to get a vaccine?[123] While I am supportive of efforts to convince health care workers to voluntarily get the vaccine,[124] I do believe that health care workers should be required to get the vaccine. I cannot work without the flu vaccine. The same should eventually apply to the COVID vaccine.

On April 6, researchers documented in a paper[125] undergoing peer review that vaccination not only protects the person being vaccinated but leads to lower community infection rates. I spend about a quarter of my time with each patient discussing the pros and cons of the vaccine; and yes, patients have asked me about the computer chip that they are sure is being implanted when someone gets the vaccine. A recent excellent article[126] reviews vaccine hesitancy among marginalized populations.

We can now travel – at least according to the CDC. I am going to take a wait-and-see attitude. Certainly, unless I have an emergency, I am not getting on a plane anytime soon. But if you do have to travel here are suggested tips.[127]

The COVID pandemic has resulted in the death of more than 3,600 health care workers. Maritza Beniquez, an emergency room nurse at Newark's University Hospital in New Jersey, watched 11 colleagues die[128] in the early months of the pandemic. Like the patients they had been treating, most were Black and Latino. "It literally decimated our staff," she said.

This pandemic has revealed our true inequities. We have failed in one of the most basic functions of society – protecting the vulnerable.

April 20, 2021. Vaccine Acceptance; WHO Challenges

On Saturday, we had a vaccine clinic at our practice! Together with another physician, I was the medical backup for emergencies. Happily, nothing untoward occurred. We had a few extra doses. I called several patients. Two immediately said yes and one brought her 20-year-old son. One person I had already convinced a couple of weeks before to get it. One said she was too anxious. This non-scientific sample is about right – at least 20% of my patients at this point are not ready. At the same time, I am still getting plenty of COVID-positive patients, including one who was exposed to his daughter Sunday found out that she was positive on Monday; the father received the COVID vaccine Tuesday and developed symptoms/found out he was positive on Wednesday. He was just a little late on the vaccine. But he is fine otherwise.

The World Health Organization (WHO) started in 1948. In its first two decades, the WHO was dominated by a few largely industrialized countries split between Soviet and U.S. camps. Despite this tension, the WHO worked hard and largely unsuccessfully to eliminate TB and malaria but much more successfully to eliminate smallpox. Interestingly, the Soviet Union left for a brief period of time for political reasons. Decolonization resulted in a large increase in UN membership and WHO membership. In an era of populist nationalist governments, the WHO has had a very significant challenge leading a global response to the COVID pandemic.[129] The real challenge confronting a global response to the COVID pandemic is the conflict between China and the U.S. U.S. world standing has diminished from its own abysmal response to the COVID tragedy, in combination with the U.S. decision to hoard many treatments/vaccines.

So, we have arrived at a point where vaccination is available for all who want it and I still have patients getting sick and others continue to tragically die (don't forget the vaccine isn't 100% effective!).

April 28, 2021. COVID Projections Informed by My Patients' Reality

COVID "scars" are at the emotional and physical surface. I had one patient yesterday whose diabetes went from perfectly controlled to completely uncontrolled during the pandemic. He began to cry when speaking about his father who died of COVID. He couldn't be with him before he died.

In the U.S., under Biden the vaccine distribution effort has shined; the supply chain[130] has dramatically improved.[131] Yet there could be an improved organizing effort[132] behind the current modest efforts[133] to encourage vaccination. The federal government, together with the private sector, should make a full-court press and engage with national physician and nurses' organizations. The objective would be to get out asap nurse and physician videos, tweets, meetings, and individual phone calls to individuals least likely to be vaccinated or follow CDC guidelines.

We can't forget that we had a president who just a year ago recommended we ingest bleach as a treatment against COVID.[134] Health systems, including my own, were negotiating with anyone to get desperately needed PPE. Republicans are the most likely group to refuse the vaccine.[135] Some Republican presidential candidates[136] are simply against science;[137] others inappropriately frame the argument as freedom vs science.[138] Yet, to be fair, Republican physician members of Congress are encouraging vaccination.[139]

We need to keep in mind the tragedy occurring right now in India (with people literally gasping for air on the street[140]). We also need to imagine the eventual end to this pandemic;[141] Mark and Paul Engler, among others, recently detailed ways of addressing our political divide.[142] This is our and AND's long-term challenge.[143]

May 12, 2021. Breakthrough COVID Infections; Vaccine Hesitancy; Vaccines for All?

Tragically, the 20-year-old granddaughter of one of my patients, died of COVID. I also dealt with patients opposed (I was trying to keep the door open) to the vaccine. That should not be surprising considering that a U.S. Senator inappropriately connects the vaccine to thousands of deaths.[144] The CDC has no evidence establishing vaccination as the cause of any death. If herd immunity is not attainable, rate of hospitalizations and deaths after pandemic restrictions are lifted are the critical numbers. At my hospital last week: 50 patients hospitalized with COVID, 20 in the ICU. This week, I had my second COVID-positive patient post-vaccine; pleased that they had minor symptoms.

Much has been made of the recent revision of CDC guidelines. The bottom line is to use common sense. The following factors are problems: *Enclosed spaces with inadequate ventilation or air handling; Increased exhalation of respiratory fluids* if the infectious person is engaged in physical exertion or raises their voice (e.g., exercising, shouting, singing). *Avoid prolonged exposure* (typically more than 15 minutes) to these conditions.

What does it mean that Biden has waived the vaccine patents that Pfizer, for example, currently enjoys? Many say the impact will be marginal[145]; if nothing else, European countries are lukewarm, demanding that the U.S. share its excess vaccine supply first. The pharma lobby is so strong that it is unlikely that we will see any meaningful reduction in U.S. drug prices, the highest by far of any country in the world.

COVID has had a disproportionate impact on impoverished socioeconomic groups.[146] One of the many challenges is that the medical profession is overwhelmingly White. The American Medical Association has just issued a plan on how to address structural racism and some activists have expressed support.[147]

July 7, 2021. Worldwide Vaccine Access Initiative; New Legislative Push

Most importantly, without global vaccination we cannot begin to end this pandemic. Do you want to end vaccine apartheid globally? Do you know people who would come to NYC for a daytime, weekday action? People's Action, ACT UP, Rise and Resist, and others are organizing a big direct action on 7/14 10 am–12 pm and they need help with turnout. I plan on going – hope to see some of you there.

An important question confronting immunocompromised individuals: Should they get a third dose? French individuals get a third vaccine. The bottom line is that we don't know.[148]

Fauci quote: more than 99% of people who die of COVID in June weren't vaccinated,[149] every person who died of COVID in Maryland in June was not vaccinated,[150] even Mitch McConnell endorses the COVID vaccine![151] I've had few patients who developed COVID despite being vaccinated; all minor illness. Yet Delta is rapidly increasing. CHECK Vaccine lessons learned (thus far) from COVID[152]; in the U.S., the issue is vaccine hesitancy. This week, I gave a vaccine Q&A – in Spanish.[153]

July 21, 2021. I Want the Vaccine – Too Late; Vaccine Patent Protests

I am still hoping that the Biden administration works together with national associations of doctors, nurses, and others to have a countrywide mobilization of health professionals. With high social credibility, health professionals can effectively communicate scientific information, as recently demonstrated by an excellent recent issue of the *Proceedings of the National Academy of Sciences.*[154]

More than 99% of the deaths and 97% of the hospitalizations are among the unvaccinated. I see the impact with my own patients. I convinced four patients just yesterday! With very rare exceptions, I can turn the vaccine hesitant into vaccine acceptors. Sadly … "I'm admitting young healthy people to the hospital with very serious COVID infections," wrote Cobia, a hospitalist at Grandview Medical Center in Birmingham, in an emotional Facebook post Sunday,[155] "One of the last things they do before they're intubated is beg me for the vaccine. I hold their hand and tell them that I'm sorry, but it's too late."

I am in favor of universal free access to vaccines. That is why I went to NYC last week to join a demonstration and an act civil disobedience (I did not participate in this) against Pfizer and the German government – both of whom are against the release of the patent. It received a good media play.[156]

August 11, 2021. Great to See Old Patients Face to Face

On Friday, I had a joyous twofer. I saw a patient face-to-face whom I had not seen in one and a half years. While she was vaccinated, she told me that her fiancé (who was not a patient) was vaccine resistant. We got him on the phone right then and there and after responding nonjudgmentally to many questions we scheduled the COVID vaccine for today, Monday! About 80% of my patients have received the vaccine. Those who do not want the vaccine are aided and abetted by politicians,[157] clergy,[158] and the media.[159] What can you say when states like Tennessee strongly encourage the vaccination of cows but not of humans?[160]

The United States accounts for more than one-fifth of the total global COVID cases for the first time since mid-February, before vaccines were widely available.[161] The country reported more than 900,000 cases in a week for the first time since February 4, while deaths surpassed 4,500 a week. Cases are rising in 46 states. Florida, Hawaii, Louisiana, and Mississippi broke all-time case count highs last week, based on data reported Friday. Most politicians in Mississippi don't believe in science resulting in low vaccination rates in this state and the worst COVID suffering in the nation.[162] Amazingly, considering the increasing cases among children, "The Texas Education Agency has said schools no longer need to conduct contact tracing, **nor are they required to notify parents of positive cases in the classroom** [emphasis added]."[163] With respect to children and COVID, this same article provides an excellent guide for parents.

August 25, 2021. After FDA Vaccine Approval, Several Said Yes! Universal Vaccines!

The FDA approval of the Pfizer vaccine has definitely had an impact. I had several patients yesterday who were immediately willing to get the vaccine – all wanted Pfizer. But I still have holdouts – including one patient who I thought had received the vaccine. Unfortunately, he now has had day after day of fevers of 103 but no shortness of breath, and now wants the vaccine. He is lucky, as he is otherwise pretty healthy, and he will get the vaccine shortly. Another patient of mine explained that he is not ready and instead sent me "information" espousing false theories under the veneer of science.[164] As I explained to him in a nonjudgmental manner, this research is important but right now he is in the highest risk group – he is morbidly obese.

The Biden administration response to the pandemic has thus far failed on three fronts: an inadequate vaccine push; not pushing aggressively on worldwide access to vaccines[165]; and standing by while our public health infrastructure continues to deteriorate.

Pediatric cases have surged significantly.[166] Louisiana reported 139 COVID-related deaths yesterday[167] – the state's highest reported number of deaths in a single day since the pandemic began. Seventy-five doctors in Palm Beach Gardens staged a symbolic walkout[168] to protest unvaccinated people who are flooding Florida hospitals.

September 1, 2021. More Accept Vaccines, More COVID Infections; Mandates Now

With Delta spreading everywhere, including classrooms,[169] more but not all of my patients are willing to get the vaccine. Thus far, all my infected vaccinated patients have had mild illnesses; unvaccinated ones are much sicker; all clamor for the vaccine as soon as their infection is over. Currently, my hospital has about 75 COVID patients, ten times the number from a month ago. We are beginning to understand[170] the long-term effects of COVID.

Despite the controversies[171] over vaccine equity, a number of my friends have already received the vaccine booster although not yet eligible from pharmacies that claim that they have expiring doses. Even though infection is already widespread, vaccine mandates are absolutely necessary.

A group of physicians in Atlanta recently pleaded with Georgians to get vaccinated.[172] As reported in the same article, "Hours later, Gov. Brian Kemp announced he had signed an executive order blocking cities from forcing private businesses to enact mask rules, mandate vaccines or take other actions to mitigate the coronavirus." Would the outcome have been the same if Georgian health professional societies had been politically engaged in a sustained manner?

September 14, 2021. I Got the Vaccine Instead of Being Fired;

Last week, one of my patients, who I never thought would get the vaccine, got it. I asked why she changed her mind: Her non-health care employer said get the vaccine or be fired. The mandate will not work for all. But there is extensive testing of the vaccine's safety. Vaccines save lives. I always tell my patients: the vaccine is new, but it has been tested extensively. One always needs to ask the question, compared to what?[173] The critical part of the Biden plan[174] to increase vaccinations is to ramp them up through an employer vaccine mandate that also includes the appropriate use of masks.

But we still need leaders with common sense, as the Sturgis motorcycle rally in South Dakota was yet again another super-spreader event. The conclusion from the avoidable Sturgis rally COVID tragedy[175]: ensure a vaccinated population before a major event; verify people's vaccination status; require rapid and frequent testing during the event, especially for the unvaccinated; improve indoor air quality and use masking when indoors.

Republican opposition to the COVID vaccine could spread to other vaccines.[176] No other country[177] in the world is confronting this level of chaos. Dylan Scott of Vox tells us that more than 97 percent of Portuguese children are vaccinated against the measles these days. ... But in the U.S., the share is lower, closer to 90%. This article gives additional behavioral guideposts on what we can and can't do after being vaccinated[178]; another provides more detailed, scientifically based suggestions on risk factors for COVID after vaccination.[179]

Over the next few weeks, in addition, to promulgating the executive order on vaccine mandates, the country will decide, via a massive reconciliation bill, which, if any, changes in the American government will pass into law – with no Republican support.[180] There are critical health care proposals AND is working on, including, most importantly, allowing, the federal government to negotiate prices with pharmaceutical companies. Such a "package could plug some of Medicare's biggest coverage holes while reducing what patients pay for prescription drugs – policies that are popular across party lines."[181] Pharma is unalterably opposed and banking on its lobbying clout to eliminate all drug pricing proposals.[182]

September 29, 2021. Vaccine Mandates Work, but Not for All

Despite the worries about mass firings,[183] vaccine mandates for health care workers in New York state gave us the results[184] we needed to hear – in short, vaccine mandates work.[185] Vaccination status is impacting hiring/firing[186]; yet the absence of mandates in some parts of the country will simply prolong the pandemic for *all* of us. The mandates, however, need to be stronger.[187] "The Biden administration needs to give companies and jurisdictions incentives to require proof of vaccination for entry into restaurants and other businesses" – as in most countries in western Europe. Or to put it simply, the article continues, quoting Dr. Leana Wen: "That would send the message of 'You don't get to enjoy the privileges of pre-pandemic life unless you're vaccinated. Right now, the vaccinated are being held hostage by the unvaccinated. The vaccinated are having breakthrough infections and the unvaccinated are endangering those who cannot get vaccinated, like kids."

In the meantime, most are willing to be vaccinated. I had one patient last week who just needed to be "nudged"; we just need to reach them.[188] Instead, politicians in states with low vaccination rates are dismantling public health services[189] and discouraging vaccines.[190] They are influencing patients of mine who believe that COVID is a government conspiracy. The impact: Alabama,[191] which has one of the country's lowest COVID vaccination rates, recorded more deaths in 2020 than births – a first in state history.

Masks continue to be critical,[192] despite Abbott/DeSantis and company. "Not only is layering important to improve filtration but so is fit. A CDC-recommended technique for improving the fit of either a cloth or surgical mask is knotting the straps and tucking the sides.[193] A mask is generally a good fit if you feel warm air coming through the mask as you inhale and exhale."[194] Precautions are truly needed, as this reporter's personal story of what he wished he had known attests.[195]

October 15, 2021. Death Rates Finally Fall[196]; Facebook; Vaccine Marvels, Hesitancy, and Mandates

The Facebook whistle-blower testified to Congress on the same day that I received my COVID booster and three patients declined the vaccine.[197] *"When we realized tobacco companies were hiding the harms it caused, the government took action. … When we figured out cars were safer with seat belts, the government took action. And today, the government is taking action against companies that hid evidence on opioids. I implore you to do the same here."* – Frances Haugen, about Facebook's knowledge of the mental health harms Instagram poses to youth.[198] At the same time, research has also demonstrated how one can use social media to engage and convince people to get the vaccine.[199]

The COVID vaccines are truly a marvel of modern science.[200] The consequences of not getting the vaccine are unfathomable.[201] Despite data challenges, achieving a 75% vaccination rate in Florida would have averted 600,000 cases, 60,000 hospitalizations, and 16,000 deaths![202] This graphic demonstrates COVID's negative impact on life expectancy in rich countries.[203] Vaccination continues to be key, and mandates work and save lives.[204]

It is hard for AND and others[205] to grapple with the idea that Facebook is the same as tobacco, but I confront that reality every day. While most of my patients have willingly accepted the vaccine, not all have; mandates work, but these only apply to specific employer situations.[206] In contrast, in Italy, my birthplace, while to be sure there is opposition, one needs a "Green Pass" to do virtually anything. Why is Italy so different? We have a major political party in the U.S. (as opposed to fringe parties in Europe) that is essentially opposed[207] to the COVID vaccine and embraces conspiracy theories[208] – thus explaining Republican voter refusal to be vaccinated. One's party is a greater predictor than race![209]

October 29, 2021. Future Pandemic Preparedness; COVID Endemic?

Is COVID becoming like the flu? Not by a long shot. COVID is much more serious, and there are many states where COVID is still rampant. Yet in some states, people think of COVID as endemic,[210] present, but not overwhelming. Two points: we've felt like this before the Delta variant arrived. Despite everyone's prognostications, we simply don't know. For now, I have few COVID-positive patients.

The U.S. has one-seventh of the world's COVID deaths! A *new Axios/Ipsos poll* finds Americans are uncertain about how well the COVID-19 vaccines work, despite reams of data about their ability to protect people from severe disease, hospitalization, and death.[211] Unfortunately, the medical profession has largely stood by as physicians continue to spread misinformation.[212] This article answers the question, why do people, from a historical and psychological perspective, wear masks?[213]

Last week I gave "medical grand rounds" at Baystate Medical Center, where I practice.[214] Entitled Peace through Health, I emphasized that the U.S. is a fragile state, a term typically reserved for countries emerging from war.

November 22, 2021. Anti-Vax Positive COVID Patient – the Day after I Got Back from Vacation in Italy

Last Thursday, I returned from my vacation in Italy, my birthplace. One of my first patients Friday was a longtime patient, an anti-vaxxer, who was having mild shortness of breath. He did a home COVID test which came back positive, but he had heard that there was cross-reactivity with this test and the one for the flu. While I said that this was not true, he could repeat the test. It came back positive, and he is about to receive monoclonal antibodies, as he is morbidly obese. His oxygen level is borderline; I told him that he should go right to the ER if his breathing deteriorates. From the time his symptoms started, he had contact with at least 100 individuals before I told him his COVID results.

As travelers in Italy, my wife and I had to show our CDC vaccination card virtually everywhere we wanted to go. I saw people turned away at restaurants who could not demonstrate a "Green Pass," the Italian telephone app documenting vaccination status. In Italy, one cannot work without being vaccinated. For those who don't want to be vaccinated, they have to be tested every 72 hours – at their own expense.

December 6, 2021. My Patients, Anti-Vaxxer Couple, Both Hospitalized; Omicron; If Eligible, Please Get Your Booster

Anti-vaxxer couple, longtime patients of mine, were both hospitalized last week with COVID pneumonia. I had on numerous occasions tried to convince them to be vaccinated – to no avail.

Key points: Vaccine breakthrough cases in MA are rare but do occur; 1.6% of fully vaccinated individuals have been diagnosed with COVID-19 infection (I have one of those patients, who received monoclonal antibody Friday, as she has a risk factor – elderly like me). Since vaccines were introduced less than 1% (0.77%) of vaccine breakthrough cases have died from COVID-19 (Colin Powell, who had significant chronic illnesses, is one example of someone who died from breakthrough COVID).[215]

Vaccine-induced immunity wanes over time; this is especially noteworthy in older people. This fact and Omicron are driving the booster initiative nationally.[216] At the same time, Republicans are not only decrying efforts to increase vaccination rates but even threaten people at the individual level.[217] The result: people living in counties that went 60% or higher for Trump in November 2020 had 2.7 times the death rates of those that went for Biden. Counties with an even higher share of the vote for Trump saw higher COVID-19 mortality rates. In October, the reddest tenth of the country saw death rates that were six times higher than the bluest tenth. This is occurring in tandem with health care workers quitting.[218]

The political corollary of Republican resistance to vaccines is the benefit that Republicans accrued at last month's electoral box.[219] Vaccine mandates feed into the cultural narrative that Republicans are capitalizing on with misinformation: Trump's White House doctor, a physician, now a congressman, even claimed that Omicron is a Democratic midterm election ruse.[220]

The following picture (Image 3.1), courtesy of my wife – Sandra Matthews, who took this picture in Northampton, MA, says it all.

December 21, 2021. Ivermectin Ingestion; Changed Travel Plans

My anti-vaxxer couple, patients who were both hospitalized with COVID pneumonia survived and were discharged. Still anti-vaxxers. Their son told me that he secretly gave Ivermectin to one of his parents in the hospital and that is why his father survived. Two high-risk anti-vaxxer patients became positive this past Friday, and I've arranged for them to receive monoclonal antibodies; not clear that they will follow through.

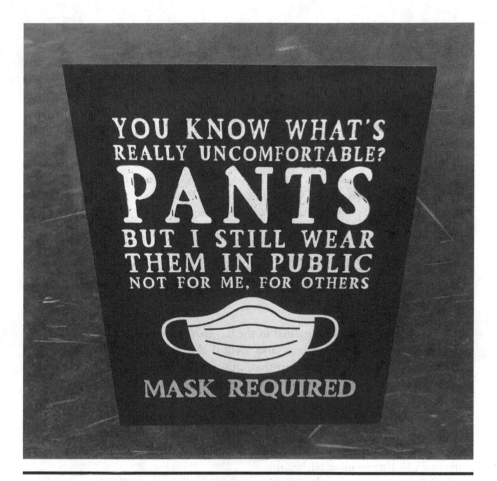

Image 3.1 A large verbal sign with a mask in the center

Source: Courtesy of Sandra Matthews.

An excellent report from the Government Accounting Office highlights the dramatic mental health consequences of the COVID pandemic and highlights six groups of people, including health care workers.[221]

Can we at least have Biden's legislative proposal affectionately called Build Back Barely instead of Build Back Better? The implications for failure are dramatic on so many aspects of health care. While hospitals and doctors are performing heroically, they sadly are also suffering; more than 100,000 health professionals have until now died of COVID.[222]

In an exit interview, Francis Collins, the retiring NIH director, stated he resisted Trump's pressures to fire Fauci and to endorse unproven therapies.[223] His one regret is a wish to better understand vaccine hesitancy and resistance.[224] For me, it is largely an issue of leadership – from politicians to pastors. Last week, Senate Republicans voted to defund vaccine mandates; Senator Johnson from Minnesota stated that gargling Listerine® kills COVID.[225] We are almost two years into this pandemic and a recent assessment indicated that we are not ready for the next one.[226] Biden has done reasonably well,[227] but we have a long way to go.[228] 70% of COVID vaccines have been distributed to the world's ten largest countries, and the world's poorest countries have received just 0.8%.[229]

My wife and I try to go to LA at this time of year – to celebrate our anniversary (42 this year!). We missed last year because of COVID. Yesterday, I canceled this year's trip because of rising COVID rates. As an AP headline stated, "One Year of Vaccines: Many Lives Saved, Many Needlessly Lost."[230]

January 3, 2022. My Hospitalized Patients, All Unvaccinated; Vaccine Protects against Omicron, but …

I have had three patients hospitalized in the last two weeks – all unvaccinated; large numbers of my vaccinated patients (and friends) also turned positive – none hospitalized. While it is preliminarily clear that Omicron is "milder," likely because of less lung impact than Delta, the reality is that the hospital where I admit patients now has the highest number of COVID patients since the onset of the pandemic. As of today, the hospital has implemented several measures, including pop-up booster clinics (98% of employees are vaccinated); rapid testing for employees; reducing some nonemergency procedures such as most colonoscopies that are done for prevention purposes; pivoting to more telehealth.

In Michigan for example, Michigan's death toll from COVID in 2022 has eclipsed 2020, when there was no vaccine and fewer treatment options, and no one had heard of the Omicron variant.

We need to remember basics that many take for granted. Last week, I had a substance abuse patient who really turned himself around. I asked him what made the difference. In two words: health insurance. Biden has really made a difference on this score, particularly impacting red states in a positive way.[231]

The anti-vax political and religious leaders are the principal problem on this pandemic.[232] Lamentably, many of these leaders around the world, including from Israel,[233] compare coronavirus restrictions to Nazi anti-Jewish laws; in the U.S.,[234] Fauci has been compared to the concentration camp doctor Josef Mengele. We read about frequent deaths among their number; the evangelist Marcus Lamb died of COVID-19 after his network discouraged vaccines, but some Christian evangelists don't want to talk about it.[235] By asking for delays in vaccine mandates, corporations are not helping.[236]

Needed: easy availability/low cost of N-95, KN-95 masks, home testing, and boosters (which may dent universal vaccine access[237]) and, yes, consistent accurate messaging from R&D politicians.

January 11, 2022. Ten Positive Patients in 24 Hours, All Vaccinated

Patient after patient of mine, all vaccinated, became COVID-positive in the last 24 hours. All of them are eligible for treatment, as they have significant chronic illnesses, but no one needed hospitalization. To avoid hospitalization, several were lucky to get outpatient anti-COVID medication. The rest received nothing, as we've run out of the medication in our part of the state.

With Massachusetts hospitalization rates now climbing higher than last winter, four leaders of hospitals and health systems asserted that their workers have done their part – and now it's time for the public to do its part by getting vaccinated, boosted, and wearing masks. COVID-19 deaths are up 33% in past 14 days, averaging 42 per day. The only positive feature of Omicron is that in a recent Axios survey 30% of unvaccinated respondents said Omicron makes them more likely to get the vaccine including one patient of mine yesterday, up from 19% in December.[238] The net result could follow what has just occurred in Arizona and elsewhere[239] throughout the country: a major health care system in Arizona announced that it will allow employees who are experiencing mild COVID symptoms or are asymptomatic to keep working.[240]

On January 6, 2021, a mob attacked the U.S. Capitol. On January 6, 2022, the *Journal of the American Medical Association* (*JAMA*) published a set of articles (pandemic preparedness,[241] new therapeutics,[242] and reimagining public health[243]) that amounted to an "extraordinary, albeit polite critique"[244] of much of President Biden's COVID policy. Others[245] document how the *JAMA* articles simply do not go far enough in their public health recommendations.

January 22, 2022. Many COVID Patients; The Vaccine Works; Political Supreme Court

I have many new COVID-positive patients every day, yet overall case rates are declining. But the truly good news is protection against omicron-related hospitalization was nearly 90 percent four months after a booster.[246]

There has been a blizzard of CDC guidance. If you are truly worried about exposing a high-risk person to COVID, it is best to just repeat the test if the home test is negative. This is a nice article on safely reusing N-95 or KN-95.[247]

The sad consequence of today's federal court decision on government employees and the recent Supreme Court decision against vaccine mandates, which had no firm legal basis,[248] is the unnecessary deaths of thousands of people. The GOP continues to endanger people's lives by resisting vaccination efforts, going so far as to place health officials on leave for encouraging vaccination.[249]

February 1, 2022. Many Vaccinated Hardly Sick COVID Patients; Endemic vs Pandemic?

The COVID-positive patients keep rolling in. Had several new patients on Friday. Some of my small number of vaccine-resistant patients are ready for the jab.[250] Hospitalizations at my hospital are going down but still a large number – well over 200 but down from almost 300 just a week ago. Still, elective procedures are mostly on hold.

Echoing what I have found for most of my long COVID patients: One year after 246 COVID-19 survivors were treated in one of 11 intensive care units (ICUs) in the Netherlands, nearly 75% reported lingering physical symptoms, more than 26% said they had mental health symptoms, and upward of 16% still had cognitive symptoms.[251] The COVID impact on health workers both in the U.S. and abroad, especially low-income countries,[252] is staggering. One newspaper account was spot-on[253]: we are living in a split-screen pandemic with many people resuming "normal" lives while hospitals are still overloaded. Starting next week, most of my patient care is face to face.

What does the future hold in store for us at a national level as we think about continuing to handle this and future pandemics? Government Accounting Office investigators "found persistent deficiencies" in how the CDC has led the response to the coronavirus pandemic and past public health emergencies dating to 2007 citing "continued problems coordinating among public health agencies, collecting infectious-disease surveillance data, and securing appropriate testing and medical supplies, among areas it said are unresolved."[254]

While the conclusions are sobering, I am heartened by the fact that we are at least having this conversation out in the open. The *NYT* had an excellent article reviewing Biden's first year,[255] echoing my belief that we can do much better. In 2020, the Senate released a report on preparing for the next pandemic[256] and there has been no follow-up.

February 15, 2022. Fewer COVID Patients; 150 People Still Hospitalized; Wear a Mask?

I am having fewer COVID-positive patients. But they are still coming. I sent one patient, fully vaccinated, this morning to the ER who couldn't walk the five steps to her bathroom without getting winded. I had one symptomatic (vaccinated) patient this week who was the first patient I put on the oral anti-COVID medication Paxlovid. He is fine. No one hospitalized in the last month. Still almost 150 people hospitalized at the local hospital.

So, are we now in an endemic situation?[257] And what does that mean anyways? Leanne Wen MD from the *Washington Post*:

> I'd encourage vaccinated people to consider three factors when deciding which activities to bring back to your lives: medical risk of your household; personal risk tolerance; and circumstances involved.[258]

Vaccine work and jab rate is an important measure of quality. The federal government should compare physicians, nursing homes, and HMOs by COVID vaccine rate, as it already does with the pneumococcal vaccine. Here is info on an excellent program.[259]

What the future will bring is anyone's guess. But there was a fourth wave in 1920 during the "1918" flu that killed many.[260] "The country's experience a century ago suggests that we could be in for a lot more pain – especially if we let our guard down."

What to make of these two headlines: *Kaiser Permanente broke its own profit record in 2021.* And *Why are millions on Medicaid at risk of losing coverage in the months ahead?* The answer is straightforward: culturally, we do not consider health care a common good. The result: a fragmented health care system. The reality is that each of the fragments has distinct economic interests.

March 1, 2022. AND on Podcast; Webinar in Preparation for 2022 Elections; Four First-Time Vaccinations in One Day!

AND continues to build up health professional networks in preparation for the 2022 elections. As part of this effort, Jeff Lerner (AND lead in Pennsylvania) and I appeared on the Robert Hubbell podcast last week.[261]

It never happened to me before during this pandemic – out of the 23 patients I saw last Tuesday I had four who I convinced to get the vaccine! I failed at two others. But I felt an incredible high; what a strange idea – again, unique during my lifetime, that I feel a sense of exhilaration at the end of the day having convinced four previously unvaccinated individuals to change their minds.

The mental health and substance abuse impact is staggering. Just as I am writing this, I am working with a young mother using ten bags of heroin a day laced with fentanyl (she has Narcan) who is now in withdrawal, and we are trying to convince her to switch to suboxone.

Public health in the U.S. is deteriorating, with public health officers continuing to leave[262] their positions. Not surprisingly, private companies have stepped into this increasing void.[263] After bankruptcy, the Detroit Public Health Department was privatized, with disastrous consequences.[264] Poor public health services exacerbate the social disparities impact of COVID. In Virginia, 41% of Medicaid enrollees 5 and older are vaccinated, compared with 76% of state residents in that age group. Sadly, the new surgeon general in Florida does not clearly state[265] that vaccines work and Ivermectin doesn't. A national public health system simply can't occur at this point in the U.S.

March 14, 2022. I Was Tested; Two-Year COVID Anniversary; Socioeconomic Disparities

I am primarily dealing with long COVID – very few new COVID patients. I had a patient last week who is likely to be permanently on oxygen; when she was hospitalized with COVID she was unvaccinated. She is now.

We are coming up to the two-year anniversary of COVID. A number of newspapers have had good series of articles. The bottom lines from these articles:

a. From a *New York Times* article: "What if China had been open and honest in December 2019? What if the world had reacted as quickly and aggressively in January 2020 as Taiwan did? What if the United States had put appropriate protective measures in place in February 2020, as South Korea did? Taiwan has suffered 853 deaths. If the United States had suffered a similar death rate, we would have lost about 12,000 people, instead of nearly a million. Sadly, every other industrialized country has done better than the U.S."[266]

b. COVID socioeconomic disparities are worldwide; this *New Yorker* story[267] recounts COVID's impact on Guayaquil, Ecuador, over the past two years. Today, Hong Kong is suffering from a catastrophic surge, with the poor suffering the most.[268]

c. We can fault Donald Trump and his acolytes, but we also need to work together to increase trust in public health.[269] Without strengthened public health, we will face renewed COVID dangers and exacerbate other public health crises, including overdoses and sexually transmitted diseases.[270]

d. We have made amazing progress developing therapies with many new meds and enhancing prevention against COVID using vaccines. Not surprisingly, we still have a lot to learn. I continue to wonder why some of my patients never got COVID.[271] Long COVID continues to bedevil us, especially when it impacts the nervous system.[272] While many have appropriately emphasized mental health challenges that COVID has brought on, this article emphasizes human resilience in the face of the COVID tragedy.[273]

e. There will be more surges. And there will be other pandemics. Our system has proved to be unprepared to deal with them.

On a more positive note, we continue to have good information on common-sense diet and exercise practices. A recent large study[274] examined how the more physically fit one is, the less likely one develops Alzheimer's. I went for a bike ride today!!

April 5, 2022. Avoiding COVID in the Middle East; A New COVID Wave in the U.S.?

I doubt that we will ever return to lockdowns. Mask requirements will be tough to enforce even in Democratic areas. In addition, the mental health and substance abuse toll is too high. The absence of mask requirements places a greater burden on individuals at higher risk (such as the immunocompromised, obese individuals, elderly, or diabetics) to care for themselves by wearing masks and avoiding large crowds, especially as COVID rates rise. The unvaccinated are the other major at-risk group; they are 97 times[275] more likely to die than the vaccinated (see this important article in which an excerpt of a TV clip of Trump touting the vaccine made a difference).[276] Importantly, today we have treatment options.

There continue to be excellent reviews of what went wrong in the pandemic response throughout the world from NYC[277] to Sweden.[278] The bottom-line conclusion of this article on Sweden, where the death rate was extremely high:

> The Swedish response to this pandemic was unique and characterised by a morally, ethically, and scientifically questionable laissez-faire approach, a consequence of structural problems in the society. There was more emphasis on the protection of the "Swedish image" than on saving and protecting lives or on an evidence-based approach.

Sound familiar? The U.S. is thus not the only country to fail in its COVID response. Sadly, we are the worst and continue to struggle in our efforts. Health professional organizations such as the AMA have not, for example, vigorously defended public health officials who have been threatened.[279] In response, AND continues to work on state-level public health responses, electoral engagements, strengthening the ACA (including Medicaid, which is facing significant financial threats), and fighting for international vaccine equity, where we continue to lag.

On April 28, there will be a demonstration at the Moderna shareholder meeting in Boston to point out Moderna's part in the drastic inequities in worldwide vaccine distribution. Please spread the word.

April 18, 2022. Life Expectancy Dropped by Two Years; Nurses as Diplomats

Due to the COVID pandemic, life expectancy in the U.S. fell by two years in 2020 to about 77 years – a drop greater than in any other high-income country.[280] Hispanics and Blacks, especially men, suffered the most (each about 3.5 years). Drug overdoses are an important part of this tragic story: there were at least 105,000 overdose deaths in 2021 – up from 93,000 the year before, with a jump in overdose deaths among 14–18-year-olds.[281] An article on the NJ county with the highest COVID death rate reaffirms that Republicans are at the greatest risk of death.[282]

However, health professionals are key first responders in every respect for this pandemic. This article which just came out in *American Nurse* (circulation 125,000) highlights the role of nurses as diplomats in the COVID culture wars.[283] AND is highlighted.

COVID cases – but not hospitalizations – are rising again. I had a patient last week, an emergency medical technician who went to work with "a cold"; his co-workers insisted that he get tested and he was positive. As we caught it early, I prescribed him one of the new COVID oral medications. The booster vaccine that I received last week does protect me from the serious consequences of COVID. But for how long is a question that still needs more research.

The mental health consequences of the COVID pandemic continue to be in the news. Four in ten adults reported significant mental health issues in 2020.[284] I had another patient last week who spoke to me about his anger caused by isolation during the pandemic. He was proactive and has taken anger management classes at the VA.

May 1, 2022. COVID Hospitalizations Rising; Family Members with COVID; Executive Regulation

COVID rates and hospitalizations are rising again. I have little confidence in rates (home testing results are not reported). Family members and friends all around me are testing positive. More importantly, 17,000 individuals are currently hospitalized in the U.S., a 16% increase over the past two weeks. For myself, I am most concerned about long COVID – a complication that continues to be poorly understood, though it appears that vaccinations do help prevent the progression to long COVID. This connection convinced one of my anti-vaxxers yesterday to agree to get the vaccine. Most children from 5 to 11 years old hospitalized with COVID-19 during the U.S. surge driven by the Omicron variant were unvaccinated, per a CDC study.[285]

The polarization on health system reform at a state level was recently on full display with California[286] opening its Medicaid rolls to older undocumented individuals while states like Tennessee[287] could see hospitals collapse and many avoidable deaths because it is one of the dozen states that has not expanded Medicaid to cover more low-income adults under the ACA.

The Government Accounting Office issued a report last week definitively documenting Trump administration's political interference with the main federal agencies.[288] More importantly, it detailed procedures on how political interference in their work should be reported and handled. Specifically, as the GAO stated, the CDC "has not defined political interference and does not have a formal process to address allegations of political interference."

May 16, 2022. More COVID Patients; Studies on Long-Term COVID; A Million Deaths

I had several COVID-positive patients this week, all vaccinated. All, relatively speaking, mild (i.e., no respiratory distress), including members of my family. COVID is constantly mutating. It would appear that one of the mutations is responsible for the new wave; but for sure it is all propelled by the widespread disappearance of masks from indoor use and low vaccination rates. We are beginning to understand the long-term consequences, with a large percentage, for example, of those on respiratory support developing chronic lung problems.[289]

We hit a tragic milestone since the last COVID Notes: a million (likely an undercount) COVID deaths. It is an unfathomable tragedy. I met with one of my diabetic patients whose son died of COVID. The son was in his 30s and had a family of his own. My own patient has suffered terribly with ongoing chest pain, necessitating an ER visit. I am currently evaluating the cause, but emotional "heartbreak," especially for women, is real.[290]

Cruises are back in style. That doesn't mean that COVID has left cruise ships alone. The CDC's cruise ship status report shows that 76 of 92 ships have reported cases of the coronavirus on board.[291]

Building on an article that nurses and AND leaders recently published,[292] AND approached a state medical society last week suggesting that Democratic and Republican physicians appear together throughout the state.

May 31, 2022. Paxlovid; Vaccinated Hospitalizations; Extra Work Sessions

Elderly patient this past Thursday tested herself; classic symptoms; positive at home. A few hours later she was on Paxlovid – after I checked all the many possible medication interactions using the very helpful University of Liverpool COVID-19 Drug Interaction software!![293] Then Saturday, despite her wearing a mask and implementing preventive measures, her husband came down with it also and in a few hours was also on Paxlovid. Both definitely doing better within 24 hours. Don't forget that there is a slight possibility of return of symptoms after finishing a course of Paxlovid. Lots more COVID patients.[294] They asked for staff volunteers to take on more telephonic sessions to ease the ER burden. Am doing an extra session this week.

I've written before about the high death rates and decreased life expectancy in the U.S. The variation throughout the world is astounding: Peru and Argentina, 97% greater than the expected death rate in Peru and 12% in Argentina.

Growing vaccine hesitancy is one of the WHO's top ten threats to global health.[295] Anti-vaxxers are extending their reach to all vaccines, not just COVID. Paraphrasing the conservative columnist Michael Gerson: Let's stop our complacency – about vaccine hesitancy.[296]

AND's electoral focus right now is on Pennsylvania. We are working on op-eds, LTEs, and other electoral issues.

June 15, 2022. Political Party Matters; Mother/Son with Mild COVID; June 29 AND Training Session

I called a male patient in his 30s last week for a phone visit (symptoms were cough and sore throat) and asked the woman who answered if I could speak to him. "He is severely autistic, can't speak, I am his mother and both of us are COVID positive," she said. Their cases were mild. My oldest friend (from 5th grade!) came down with COVID over the weekend. He got it at the Special Olympics in Florida, where he was officiating. According to my friend, Governor DeSantis threatened Special Olympics officials with a multimillion-dollar lawsuit if they required vaccines and/ or masks.

I've written before about differences between Republican and Democratic voters on willingness to be vaccinated against COVID. Last week, the *British Medical Journal* published an article[297] with an accompanying editorial that concluded: "The mortality gap between Republican voting counties and Democratic voting counties has grown over time, especially for white populations, and that gap began to widen after 2008."

COVID-19 caused 62% of duty-related deaths of U.S. police officers in the first year of the pandemic – a rate that rose to 77% to 82% among minority officers – according to a new study published in *Policing: An International Journal.*[298]

During the first 12 months of the pandemic, at least 34% of the people killed by the virus lived in nursing homes and other long-term care facilities even though residents of those facilities make up fewer than 1% of the U.S. population. Recent research has found that resident outcomes are significantly worse at private equity-owned (i.e., for-profit) nursing homes.[299] Sufficient staffing is key.

Few studies have examined the relationship between long COVID and mortality. A study of European cancer patients, published in the *Lancet* in July 2021, found that about 15 percent of those who survived COVID-19 had long COVID symptoms, and their survival outcomes were significantly worse.[300]

July 5, 2022. Housing; Medical Debt; Mental Health; Choice; 33K Hospitalized COVID Patients

This past two weeks I had more homeless[301] patients than new patients with COVID. Simply put, no home, no health, no stability in life. Veronica sleeps in her car in a Walmart parking lot; she is almost 70. Frank sleeps on a mattress that he carries around with him to the home of different friends. But he can't use his sleep apnea machine, thus worsening his high blood pressure and asthma. Sadly, many more of my patients are confronting the real possibility of losing their housing, a crisis that, as Vox has documented,[302] we could have at least mitigated. This type of trauma can have both short- and long-term physical and mental health impacts.[303]

Medical debt is making the housing crisis worse. 100 million Americans[304] are carrying medical debt, especially the uninsured, Black, and Hispanic adults, those with lower Incomes, and women.

Even though Massachusetts has almost universal coverage (3% uninsured), it does take effort to get health insurance. I had a patient last week who postponed seeking care because she had trouble arranging for health insurance. Her blood pressure was sky high – 200/100 – and it took a while in the office to bring it down. In contrast, Texas, for example, has an uninsured rate of 18% – twice the national average.

In the shadow of the recent antichoice Supreme Court decision, this 4th of July brings home sadly who is not independent; you will not be surprised.[305]

July 19, 2022. Patient Vaccine Anger

The coronavirus pandemic caused the worst backslide in global vaccination coverage in a generation.[306] I am relentless, and my own few vaccine-resistant patients are appreciative of my concern. But some patients who are not mine are different: After bringing up the vaccine at the end of a recent visit, one patient accused me of being paid extra for every patient who I convince to get vaccinated. I told this person that I found the comments insulting. I could feel the anger of another unvaccinated pregnant patient when I brought up the issue; I could easily imagine her committing acts of violence similar to what occurred on January 6, 2020.

Conservatives continue to advocate limiting the power of public health officials.[307] On the other hand, credit where credit is due: the Biden administration has facilitated masks, medication, and vaccines – for those who want it.[308] More evidence of vaccine impact: 20 million lives saved.[309] Despite this, COVID-19 was the third leading cause of death between March 2020 and October 2021.[310]

August 1, 2022. Many New COVID Cases; Wednesday Webinar – See You There!

Ever wonder why some people don't get COVID? We still don't know.[311] I haven't had COVID – to my knowledge. I have had several new COVID patients in the last ten days; none had to go to the hospital. I was pleased that I was able to convince one unvaccinated person last week to take "the jab."

If the Republicans take over either house of Congress, it is likely that the polarization around COVID (with, as I've pointed out before, Republicans dying at a higher rate than Democrats) will only get worse. According to one expert,[312] a nakedly partisan investigation of Fauci would do even more damage to the fraying public trust in public health officials.[313] Vaccine skeptics have touted Biden's recent COVID infection despite his four vaccines, using "a tactic that vaccine skeptics have used to question the effectiveness of vaccines or mandates."[314]

Schools are playing catch-up while trying to address the traumas and challenges from the pandemic.[315] According to this report,[316] patterns in 2021–22 show some encouraging evidence of rebounding: "The gains made during the 2021–22 school year are at least parallel to the pre-pandemic sample, and in some cases actually steeper." School efforts range from lengthening the school year, food drives, after-school offerings, and even health screenings. Significant teacher shortages still exist, despite efforts at boosting pay and teacher recruitment.

And then we find that: "The share of US adults believing that harassing public health officials was justified rose 5.4 percentage points from 20% (218 of 1081 respondents) in November 2020 to 25% (276 respondents) in July to August 2021 ($P = .046$)."[317] Axios highlighted that: there's so far been little evidence of success bridging partisan communication divides.[318]

We also need to begin to focus on the November elections in either a partisan or nonpartisan manner. AND is focusing on the importance of health professionals creating short (less than a minute) videos on the abortion issue similar to this.[319] Easy to create!

August 17, 2022. Three Unvaccinated Patients Jabbed; IRA

It never happened to me before – three patients were jabbed last Thursday – their first time. All were vaccine resistant; none of them were conspiracy theorists – though deep inside they must have felt some affinity to conspiracy ideas. I was high-fiving all over the office!!

The health care provisions of the Inflation Reduction Act (IRA) which awaits Biden's signature are the big news since the last COVID Note. The IRA contains significant Medicare improvement, including drug price negotiations. Please read the excellent analysis of the legislation.[320] As you might expect, there may be unintended consequences[321] but not the tragedy[322] that Big Pharma claims will occur.

September 6, 2022. COVID, Strep Throat, Health Professionals Running for Office, Some Anti-science

More patients with COVID and … let's not forget strep throat. I had a pregnant patient last week who had no COVID symptoms other than a sore throat. Strep test was positive.

I agree with one newspaper assertion that "predictions about the pandemic rarely age well."[323] For sure, health professionals opposed to COVID treatment are making themselves heard.[324] A lengthy but worthwhile description about Scott Jensen MD Republican nominee for governor in Minnesota:

> Scott Jensen, who received more than 90% of the Republican vote in the primary said that Democratic Gov. Tim Walz's COVID policies were comparable to Kristallnacht "the night of broken glass", that heralded the beginning of the Nazis' antisemitic mass violence. "If you look at the 1930s and you look at it carefully, we could see some things happening, little things, that people chose to push aside… And then the little things grew into something bigger,'" Jensen said at the rally, in a speech captured on video…. Well, in a way, I think that's why you're here today. You sense that something's happening, and it's growing little by little."

I wonder what Jensen would say about the polio vaccine – the U.S. just had its first case in a decade.[325]

Pregnant women continue to have lower rates of vaccination, despite its demonstrated safety, once again.[326] Also depressing is the largest decline in life expectancy in the U.S. over the past two years in 100 years.[327] Interestingly, the decline in White American life expectancy was more than Black Americans. At the same time, racism is a very important factor for Black mortality and some health systems are attempting to face the issue.[328] This database could not distinguish between Republicans and Democrats.

Native Americans had the worst outcomes: Carol Schumacher, 56, who was raised in the remote community of Chilchinbeto in the Navajo Nation, has lost 42 family members to COVID-19 over the last two years. The dead included two brothers aged 55 and 54, and cousins as young as 18 and 19… The nearest hospital was a long drive away on dirt roads, she said, "and there's no guarantee about the quality of care there even if you make it in time. Some families don't even have transportation or running water."[329]

September 22, 2022. More COVID Patients; Pandemic/Endemic? COVID Third Leading Cause of Death in the U.S. Last Week

I had four patients with COVID last week. All three were treated with Paxlovid and all did well – so far. Key is to get the medication to them quickly. One was diagnosed the day after his symptoms began, including some with respiratory difficulty. I called him the following day and he was doing better. I had another patient yesterday, an elderly woman, COVID-positive with a myriad of problems, who I elected not to treat because there is a serious interaction with some of her other medications. In addition, she was feeling well. I am calling her twice a day to check in.

Re endemic vs pandemic. For me, the key issue is one's behavior – and ... I haven't changed. N-95 masks when I am indoors with many other people unless eating. One expert pointed out these facts: "We still have a disease in this country that is hospitalizing over 32,000 people a day, with over 3,000 ICU admissions, and over 450 cases on average per day are dying."[330] Long COVID, especially "brain fog,"[331] is of great concern. In preliminary work, COVID vaccine may cut down on long-term symptoms.[332]

Despite the challenges, many health professionals take a stand. Senator Richard Pan, State Senator in California, who was firm on vaccines and had menstrual blood thrown at him in response, has reached his term limit, and is retiring.[333]

An unfathomable number: 10. 5 million children[334] were orphaned or lost a primary caregiver to COVID. Anti-vaxxer attitudes will likely prolong COVID but also create spikes in other avoidable illnesses.[335]Burnout and nursing strikes are still occurring among health care professionals.[336] Infection control and prevention in nursing homes continues to be a major challenge according to this published Government Accounting Office report.[337]

A humorous line in the *New Yorker*: "As a cost-saving measure for our valued customers, we, the HEALTH INSURANCE COMPANY,™ have kindly merged our eye and psychological exams."[338]

AND continues to work and publish op-eds and LTEs [letters to the editors] in Florida,[339] Maine, and Pennsylvania.[340] The November election stakes are high, with Dr. Mehmet Oz saying that "uninsured Americans have no right to health."[341]

October 12, 2022. COVID Patient in the Hospital (or Is It COVID?); Dr. Ladapo, Florida Surgeon General – A Test of Organized Medicine

I hospitalized an immunocompromised patient on Sunday. She developed COVID ten days before, shortly after going maskless to a large event. For the first few days, she was completely asymptomatic. My clinical challenge was whether or not to treat her. I couldn't give her the standard medication as she had several clinical problems that wouldn't allow me to prescribe Paxlovid. What to do? I was possibly lulled into a false sense of security as she was completely asymptomatic for the first week. And then within 24 hours, her clinical condition went south, she had significant difficulty breathing. She called me this past Sunday and I right away told her to go to the emergency room. Should I have treated her with one of the IV COVID meds? Possibly, but in discussing this with an infectious disease specialist yesterday, we both highlighted that Omicron does not take the same the course as the original COVID virus. In the meantime, I've had, in addition, at least five new COVID patients in the last ten days – all did fine, some with medication and others who could not get the medication.

What both the AMA and the Florida licensure board do regarding the Florida Surgeon General Ladapo's outright fabrications about COVID vaccines will be a real test of organized medicine. I assume that the AMA and the Florida licensure board will do nothing. Yet, health professionals can make a positive difference!! Please read this article about the impact of the director of public health for Marin County in CA – "Once known for vaccine skeptics, Marin now tells them 'you're not welcome,'" a recent newspaper headline.[342] While the Ladapos of the world are not helping, federal health professionals and politicians are still not doing enough to boost the new vaccine.[343] In short, we continue to be ill-prepared for both this and future pandemics.[344]

Oct 31, 2022. Two Patients Hospitalized in Last Two Weeks

I hospitalized two patients with COVID in the last two weeks. The first a fairly unusual scenario – COVID pneumonia – unusual in the sense that the Omicron variant typically causes less pulmonary damage than the predominant COVID variety at the start of the pandemic. The second patient had dehydration from her diarrhea and needed intravenous fluid replacement. In the U.S., there are more than 25,000 people in the hospital right now with COVID and more than 350 deaths per day.

Politico published an excellent article interviewing CDC Director Rochelle Walensky on CDC challenges in a pandemic era.[345] Bottom lines, the CDC

- Is unable to force states to share information on disease outbreaks.
- Needs greater funding "to draw in new talent and train the public health workforce to speed up the information flow to the public."
- Needs to "steer the agency toward the 'sweet spot' between its old way of publishing its findings, which can take weeks or months, and ensuring that the science going out to the public is safe and reliable."
- "Announced a … spate of reforms in August, including speeding up data delivery, making public health guidance easier to understand, building up its communications team, strengthening the CDC's national laboratory system and shifting internal incentives for staff away from publishing in scientific journals and toward making practical policy recommendations."[346]

Scholars continue to author articles on, for example, the impact of liberal vs conservative state health care policies on mortality.[347] Other researchers demonstrated that "The gap in excess death rates between Republicans and Democrats is concentrated in counties with low vaccination rates and only materializes after vaccines became widely available."[348] In a similar vein, AND has worked with local health care professionals to publish LTEs and op-eds in the last few weeks in local conservative newspapers in PA[349] and Florida.[350] We hope that AND can make a difference in some of the tight election races.

January 3, 2023. Many COVID-Positive Patients; Two Hospitalized; An Anti-Vaxxer Patient Flips

New patients with COVID every week but by the time I find out their diagnosis it is too late to treat 50% of them. I haven't had any patients not willing to take Paxlovid. The few patients of mine who are anti-vaxxer are going to stay that way. But I still bring it up each time I speak with them. And one of them folded yesterday. I had discussed vaccination with him at least 20 times (he is in his 90s and has significant comorbidities). For him, Tuskegee was the main reason for his anti-vax philosophy. Why did he flip – I just don't know.

This remarkable article tells the story how physicians practicing in a rural North Caroline made a difference.[351]

Only 15% of eligible Americans (including less than 50%[352] of nursing home residents!) are boosted, despite research showing that it cuts hospitalizations in half.[353]

There continues to be turmoil among health care workers. Nurses just went on strike (and settled a few days later) at a number of NYC hospitals.[354] Health professionals continue to be under tremendous stress. According to a NYT investigation, "hospitals helped lay the groundwork for the labor crisis long before the arrival of the coronavirus. Looking to bolster their bottom lines, hospitals sought to wring more work out of fewer employees … moved away from their charitable mission … and skimped on free care."[355] The allergist of one of my patients quit last week. Most important of all, hundreds of thousands of health care workers have lost their lives or are permanently disabled from COVID.[356]

Flu and RSV are rampant. I had a patient hospitalized and almost immediately intubated with RSV pneumonia. He was in the hospital for two months.

With 40,000 hospitalized patients and 750 deaths per day in January 2023, this country still doesn't realize, as Eric Topol said, that COVID is not done with us.[357] Congress has provided little leadership on COVID or on the next pandemic.[358] Or as Rachel Cohrs opines: "After 9/11, Congress created an entirely new government agency to address the threat of terrorism, and Americans are still taking off their shoes in airports more than 20 years later. After a pandemic that killed more than 1 million people in the United States alone, very little about the federal government has changed at all, and it may not for a long time."[359]

Social media continues to be rife with COVID misinformation.[360] In response to an avalanche of COVID misinformation after the collapse and death of the journalist Grant Wahl at the World Cup in Qatar, his wife and notable infectious disease specialist, Celine Gounder, responded in a dignified manner.[361] Quoting at length

> The vaccine disinformation playbook includes the use of fake experts, logical fallacies, impossible expectations, cherry-picked data and conspiracy theories. … Merchants of disinformation argue that vaccines killed my husband, but they're also at least in part responsible for the return of polio to the United States and the fact that so many children

in Ohio are suffering from measles right now.... I will continue to honor Grant by living by our shared values. I'm channeling my grief into something productive: protecting the public's health against those who would profit from the suffering of others.

The Florida Medical Licensure Board is not meeting its responsibilities by refusing to censure or discipline Florida Surgeon General Joseph Ladapo for recommending that young men not receive the COVID vaccine.[362] Even though he wasn't always anti-vaxx,[363] Governor Ron DeSantis is in charge of misinformation[364] (this despite the fact that this approach is killing Republicans more than Democrats[365]!). In contrast, GOP Governor Asa Hutchison of Arkansas defends science!![366]

Availability of affordable health insurance will likely be one winning issue in 2024. Republican-leaning Miami residents are wildly in favor of Obamacare.[367] For sure, AND in 2024 will also raise up the fact "Covid is still not done with us."

February 7, 2023. Two More Patients; End of Pandemic? We Need to Plan Now for Next One!

Two more patients this week – both doing well on Paxlovid. Several of my patients have highlighted the news reports of increased risk of stroke from COVID vaccines. Yet, the CDC continues to recommend the vaccine, and a recent article reported that "no increased risk was found for non-COVID-19 mortality among recipients of three COVID-19 vaccines used in the US."[368] Had another first-time vaccine success last week – never give up – we all should engage!!

Governor DeSantis would like[369] to enshrine into Florida law the right of health professionals to spread misinformation about a vaccine, which only 11% of Floridians have taken up. This at a time that COVID in Florida still has more than 2000 people in the hospital and 50 deaths per day.

Biden announced the end of the pandemic (technically the end of the public health emergency[370]) a few days ago. I am one of those that agrees with the declaration but we must plan for the next pandemic. The reality is that Americans have moved on. I still wear a mask indoors in public and I am not going to Broadway musicals, but I am a vanishing breed. I do it in an effort to avoid long COVID.[371]

Where I disagree with the Biden administration is that we have little in place for the next pandemic and/or if COVID comes back. If we actually had efforts in place for the next pandemic, we would be also dealing with this pandemic. AND will continue to try – both at a national and a state level – to address this and the next pandemic. You might expect that legislators in a state like Massachusetts, controlled by Democrats at all levels of the government, would be open to planning for the next pandemic. But the reality is that they are not. Advocacy groups are not interested – yet.

The U.S. continues to have a shortage of primary care health professionals. Primary care health professionals have quit at a high rate.[372] Demoralization is rampant.[373] Others strike.[374]

Along with Medicare, abortion is almost certainly a top election issue in 2024. Hard to know how COVID politics will play in the election but AND will push for effective policies.

Despite Biden's declaration, our engagement with COVID and other infections is not over. This week there is nationally an average of almost 30,000 patients in the hospital and 450 daily deaths. This diary hopefully gives a sense of one health professional's journey as I tried to respond to the needs of my patients while aiming to constructively engage with COVID policies. Our work as health professionals has the potential to be lifesaving for both the individual patient and our fragile society.

Notes

1 Telford, T. (2022) Rejoice! Despair! The office holiday party is back in person. *Washington Post*. Available at: https://www.washingtonpost.com/business/2022/12/10/office-holiday-party-in-person-pandemic/. Accessed: December 13, 2022.

2 Cameron, B. (2020). I ran the White House Pandemic Office. Trump closed it. *Washington Post*. Available at: https://www.washingtonpost.com/outlook/nsc-pandemic-office-trump-closed/2020/03/13/a70de09c-6491-11ea-acca-80c22bbee96f_story.html. Accessed: September 12, 2022

3 Goldstein, A. (2020) https://medium.com/@Andrew.Goldstein/as-coronavirus-transmission-accelerates-we-need-boldgovernment-action-to-halt-transmission-and-5259482e65dc. Accessed: December 13, 2022.

4 #StaytheFuckHome (2020). Available at: https://staythefuckhome.com/?fbclid=IwAR3jrs06ruXNhJxBEGQavCjJWURT78lceNDML33xLqY8DIjN6b9DXkDS7g. Accessed: September 12, 2022.

5 Sargent, G. (2020) A new poll shows Trump's magical lying powers are failing him. *Washington Post*. Available at: https://www.washingtonpost.com/opinions/2020/03/17/new-poll-shows-trumps-magical-lying-powers-are-failing-him/. Accessed: December 18, 2022.

   The Economist (2020) The politics of pandemics. *Economist*. Available at: https://www.economist.com/leaders/2020/03/12/the-politics-of-pandemics. Accessed: December 18, 2022.

6 Berwick, D. (2020) They don't hide from the Coronavirus, they confront it. *New York Times*. Available at: https://www.nytimes.com/2020/03/23/opinion/coronavirus-doctors.html. Accessed: September 12, 2022.

7 Toosi, N., Lippman, D., and Diamond, D. (2020) Before Trump's inauguration, a warning: 'The worst influenza pandemic since 1918' *Politico*. Available at: https://www.politico.com/news/2020/03/16/trump-inauguration-warning-scenario-pandemic-132797. Accessed: September 12, 2022.

8 Blake, A. (2020) Trump ties Coronavirus decisions to personal grievances. *Washington Post*. Available at: https://www.washingtonpost.com/politics/2020/03/27/trump-suggests-personal-grievances-factor-into-his-coronavirus-decisions/. Accessed: September 17, 2022.

9 Sonmez, F. (2020). Trump touts TV ratings of his news conferences amid pandemic. *Washington Post.* Available at: https://www.washingtonpost.com/world/2020/03/29/coronavirus-latest-news/#link-ZABDGKSOKFBE3O2PRKHCCDXE5M. Accessed: September 17, 2022.

10 Available at: https://www.youtube.com/watch?v=e0-2XxgHIYI&feature=youtu.be. Accessed September 12, 2022

11 Ferris, S. and Caygle, H. (2020) Desperate lawmakers hunt for medical supplies as Trump takes hands-off approach. *Politico*. Available at: https://www.politico.com/news/2020/04/01/lawmakers-desperate-hunt-supplies-health-workers-157883. Accessed: September 17, 2022.

12 Martin, J., Haberman, M., Baker, M. (2020) Trump suggests lack of testing no longer a problem. Governors disagree. *New York Times*. Available at: https://www.nytimes.com/2020/03/30/us/politics/trump-governors-coronavirus-testing.html. Accessed: September 17, 2022.

13 Rosenthal, E. (2020) Analysis: He got tested for Coronavirus. Then came the flood of medical bills. *Kaiser Health News*. Available at: https://khn.org/news/covid19-coronavirus-test-surprise-medical-bill/. Accessed: September 17, 2022.

14 Noack, R., Wagner, J., Beachum, L., Horton, A. et al. (2020) As U.S. death toll surpasses 4,600, Fauci says the real turning point in coronavirus mitigation won't happen until there's a vaccine. *Washington Post.* Available at: https://www.washingtonpost.com/world/2020/04/01/coronavirus-latest-news/#linkPEBH57JZTRAA7M24XWM3J3VLIU. Accessed: December 18, 2022.

15 Fineberg, H. (2020) Ten Weeks to Crush the Curve. *New England Journal of Medicine.* Available at: https://www.nejm.org/doi/full/10.1056/nejme2007263. Accessed: September 17, 2022.

16 Pick, J. (2020) An open letter to Dr Anthony Fauci asking for Passover Seder advice Available at: https://www.mcsweeneys.net/articles/an-open-letter-to-dr-anthony-fauci-asking-for-passover-seder-advice. Accessed: December 18, 2022.

17 Sheridan, M., Masih, N., and Cabato, R. (2020) As Coronavirus fears grow, doctors and nurses face abuses, attacks. *Washington Post.* Available at: https://www.washingtonpost.com/world/the_americas/coronavirus-doctors-nurses-attack-mexico-ivory-coast/2020/04/08/545896a0-7835-11ea-a311-adb1344719a9_story.html. Accessed: January 16, 2023.

18 Mozingo, J. (2020) From the Black Death to AIDS, pandemics have shaped human history. Coronavirus will too. *Los Angeles Times.* Available at: https://www.latimes.com/california/story/2020-04-12/coronavirus-pandemic-black-death-aids-shape-history. Accessed: November 28, 2022.

19 Samuels, E. and Kelly, M. (2020) Why false hope spread about hydroxychloroquine to treat Covid-19 – and the consequences that followed. *Washington Post.* Available at: https://www.washingtonpost.com/politics/2020/04/13/how-false-hope-spread-about-hydroxychloroquine-its-consequences/. Accessed: November 28, 2022.

20 Blake, A. (2020) Why the Trump Fauci tension matters. *Washington Post.* Available at: https://www.washingtonpost.com/politics/2020/04/13/why-trump-fauci-tension-matters/. Accessed: November 28, 2022.

21 Gottlieb, S., Rivers, C., McLellan, M., Silvis, L., and Watson, C. (2020) National Coronavirus Response: A roadmap to reopening. *American Enterprise Institute*. Available at: https://www.aei.org/wp-content/uploads/2020/03/National-Coronavirus-Response-a-Road-Map-to-Recovering-2.pdf?x91208. Accessed: September 12, 2022.

22 Gadarian, S., Goodman, S., and Pepinsky, T. (2020) Partisanship, health behaviors, and policy attitudes in the early stages of the Covid-19 pandemic. *SSRN* Available at: https://papers.ssrn.com/sol3/papers.cfm?abstract_id=3562796. Accessed: November 28, 2022.

23 Rosenbeg, M. and Rogers, K. (2020) For Charlie Kirk, conservative activist, virus is a cudgel. *New York Times.* Available at: https://www.nytimes.com/2020/04/19/us/politics/charlie-kirk-conservatives-coronavirus.html?action=click&module=Top%20Stories&pgtype=Homepage. Accessed: November 28, 2022.

24 Fukuyama, F. (2020). The thing that determines a country's resistance to the coronavirus. *The Atlantic.* Available at: https://www.theatlantic.com/ideas/archive/2020/03/thing-determines-how-well-countries-respond-coronavirus/609025/. Accessed: November 27, 2022.

25 Tankersley, J. and Cochrane, E. (2020) Congress shovels trillions at virus, with no end-game in sight. *New York Times.* Available at: https://www.nytimes.com/2020/04/24/business/congress-coronavirus-stimulus-bill.html?action=click&module=Top%20Stories&pgtype=Homepage. Accessed: November 28, 2022.

26 Richardson, S., Hirsch, JS., Narasimhan, M., Crawford, JM. et al. (2020) Presenting Characteristics, Comorbidities, and Outcomes among 5700 patients hospitalized with COVID-19 in the New York City area. *JAMA.* 323: 20: 2052–59. Available at: https://jamanetwork.com/journals/jama/fullarticle/2765184?guestAccessKey=906e4 74e-0b94-4e0e-8eaa-606ddf0224f5. Accessed: November 27, 2022.

27 Cha, AE. (2020) A mysterious blood-clotting complication is killing coronavirus patients. *Washington Post* Available at: https://www.washingtonpost.com/health/2020/04/22/coronavirus-blood-clots/. Accessed: November 27, 2022.

28 Bennhold, K. A (2020) German exception? Why the country's coronavirus death rate is low. *New York Times.* Available at: https://www.nytimes.com/2020/04/04/world/europe/germany-coronavirus-death-rate.html. Accessed: November 27, 2022.

29 https://www.washingtonpost.com/nation/2020/04/24/disinfectant-injection-coronavirus-trump/

30 Health Management Associates. (2020) Covid-19 impact on Medicaid, marketplace and the uninsured by state. *Health Management Associates.* Available at: https://www.healthmanagement.com/wp-content/uploads/HMA-Estimates-of-COVID-Impact-on-Coverage-public-version-for-April-3-830-CT.pdf?mod=article_inline. Accessed: November 27, 2022.

31 Goldberg, D. and Ollstein, A. (2020) Tracking the virus may require 300,000. We're nowhere close *Politico.* Available at: https://www.politico.com/news/2020/04/21/tracking-coronavirus-workforce-does-not-exist-197622. Accessed: November 27, 2022.

32 Gabriel, T. (2020) Ohio's GOP governor splits from Trump and rises in popularity. *New York Times.* Available at: https://www.nytimes.com/2020/04/28/us/politics/mike-dewine-ohio-coronavirus.html. Accessed: November 27, 2022.

33 Hohmann, J. (2020) The Daily 202: Barr memo threatening lawsuits against coronavirus restrictions is a warning shot. *Washington Post.* Available at: https://www.washingtonpost.com/news/powerpost/paloma/daily-202/2020/04/28/daily-202-barr-memo-threatening-lawsuits-against-coronavirus-restrictions-is-a-warning-shot/5ea7a78e88e0fa3dea9c4414/. Accessed: November 27, 2022.

34 Colllier, P. (2020) The problem of modelling. *Times Literary Supplement.* Available at: https://www.the-tls.co.uk/articles/problem-modelling-public-policy-coronavirus-paul-collier/. Accessed: November 27, 2022.

35 Beech, H., Rubin, A., Kurmanaev, A., and Maclean, R. (2020) The Covid-19 riddle: Why does the virus wallop some places and spare others. *New York Times.* Available at: https://www.nytimes.com/2020/05/03/world/asia/coronavirus-spread-where-why. html?searchResultPosition=2. Accessed: November 27, 2022.

36 O, Toole, F. (2020) Donald Trump has destroyed the country he promised to make great again. *Irish Times.* Available at: https://www.irishtimes.com/opinion/fintan-o-toole-donald-trump-has-destroyed-the-country-he-promised-to-make-great-again-1.4235928. Accessed: November 27, 2022.

37 White House. (2020) United States Daily Covid Deaths. *White House Archive.* Available at: https://twitter.com/WhiteHouseCEA45/status/1257680258364555264? s=20. Accessed: November 27, 2022.

38 Rosenberg, M. and Rutenberg, J. (2020) Fight over virus's death toll opens grim new front in election battle. *New York Times.* Available at: https://www.nytimes.com/2020/05/09/ us/politics/coronavirus-death-toll-presidential-campaign.html?action=click& module=Top%20Stories&pgtype=Homepage. Accessed: November 27, 2022.

39 Dawsey, J., Parker, A., Rucker, J., and Abutaleb, Y. (2020) As deaths mount, Trump tries to convince Americans it's safe to inch back to normal. *Washington Post.* Available at: https://www.washingtonpost.com/politics/as-deaths-mount-trump-tries-to-convince-americans-its-safe-to-inch-back-to-normal/2020/05/09/bf024fe6-9149-11ea-a9c0-73b93422d691_story.html. Accessed: November 27, 2022.

40 Gearan, A., DeBonis, M., and Dennis, B. (2020) Trump plays down coronavirus testing as U.S. fall far short of level scientists say is needed. *Washington Post.* Available at: https://www.washingtonpost.com/politics/trump-plays-down-coronavirus-testing-as-us-falls-far-short-of-level-scientists-say-is-needed/2020/05/08/d9241454-913f-11ea-a9c0-73b93422d691_story.html. Accessed: November 27, 2022.

41 Facher, L. (2020) A bipartisan group of health officials seeks to sell a 46.5 billion coronavirus plan to the White House *Stat News.* Available at: https://www.statnews. com/2020/04/29/gottlieb-slavitt-coronavirus-plan-white-house/. Accessed: November 27, 2022.

42 Altucker, K. and O'Donnell, J. (2020) Fifty states and fifty different approaches: States scramble to hire contact tracers. *USA Today.* Available at: https://www.usatoday.com/ story/news/health/2020/05/13/coronavirus-states-scramble-hire-covid-19-contact-tracers/3088014001/. Accessed: November 27, 2022.

43 Garfield, R., Claxton, G., Damico, A., and Leavitt, L. (2020) Eligibility for ACA health coverage following job loss. *Kaiser Family Foundation.* Available at: https:// www.kff.org/coronavirus-covid-19/issue-brief/eligibility-for-aca-health-coverage-following-job-loss/?utm_campaign=KFF-2020-Health-Reform. Accessed: November 27, 2022.

44 Ollstein, AM. (2020) Sanders rekindles Democrats health coverage feud before key House vote. *Politico.* Available at: https://www.politico.com/news/2020/05/15/ bernie-sanders-medicare-for-all-coronavirus-relief-bill-260183. Accessed: November 27, 2022.

45 Kaiser Health News. (2020) Lost on the frontline. *Kaiser Health News.* Available at: https://khn.org/news/lost-on-the-frontline-health-care-worker-death-toll-covid19-coronavirus/. Accessed: November 27, 2022.

46 Winton, R. (2020) We don't want another Gabriel Fernandez: Coronavirus leads to "alarming" drop in child abuse reports. *Los Angeles Times.* Available at: https://www. latimes.com/california/story/2020-04-21/coronavirus-child-abuse-reports-decline. Accessed: November 27, 2022.

47 Bernstein, L. (2020) More evidence emerges on why Covid-19 is much worse than the flu. *Washington Post*. Available at: https://www.washingtonpost.com/health/more-evidence-emerges-on-why-covid-19-is-so-much-worse-than-the-flu/2020/05/21/e7814588-9ba5-11ea-a2b3-5c3f2d1586df_story.html. Accessed: November 27, 2022.

48 Zwirner, D. (2020) Art is how we justify our existence. *New York Times*. Available at: https://www.nytimes.com/2020/05/22/opinion/david-zwirner-museums-coronavirus.html. Accessed: November 27, 2022.

49 Scott, D. (2020) Two public health crises have collided in the protests over George Floyd's death. *Vox*. Available at: https://www.vox.com/2020/6/1/21276957/george-floyd-protests-coronavirus-police-brutality-racism. Accessed: November 27, 2022.

50 Keehn, E., Boyd, J. (2020) How mass incarceration harms US health, in five charts. *The Conversation*. Available at: https://theconversation.com/how-mass-incarceration-harms-u-s-health-in-5-charts-90674. Accessed: November 27, 2022.

51 Barclay, E. (2020) How to more safely protest in a pandemic. *Vox*. Available at: https://www.vox.com/2020/5/31/21276082/what-to-bring-to-a-protest-coronavirus-covid-19-risk-safety. Accessed: November 27, 2022

52 Christensen, j. and Crespo, G. (2020) Covid-19 is Dr Anthony Fauci's "Worst Nightmare." *CNN Health* Available: https://www.cnn.com/2020/06/09/health/fauci-coronavirus-worst-nightmare/index.html?utm_campaign=wp_todays_worldview&utm_medium=email&utm_source=newsletter&wpisrc=nl_todayworld. Accessed: November 27, 2022

53 Fisher, M., Hernandez, A., and Sellers, F. (2020) "People are looking at me": For many who lost jobs in the corona virus pandemic, hunger comes with shame. *Washington Post*. Available at: https://www.washingtonpost.com/national/coronavirus-food-insecurity/2020/06/04/c48bba48-a0fc-11ea-b5c9-570a91917d8d_story.html?_. Accessed: November 27, 2022.

54 Cha, A. (2020) We don't get justice: When a black girl's death from Covid-19 feels like a collision of two crises. *Washington Post*. Available at: https://www.washingtonpost.com/health/2020/06/05/coronavirus-baltimore-race-police-violence/. Accessed: November 27, 2022.

55 Luthi, S. The 7,000 Covid Test. (2020) *Politico*. Available at: https://www.politico.com/news/2020/06/08/coronavirus-test-costs-304058. Accessed: November 27, 2022.

56 Deng, X., Gu, W., Federman, S., and du Plessis L. (2020) Genomic surveillance reveals multiple introductions of SARS-CoV-2 into Northern California. *Science*. 31: 369: 6503: 582–87. Available at: https://www.science.org/doi/10.1126/science.abb9263. Accessed: November 27, 2022.

57 Resnick, B. (2020) The US badly needs a wake-up call on the Coronavirus pandemic. *Vox*. Available at: https://www.vox.com/science-and-health/2020/6/23/21299109/covid-19-pandemic-years-potential-life-lost. Accessed: November 27, 2022.

58 Basset, M., Chen, J., and Krieger, N. (2020) The unequal toll of Covid-19 mortality by age in the United States: Quantifying racial/ ethnic disparities. *Harvard Center for Population and Development Studies. Working Paper Series*. Available at: https://cdn1.sph.harvard.edu/wp-content/uploads/sites/1266/2020/06/20_Bassett-Chen-Krieger_COVID-19_plus_age_working-paper_0612_Vol-19_No-3_with-cover.pdf. Accessed: November 27, 2022.

59 Rubin, A and Golden, T. (2020) Inside the U.S.'s largest maximum-security prison, Covid-19 rages. Outside, officials called their fight a success. *Pro Publica*. Available

at: https://www.propublica.org/article/inside-the-uss-largest-maximum-security-prison-covid-19-raged?utm_source=pardot&utm_medium=email&utm_campaign=majorinvestigations&utm_content=feature. Accessed: November 27, 2022.

60 Aron-Dine, A., Huang, C., and Washington. S. (2020) ACA repeal lawsuit would cut taxes for top 0.1% by an average of $198,000 *Center for Budget and Policy Priorities*. Available at: https://www.cbpp.org/research/health/aca-repeal-lawsuit-would-cut-taxes-for-top-01-percent-by-an-average-of-198000. Accessed: November 27, 2022.

61 Rosenthal, EL., Menking, P., and Begay, MG. (2020) Fighting the COVID-19 Merciless Monster: Lives on the Line-Community Health Representatives' Roles in the Pandemic Battle on the Navajo Nation. *J Ambul Care Manage*. 43: 4: 302. Available at: https://journals.lww.com/ambulatorycaremanagement/Abstract/2020/10000/Fighting_the_COVID_19_Merciless_Monster__Lives_on.7.aspx. Accessed: November 27, 2022.

62 Kuhn, C. and Rose, A. (2020) Tall pines healthcare COVID-19 outbreak experience in rural Waldo County, Maine. *Journal of Ambulatory Care Management*. 43: 4: 295. Available at: https://journals.lww.com/ambulatorycaremanagement/Abstract/2020/10000/Tall_Pines_Healthcare_COVID_19_Outbreak_Experience.6.aspx. Accessed: November 27, 2022.

63 Florida Ask Nurses and Doctors Representatives. (2020) Letter to the Editor *Florida Times-Union*. Available at: https://www.jacksonville.com/story/opinion/2020/07/09/letters-police-shooting-wasnrsquot-profiling-doctors-call-on-retailers-to-require-masks/41716701/. Accessed: January 16, 2023.

64 Parker-Pope, T. (2020) Tips on making your mask work. *New York Times*. Available at: https://www.nytimes.com/interactive/2020/06/25/burst/how-to-get-the-most-out-of-your-mask.html?action=. Accessed: November 27, 2022.

65 Lerner, J. (2020) To fight coronavirus disinformation, health care professionals must speak out *Philadelphia Inquirer*. Available at: https://www.inquirer.com/health/expert-opinions/coronavirus-disinformation-health-care-workers-speak-out-20200717.html. Accessed: November 28, 2022.

66 Martin, N. (2020) No one tracks health care workers lost to Covid-19. So she stays up at night cataloguing the dead. *Pro Publica*. Available at: https://www.propublica.org/article/nobody-accurately-tracks-health-care-workers-lost-to-covid-19-so-she-stays-up-at-night-cataloging-the-dead?utm_source=sailthru&utm_medium=email&utm_campaign=majorinvestigations&utm_content=feature. Accessed: November 28, 2022.

67 Brennan, Z. and Owermohle, S. (2020) FDA authorizes plasma treatment despite scientists' objections. *Politico*. Available at: https://www.politico.com/news/2020/08/23/plasma-treatment-coronavirus-fda-trump-400390. Accessed: November 28, 2022.

68 Thomas, K. and Fink, S. (2020) FDA "grossly misrepresented" blood plasma data, scientists say. *New York Times*. Available at: https://www.nytimes.com/2020/08/24/health/fda-blood-plasma.html?action=click&module=Top%20Stories&pgtype=Homepage. Accessed: November 28, 2022.

69 Goldfield, N., Goldstein, A., and Crittenden, R. (2020) It's time for Trump administration doctors to speak up – whatever the consequences *The Hill*. Available at: https://thehill.com/opinion/white-house/508508-its-time-for-trump-administration-doctors-to-speak-up-whatever-the/. Accessed: November 28, 2022.

70 We can do better vote. (2020) Informed Citizenry. Available at: https://youtu.be/ScoqVEqQBac. Accessed: November 28, 2022.

71 Vot-ER Available at: https://vot-er.org/. Accessed: February 13, 2023.

72 Gay Stolberg, C. (2020) Top U.S. officials told CDC to soften Coronavirus testing guidelines. *New York Times.* Available at: https://www.nytimes.com/2020/08/26/us/politics/coronavirus-testing-trump-cdc.html?searchResultPosition=1. Accessed: November 28, 2022.

73 Finkenstadt, D., Handfield, R., and Giunto, P. (2020) Why the U.S. still has a severe shortage of medical supplies. *Harvard Business Review.* Available at: https://hbr.org/2020/09/why-the-u-s-still-has-a-severe-shortage-of-medical-supplies?ab=hero-main-text&utm_campaign=KHN%3A%20First%20Edition&utm_medium=email&_hsmi=95538994&_hsenc=p2ANqtz–I2QDWLFrVDNcNMWnI1YnVoO6EjsqK-DTiI5lM_58cw3z_9Tn-c2tIW3FUNdmM-Uh6yfXMndV2QUtBMrccZRUut9T6uw&utm_content=95538994&utm_source=hs_email. Accessed: November 28, 2022.

74 Goldfield NI, Crittenden R, Fox D, McDonough J,. (2020) COVID-19 Crisis Creates Opportunities for Community-Centered Population Health: Community Health Workers at the Center. *J Ambul Care Manage.* 43: 3: 184–90. Available at: https://journals.lww.com/ambulatorycaremanagement/Abstract/2020/07000/COVID_19_Crisis_Creates_Opportunities_for.2.aspx. Accessed: November 28, 2022.

75 Luthi. L. (2020) Biden wants to restore Obamacare. He may have trouble *Politico.* Available at: https://www.politico.com/news/2020/09/15/biden-obamacare-health-agenda-415482. Accessed: November 28, 2022.

76 Goldfield NI, Crittenden R, Fox D, McDonough J,. et al (2020) COVID-19 Crisis Creates Opportunities for Community-Centered Population Health: Community Health Workers at the Center. *J Ambul Care Manage.* 43: 3: 184–90. Available at: https://journals.lww.com/ambulatorycaremanagement/Abstract/2020/07000/COVID_19_Crisis_Creates_Opportunities_for.2.aspx. Accessed: November 28, 2022.

77 Fouche, S., Entel, K., Nelson, C., Bird, C. et al. Out of the ashes: Forging the post pandemic U.S. health care system. *The RAND Blog.* Available at: https://www.rand.org/blog/2020/07/out-of-the-ashes-forging-the-post-pandemic-us-health.html. Accessed: November 28, 2022.

78 Perez, J. (2020) Campus life sans Covid: A few colleges write the playbook for success. *Politico.* Available at: https://www.politico.com/news/2020/09/28/campus-life-sans-covid-a-few-colleges-write-the-playbook-for-pandemic-success-422010. Accessed: November 28, 2022.

79 Reuters Staff. (2020) New advisor giving Trump bad information on the virus, top US officials say. *Reuters.* Available at: https://www.reuters.com/article/health-coronavirus-usa-cdc-idUSKBN26K07E?utm_campaign=KHN%3A%20First%20Edition&utm_medium=email&_hsmi=96262156&_hsenc=p2ANqtz-9mK9khVmxf2OZQtdYhgtcjIHrOMaqfhUhBGaPe72pr9jaLPyJjwwhIecKL5f-RV_arMRQu_3bUYb0t9SRQdES5XuLb7A&utm_content=96262156&utm_source=hs_email. Accessed: November 28, 2022.

80 Contrera, J. (2020) The N95 shortage the America can't seem to fix. *Politico.* Available at: https://www.washingtonpost.com/graphics/2020/local/news/n-95-shortage-covid/?utm_campaign=wp_to_your_health&utm_medium=email&utm_source=newsletter&wpisrc=nl_tyh&wpmk=1&pwapi_token=eyJ0eXAiOiJKV1QiLCJhbGciOiJIUzI1NiJ9.eyJjb29raWVuYW1lIjoid3BfY3J0aWQiLCJpc3MiOiJDQXJ0YSIsImNvb2tpZVZhbHVlIjoiNTk2YjYxNTNhZGU0ZTI0MTE5YjI4MmIzIiwidGFnIjoiNWY2OTBiOGE5ZDJmZGEyYzM2OWNhNDRkIiwidXJsIjoiaHR0cHM6Ly93d3cud2FzaGluZ3RvbnBvc3QuY29tL2dyYXBoaWNzLzIwMjA

vbG9jYWwvbmV3cy9uLTk1LXNob3J0YWdlLWNvdmlkLz91dG1fY2FtcGFpZ24
9d3BfdG9feW91cl9oZWFsdGgmdXRtX21lZGl1bT1lbWFpbCZ1dG1fc291cmNl
PW5ld3NsZXR0ZXImd3Bpc3JjPW5sX3R5cCZ3cG1rPTEifQ.NzOiwvz7wvLG
CST5OnDHIyI0zZwPVkR67ZZEZscw9Ps. Accessed: November 28, 2022.

81 Sherer, M. and Sun, L. Trump plans big Wisconsin rallies despite White House task force
calls for "maximal" social distancing in the state. *Washington Post*. Available at: https://
www.washingtonpost.com/politics/trump-wisconsin-rallies-coronavirus/2020/
09/30/edf25c70-027c-11eb-b7ed-141dd88560ea_story.html. Accessed: November
28, 2022.

82 Scott, Dylan (2020) Joe Biden's plan to beat Covid-19 in the U.S. *Vox*. Available at:
https://www.vox.com/coronavirus-covid19/2020/9/28/21451418/joe-biden-covid-
19-plan-policy?_hsmi=96357001&_hsenc=p2ANqtz-_iyTZQfQX-yZvfKDH4
EBEkDImsxV0qQRbZIO-6fN3P8Gg8Bt4iVDhlvZV-Pyr2Y9i_Mb3HkKSTdq
pKnqGACU3RpKY7kA. Accessed: November 28, 2022.

83 Abelson, R. (2020) Some workers face looming cutoffs in health insurance *New York
Times*. Available at: https://www.nytimes.com/2020/09/28/health/covid-19-health-
insurance.html. Accessed: November 28, 2022.

84 Brownstein, R. (2020) Republicans are trapped on pre-existing conditions. *The
Atlantic*. Available at: https://www.theatlantic.com/politics/archive/2020/09/why-
trump-has-no-real-health-care-plan/616523/?utm_campaign=KHN%3A%20
First%20Edition&utm_medium=email&_hsmi=96357001&_hsenc=p2AN-
qtz-_e7jlYSWfOPbbcl7_K75dvxz26KkbZgEB2zCxsG7663DjzDDIHqLdCW16l6
xb0HN2xBOpeTKMAJz3w-ShVUlebtchZFw&utm_content=96357001&utm_
source=hs_email. Accessed: November 28, 2022.

85 Scott, D. (2020) If Trump wins, 25 million could lose health insurance. If Biden
wins, 20 million could gain it. *Vox*. Available at: https://www.vox.com/policy-and-
politics/21493251/presidential-debate-2020-biden-trump-health-care-plan.
Accessed: November 28, 2022.

86 Abutaleb, Y., Rucker, P., Dawsey, J., and Costa, R. (2020) Trump's den of dissent: Inside
the White House Task Force as Coronavirus surges. *Washington Post*. Available at:
https://www.washingtonpost.com/politics/trumps-den-of-dissent-inside-the-white-
house-task-force-as-coronavirus-surges/2020/10/19/7ff8ee6a-0a6e-11eb-859b-
f9c27abe638d_story.html. Accessed: November 28, 2022.

87 Barry, J. (2020) What fans of herd immunity don't tell you. *New York Times*. Available at: https://www.nytimes.com/2020/10/19/opinion/coronavirus-herd-immunity.
html?action=click&module=Opinion&pgtype=Homepage. Accessed: November 28,
2022.

88 Douthat, R. (2020) Trump is giving up. *New York Times*. Available at: https://www.
nytimes.com/2020/10/20/opinion/trump-campaign-.html?action=click&module=
Opinion&pgtype=Homepage. Accessed: November 28, 2022.

89 Stewart, N. and Heisler, T. (2020) 1.5 million New Yorkers can't afford food. *New
York Times*. Available at: https://www.nytimes.com/interactive/2020/10/20/nyregion/
nyc-food-banks.html?action=click&module=Top%20Stories&pgtype=Homepage.
Accessed: November 28, 2022.

90 Busewitz, C. (2020) Twitter blocks tweet from presidential advisor downplaying masks.
AP Available at: https://apnews.com/article/virus-outbreak-donald-trump-health-
us-news-b57a7b140a5c39af3f7f526e6de60953?utm_campaign=KHN%3A%20
First%20Edition&utm_medium=email&_hsmi=97699549&_hsenc=p2A
Nqtz-_qeHfwXF_gywXqnBKx3Re3Sxqclrj8IUAfW-lbH3Dp8ugVvLvYs3TNdd

Ggk_13YHd7YZjH5azpTWC-BSGhS-xAq1jWqg&utm_content=
97699549&utm_source=hs_email. Accessed: November 28, 2022.

91 BSA Health System. (2020) Help your hospitals, wear a mask. *BSA Health System.* Available at: https://www.youtube.com/watch?v=pD-i-zDTZq4. Accessed: November 28, 2022.

92 Bock Clark, D. (2020) Inside the chaotic, cutthroat gray market for N-95 Masks. *New York Times.* Available at: https://www.nytimes.com/2020/11/17/magazine/n95-masks-market-covid.html. Accessed: November 28, 2022.

93 Chiu, A and Raben, L. (2020) Light therapy lamps can ease seasonal depression. Here is what you need to know. *Washington Post.* Available at: https://www.washingtonpost.com/lifestyle/wellness/light-box-therapy-seasonal-depression/2020/11/17/4116e2a0-2914-11eb-92b7-6ef17b3fe3b4_story.html?utm_campaign=KHN%3A%20First%20Edition&utm_medium=email&_hsmi=100339382&_hsenc=p2ANqtz-wFASuyUvMeae8Uc_z6Sv4KosK-J2on9LxVjxF9lNjwhMNWh_kbJUBR6eKDLxJwbVwBPGpcNguJYraTo7VlDoBIByb1A&utm_content=100339382&utm_source=hs_email. Accessed: December 18, 2022.

94 Oster, E. (2020) Schools are not spreading Covid-19. This new data makes the case. *Washington Post.* Available at: https://www.washingtonpost.com/opinions/2020/11/20/covid-19-schools-data-reopening-safety/?arc404=true&utm_campaign=wp_week_in_ideas&utm_medium=email&utm_source=newsletter&wpisrc=nl_ideas&carta-url=https%3A%2F%2Fs2.washingtonpost.com%2Fcar-ln-tr%2F2ce6472%2F5fba53049d2fda0efb70c8f8%2F596b6153ade4e24119b282b3%2F11%2F70%2F5fba53049d2fda0efb70c8f8. Accessed: December 18, 2022.

95 https://www.vermontpublic.org/vpr-news/2020-11-09/burlingtons-wastewater-surveillance-program-detects-localized-uptick-in-covid-19#stream/0

96 Goldhill, O. (2020) 'People are going to die': Hospitals in half the states are facing a massive staffing shortage as Covid-19 surges. *Stat News.* Available at: https://www.statnews.com/2020/11/19/covid19-hospitals-in-half-the-states-facing-massive-staffing-shortage/?utm_campaign=KHN%3A%20First%20Edition&utm_medium=email&_hsmi=100339382&_hsenc=p2ANqtz-9oy91wtE6M-Z-15m4MUyxxpXnXRIqzYVsL-IYa7ceUljZSI47NSzSMfyjJGLQOgYdqmaMA5sczGnxuKsTgywgx8k-iw&utm_content=100339382&utm_source=hs_email. Accessed: December 18, 2022.

97 New York Times briefing. (2020) Doctors call for more restrictions and caution as virus surges *New York Times.* Available at: https://www.nytimes.com/live/2020/11/14/world/covid19-coronavirus-updates?referringSource=articleShare. Accessed: November 28, 2022.

98 Biden-Harris. (2020) The Biden plan to combat coronavirus. *Biden Harris Democrats.* Available at: https://joebiden.com/covid-plan/#. Accessed: November 28, 2022.

99 Rovner, J. (2020) What Biden can do to combat Covid right now. *Kaiser Health News.* Available at: https://khn.org/news/article/what-can-biden-do-to-combat-covid-right-now/?utm_campaign=KHN%3A%20First%20Edition&utm_medium=email&_hsmi=100654140&_hsenc=p2ANqtz-QdVFceO-Ra3TCmLva0sZzVxEGxhByJ4Wc-z3t8La1oS6TKP5LJMx7QH4fmK2vPIN_fB8dZ1MyY7Q7twD5OkUlLJJbzw&utm_content=100654140&utm_source=hs_email. Accessed: November 28, 2022.

100 Wolfson, B. (2020) No more ICU beds at the main public hospital in the nation's largest county. *Kaiser Health News.* Available at: Accessed: November 28, 2022.

101 Aubutaleb, Y., Parker, A., Dawsey, J., and Rucker, P. (2020) The inside story of how Trump's denial, mismanagement and magical thinking led to the pandemic's dark winter. *Washington Post*. Available at: https://www.washingtonpost.com/graphics/2020/politics/trump-covid-pandemic-dark-winter/?itid=hp-top-table-main. Accessed: November 28, 2022.

102 Lerner, J. and Goldheld, N. (2020) Communicating effectively with the public and patients will be key as Covid-19 accelerates. *Atlanta Journal-Constitution*. Available at: https://www.ajc.com/opinion/opinion-a-critical-role-now-for-health-professionals/56RC54TZAJHJHANMS2JVD6SGG4/. Accessed: November 28, 2022.

103 The Atlantic (2021) Covid Tracking Project. *The Atlantic*. Available at: https://covidtracking.com Accessed: November 28, 2022.

104 Haley, D. and Saltz, R. (2020) The opioid epidemic during the Covid-19 pandemic. *JAMA*. 324:16: 1615–77. Available at: https://jamanetwork.com/journals/jama/fullarticle/2770985. Accessed: November 28, 2022.

105 Kwai, I (2021) Australia locks down a whole city after finding a single new Coronavirus case. *New York Times*. Available at: https://www.nytimes.com/2021/01/31/world/perth-covid-lockdown.html. Accessed: November 28, 2022.

106 Eggerup, P., Olsen, F., Christiansen-Hellerung, A., Westergaard, D. et al. (2021) Severe acute respiratory distress Coronavirus antibodies at delivery in women, partners, and newborns. *Obstetrics and Gynecology* 137:1: 49–55. https://journals.lww.com/greenjournal/Fulltext/2021/01000/Severe_Acute_Respiratory_Syndrome_Coronavirus_2.7.aspx. Accessed: November 28, 2022.

107 Garger, K. (2021) Alarming numbers of health care workers are refusing Covid-19 vaccine. *New York Post*. Available at: https://nypost.com/2021/01/01/alarming-number-of-us-health-care-workers-are-refusing-covid-19-vaccine/. Accessed: November 28, 2022.

108 Tuckson, R. (2020) The disease of distrust. *Science* 370:6518: 745. Available at: https://www.science.org/doi/full/10.1126/science.abf6109. Accessed: November 28, 2022.

109 Ravindranath, M. (2021) Social media 'micro-influencers' join effort to get America vaccinated. *Politico*. Available at: https://www.politico.com/news/2021/01/30/vaccine-rollout-influencers-463917. Accessed: November 28, 2022.

110 Shots heard around the world. https://twitter.com/shotsheard?lang=en. Accessed: November 28, 2022.

111 Su, A. (2021) A year after the Covid pandemic began, Wuhan has become a city of forgetting. *Los Angeles Times*. Available at: https://www.latimes.com/world-nation/story/2021-02-14/wuhan-becomes-a-city-of-forgetting. Accessed: November 28, 2022.

112 Chiu, A. (2021) If double-masking is hurting your ears, try these tips to relieve the pain *Washington Post*. Available at: https://www.washingtonpost.com/lifestyle/wellness/double-mask-pain-ear-covid/2021/02/09/419e5340-6a30-11eb-9f80-3d7646ce1bc0_story.html?utm_campaign=KHN%3A%20First%20Edition&utm_medium=email&_hsmi=110772236&_hsenc=p2ANqtz-8nWGNFRNyTsy-gNQr9VL7vJm4QcZIIqGId4ziqohJuwBPpPzbdJdJRK2ZkvXBQoMr7aNfS8jrIAg3FV7FxbBZ1QvCjWQ&utm_content=110772236&utm_source=hs_email. Accessed: November 28, 2022.

113 Mandavilli, A., Taylor, K., and Goldstein, D. (2021) CDC draws up blueprint for reopening schools *New York Times*. Available at: https://www.nytimes.com/2021/02/12/health/school-reopenings-cdc.html?surface=home-discovery-vi-prg&

fellback=false&req_id=256001691&algo=identity&variant=no-exp&imp_id=775760114&action=click&module=Science%20%20Technology&pgtype=Homepage. Accessed: November 28, 2022.

114 Perez, J. (2021) CDC guidance on schools is coming. That might not settle a heated debate *Politico*. Available at: https://www.politico.com/news/2021/02/11/cdc-corona-virus-school-reopening-guidance-468700?utm_campaign=KHN%3A%20First%20Edition&utm_medium=email&_hsmi=110772236&_hsenc=p2ANqtz-_C0ifK 9PYRdwrDfJ96_JUdRnaWgIPPBkecd7AgD3LnKamgjbtZ5GPy-XSUoxhLezyuE 1pQZbnvBr9QeJbi19TsoYZ4lA&utm_content=110772236&utm_source=hs_email. Accessed: November 28, 2022.

115 Muller, J and Snyder, J. (2021) Why vaccine production is taking so long. *Axios*. Available at: https://www.axios.com/2021/02/12/vaccine-production-delays?utm_source=newsletter&utm_medium=email&utm_campaign=newsletter_axiosvitals&stream=top. Accessed: November 28, 2022.

116 Pfizer Vaccine funny commercial by Kimmel Valentines Day special just for fun trending advertisement. https://www.youtube.com/watch?v=r8HWYXBtEoU. Accessed: November 28, 2022.

117 Wood, S and Schulman, K. (2021) Beyond politics – Promoting Covid vaccination in the United States. *New England Journal of Medicine* 384. e(23). Available at: https://www.nejm.org/doi/full/10.1056/NEJMms2033790. Accessed: November 28, 2022.

118 Rodriguez, CH. (2021) Children's hospitals grapple with young Covid long haulers. *Kaiser Health News*. Available at: https://khn.org/news/article/children-covid-long-hauler-clinics-pediatric-hospitals/?utm_campaign=KHN%3A%20First%20Edition&utm_medium=email&_hsmi=113894542&_hsenc=p2ANqtz-82aAMTJ S6j7P-iuVzmIZDU5uOOImZ3OeFQ21EToIfkrqPWc94C3TT58FvFHg 2JV2myACIXjR3ZfA6cTocglcumhyhsuA&utm_content=113894542&utm_source=hs_email. Accessed: November 28, 2022.

119 Guardian staff and agency. (2020) Trump administration refused offer to buy millions more Pfizer vaccine doses. *The Guardian*. Available at: https://www.theguardian.com/world/2020/dec/07/trump-administration-coronavirus-vaccine-pfizer. Accessed: November 28, 2022.

120 Diamond, D. (2021) 'Its up to you': Ad campaign to encourage coronavirus vaccination gets underway. *Washington Post*. Available at: https://www.washingtonpost.com/health/2021/02/25/covid-vaccine-ad-council/. Accessed: November 28, 2022.

121 Ahmad, F. and Anderson, R. (2021) The leading causes of death in the US for 2020 *JAMA Network* 325: 18: 1829–30. Available at: https://jamanetwork.com/journals/jama/fullarticle/2778234. Accessed November 28, 2022.

122 Ahmad, FB., Cisewski, JA., Rossen, LM., and Sutton, P. (2022) Provisional drug overdose death counts. *National Center for Health Statistics*. Available at: https://www.cdc.gov/nchs/nvss/vsrr/drug-overdose-data.htm. Accessed: November 28, 2022.

123 Goldstein, A. (2021) Should health care workers be required to get health care shots. Companies grapple with mandates *Washington Post*. Available at: https://www.washingtonpost.com/health/should-health-care-workers-be-required-to-get-corona-virus-shots-companies-grapple-with-mandates/2021/04/04/2369048e-92f2-11eb-a74e-1f4cf89fd948_story.html. Accessed: November 28, 2022.

124 Goodnough, A. (2021) Getting to yes: A nursing home's mission to vaccinate its hesitant staff *New York Times*. Available at: https://www.nytimes.com/2021/03/28/health/nursing-home-covid-19-vaccine.html?action=click&module=Top%20 Stories&pgtype=Homepage. Accessed: November 28, 2022.

125 Milman, O., Yellin, I., Aharony, N., Katz R. et al. (2021) SARS-CoV-2 infection risk among unvaccinated is negatively associated with community-level vaccination rates. *Medrxiv.* Available at: https://www.medrxiv.org/content/10.1101/2021.03.26.21254 394v2.full.pdf. Accessed: November 28, 2022.

126 Quinn, S. and Andrasik, S. (2021) Addressing vaccine hesitancy in BIPOC communities – Toward trustworthiness, partnership and reciprocity. *New England Journal of Medicine.* 385: 22: 97–100 Available at: https://www.nejm.org/doi/pdf/10.1056/ NEJMp2103104?articleTools=true Accessed: November 28, 2022.

127 Compton, N (2021) You've vaccinated and ready to travel. Here's your pre-trip checklist. *Washington Post.* Available at: https://www.washingtonpost.com/travel/ tips/vaccine-passport-checklist-travel-cdc/?utm_campaign=wp_to_your_ health&utm_medium=email&utm_source=newsletter&wpisrc=nl_tyh&wpmk=1&pwapi_token=eyJ0eXAiOiJKV1QiLCJhbGciOiJIUzI1NiJ9.eyJjb29raWVVuYW1lIjoid3BfY3J0aWQiLCJpc3MiOiJDWXJ0YSIsImNvb2tpZXZhbHVlIjoiNTk2YjYxNThhZGU0ZTI0MTE5YjI4MmIzIiwidGFnIjoiNjA2Yjc4M2Q5ZDJmZGExZTU2ZTM3NWM4IiwidXJsIjoiaHR0cHM6Ly93d3cud2FzaGluZ3RvbnBvc3QuY29tL3RyYXZlbC90aXBzL3ZhY2NpbmUtcGFzc3BvcnQtY2hlY2tsaXN0LXRyYXZlbC1jZGMvIiwidXJsX2lkIjoiMjg5ZDNmZGExZTU2ZTM3NWM4IiwidGFnIjoiNjA2Yjc4M2Q5ZDJmZGExZTU2ZTM3NWM4IiwidXJsIjoiaHR0cHM6Ly93d3cud2FzaGluZ3RvbnBvc3QuY29tL3RyYXZlbC90aXBzL3ZhY2NpbmUtcGFzc3BvcnQtY2hlY2tsaXN0LXRyYXZlbC1jZGMvIn0.EpGSVp0DJAe7BUI2ejC5Qikylki2RD9G1nIGIBf_IBg. Accessed: November 28, 2022.

128 Renwick, D. (2021) Covid 'decimated our staff' as the pandemic ravages health care workers of color. *Kaiser Health News.* Available at: https://khn.org/news/article/ covid-decimated-our-staff-as-the-pandemic-ravages-health-workers-of-color-in-us/. Accessed: November 28, 2022.

129 Gostin, L., Moon, S., and Meir, B (2020) Reimagining global health governance in the age of Covid-19. *American Journal of Public Health.* https://www.ncbi.nlm.nih. gov/pmc/articles/PMC7542258/pdf/AJPH.2020.305933.pdf. Accessed: December 12, 2022.

130 Handfield, R., Finkenstadt, D., Schneller, E., Godfrey A. et al (2020) A commons for the supply chain in a post-Covid-19 era, the case for a reformed national stockpile *Millbank Quarterly.* Available at: https://onlinelibrary.wiley.com/doi/epdf/10.1111/1468-0009.12485. Accessed: November 28, 2022.

131 Florko, N. (2021) Biden officials met privately with 3M, Amerisource Bergen, PHRMA, and more to debate shoring up the national stockpile. *Stat.* Available at: https://www.statnews.com/2021/04/20/biden-met-privately-shoring-up-stockpile/?utm_source=STAT+Newsletters&utm_campaign=7658420b26-dc_ diagnosis_COPY_01&utm_medium=email&utm_term=0_8cab1d7961-76584 20b26-152403458. Accessed: November 28, 2022.

132 Daniels, E. (2021) Bidenworld fears many vaccine skeptics may be unreachable. They're trying anyway. *Politico.* Available at: https://www.politico.com/news/2021/04/21/ vaccine-skeptics-outreach-484124. Accessed: November 28, 2022.

133 Laughlin, J. and McCrystal M. (2021) Philly Vax Jawn delivers doses with tunes to combat low Covid-19 vaccination rates *Philadelphia Inquirer.* Available at: https:// www.inquirer.com/health/coronavirus/vaccine-black-doctors-covid-consortium-philadelphia-rates-20210424.html?utm_medium=referral&utm_source= android&utm_campaign=app_android_article_share&utm_content=7F7ZZZER DJHYXFW7Z5XUIEGANY. Accessed: November 28, 2022.

134 McGraw, M. and Stein, S. (2021) It's been exactly one year since Trump suggested ingesting bleach. We've never been the same *Politico*. Available at: https://www.politico.com/news/2021/04/23/trump-bleach-one-year-484399. Accessed: November 28, 2022.

135 Wright, A. (2021) Republican men are vaccine-hesitant but there's little focus on them. *Pew*. Available at: https://www.pewtrusts.org/en/research-and-analysis/blogs/stateline/2021/04/23/republican-men-are-vaccine-hesitant-but-theres-little-focus-on-them?utm_campaign=KHN%3A%20First%20Edition&utm_medium=email&_hsmi=123492827&_hsenc=p2ANqtz–j36SB_iwSSP7g-EEJIrTIRI3CnIBoToKmns-1GnWJ77h0kbbiEgnJD84Hf5jNRdUep0dBxZ37HYQ7rQrhN9TANuV2R2Q&utm_content=123492827&utm_source=hs_email. Accessed: November 28, 2022.

136 Knight, V. (2021) Censorship or misinformation? DeSantis and YouTube spar over Covid roundtable take down. *Kaiser Health News*. Available at: https://khn.org/news/article/censorship-or-misinformation-desantis-and-youtube-spar-over-covid-roundtable-takedown/?utm_campaign=KHN%3A%20First%20Edition&utm_medium=email&_hsmi=122603221&_hsenc=p2ANqtz-8VOj-3oaqtmzIvHONa4z9cJqGYiYqXR-dRNRts-Z_dLJ3Xk1Oo1L3te9JXYC_JvWR3h3RiYjF-zlReSXm7j3w6NTXI8A&utm_content=122603221&utm_source=hs_email. Accessed: November 28, 2022.

137 Thebault, R. (2021) Texas Governor Abbott says state is 'very close' to herd immunity. The data tells a different story. *Washington Post*. Available at: https://www.washingtonpost.com/politics/2021/04/11/abbott-herd-immunity-texas/?utm_campaign=wp_the_5_minute_fix&utm_medium=email&utm_source=newsletter&wpisrc=nl_fix&carta-url=https%3A%2F%2Fs2.washingtonpost.com%2Fcar-ln-tr%2F31e4252%2F6078b7bf9d2fda1dfb507cd9%2F-596b6153ade4e24119b282b3%2F23%2F48%2F6078b7bf9d2fda1dfb507cd9. Accessed: November 28, 2022.

138 Dwyer, D. (2021) Video; Dr Anthony Fauci and Representative Jim Jordan clash over Covid-19 restrictions during hearing. *Boston.com*. https://www.boston.com/news/coronavirus/2021/04/16/anthony-fauci-jim-jordan-maxine-waters-covid-hearing-video-clip/. Accessed: November 28, 2022.

139 Available at: https://www.youtube.com/watch?v=h7PB1-66ues. Accessed: November 28, 2022.

140 Gettleman, J. (2021) 'This is a catastrophe'. In India, illness is everywhere. *New York Times*. Available at: https://www.nytimes.com/2021/04/27/world/asia/India-delhi-covid-cases.html?utm_source=Nature+Briefing&utm_campaign=3a0e7aea05-briefing-dy-20210428&utm_medium=email&utm_term=0_c9dfd39373-3a0e7aea05-46273342. Accessed: November 28, 2022.

141 Carroll, AE. (2021) When can we declare the pandemic over? *New York Times*. Available at: https://www.nytimes.com/2021/04/27/opinion/covid-lockdown-end.html?action=click&module=Opinion&pgtype=Homepage. Accessed: November 28, 2022.

142 Engler, M. and Engler P. (2021) Can social movements realign America's political parties to win big change? *Democracy Uprising*. Available at: https://democracyuprising.com/2021/03/25/can-social-movements-realign-americas-political-parties-to-win-big-change/ Accessed: November 28, 2022.

143 Shepherd, S. (2021) Dem pollsters acknowledge 'major errors' in 2020 polling. *Politico*. Available at: https://www.politico.com/news/2021/04/13/dems-polling-failure-481044. Accessed: November 28, 2022.

144 Rizzo, A. (2021) Ron Johnson's unscientific use of vaccine and death data. *Washington Post.* https://www.washingtonpost.com/politics/2021/05/12/ron-johnsons-unscientific-use-vaccine-death-data/?utm_campaign=KHN%3A%20First%20 Edition&utm_medium=email&_hsmi=126703897&_hsenc=p2AN qtz-_Rt328OuIcXvueW_WLlmQPI3Zp9AeuQXvn4G7ZAWWrAzab pyUZudo1dhf29taLCDyUSaddkdUcXzmK9etqMGD2ebBasg&utm_ content=126703897&utm_source=hs_email. Accessed: November 28, 2022.

145 Pager, T., Diagmond, D., and Stein, J. (2021) 'It's pretty marginal': Experts say Biden's vaccine waiver unlikely to boost supply quickly. *Washington Post.* Available at: https:// www.washingtonpost.com/us-policy/2021/05/06/biden-patent-waiver-developing-world-long-road/. Accessed: November 28, 2022.

146 Wilkinson, M. (2021) Covid is fading, but racial gap in deaths is back in force in Michigan. *Bridge News.* https://www.bridgemi.com/michigan-health-watch/ covid-fading-racial-gap-deaths-back-force-michigan?utm_source=Bridge+ Michigan&utm_campaign=ce7d481f40-Bridge+Newsletter+05%2 F12%2F2021&utm_medium=email&utm_term=0_c64a28dd5a-ce7d481f40-82400368. Accessed: November 28, 2022.

147 Tanner, L. (2021) U.S. doctors group issues anti-racism plan for itself, field. *AP.* https://apnews.com/article/business-race-and-ethnicity-science-coronavirus-pandemic-health-bdff6225b933e47997291cd6fe7e87a5?utm_campaign=KHN%3A%20 First%20Edition&utm_medium=email&_hsmi=126703897&_hsenc=p2A Nqtz-9eaBEEgBSvEnTLGRKKMPQiBVJYWhLwo8wq85UCsgJ7 gDTkY_tZq5oVosq_DbN8qf-G36idHsQcj1ePe5PFQoV7d7fVrw&utm_content= 126703897&utm_source=hs_email. Accessed: November 28, 2022.

148 Mandavilli, A. (2021) Should people with immune problems get third vaccine doses *New York Times.* Available at: https://www.nytimes.com/2021/07/04/health/ coronavirus-immunity-vaccines.html?utm_campaign=KHN%3A%20First%20 Edition&utm_medium=email&_hsmi=138507161&_hsenc=p2ANqtz-9TLoc DlI_y-FkSj9BTZswwfscp0GoGcs1Ac43TfiEk13PTAaHFmS44DQg vg45eOzm5vAv9GszAmo7rEbnj2eGvbuepTQ&utm_content=138507161&utm_ source=hs_email. Accessed: November 28, 2022.

149 Schnell, M. (2021) Fauci: More than 99% of people who died of Covid-19 in June were not vaccinated. *The Hill.* Available at: https://thehill.com/policy/healthcare/ 561585-fauci-more-than-99-of-people-who-died-from-covid-19-in-june-were-not/?utm_campaign=KHN%3A+First+Edition&utm_medium=email&_hsmi= 138507161&_hsenc=p2ANqtz-8_yufsaTjNHwXAWlgM4ZnKs81AGpcwkyC wPlSevH5y74HuGNG4yT3z1jwV8jsgCEvIhhCDHe9jBY76M-MZ1AoQlvvsY w&utm_content=138507161&utm_source=hs_email&rl=1. Accessed: November 28, 2022.

150 Johnson, J. (2021) Maryland says 100% of residents who died of Covid in June were unvaccinated. *Common Dreams.* Available at: https://www.commondreams. org/news/2021/07/06/maryland-says-100-residents-who-died-covid-june-were-unvaccinated. Accessed: November 28, 2022.

151 Carney, J. (2021) McConnell pushes Covid vaccines amid Delta variant worries. *The Hill.* Available at: https://thehill.com/homenews/senate/561703-mcconnell-pushes-covid-19-vaccines-amid-delta-variant-worries/. Accessed: November 28, 2022.

152 Branswell, H. (2021) Twelve lessons Covid-19 taught us about developing vaccines during a pandemic. *Stat.* Available at: https://www.statnews.com/2021/06/30/12-lessons-covid-19-developing-vaccines/. Accessed: November 28, 2022.

153 Available at: https://www.facebook.com/watch/live/?v=172158281491770&ref=watch_permalink. Accessed: November 28, 2022.

154 Proceedings of the National Academy of Sciences (PNAS) Misinformation about science in the public sphere. *PNAS*. Available at: https://www.pnas.org/toc/pnas/118/15. Accessed: December 17, 2022.

155 Cobia, B. (2021) Facebook Post. Available at: https://www.facebook.com/brytneysnowcobia/posts/10200951240955876. Accessed: December 17, 2022.

156 Action Network. (2021) Pharma greed could kill us all. *Action Network*. Available at: https://actionnetwork.org/events/pharma-greed-could-kill-us-movement-meeting-for-campaign-to-end-vaccine-apartheid/?fbclid=IwAR3eTGYP7P2Oqwim-KyrkIa4j LbzUxlrxQHG3pjbSBInTyk6FFVnt55SqJI. Accessed: December 17, 2022.

157 Edwards, J. (2021) A Texas GOP railed against vaccines and masks. Then he died of Covid. *Washington Post*. Available at: https://www.washingtonpost.com/nation/2021/08/05/texas-gop-leader-antimask-antivax-dies-covid/. Accessed: December 17, 2022.

158 Peiser, J. (2021) Evangelical pastor demands that churchgoers ditch their masks. "Don't believe this delta variant nonsense.' *Washington Post*. Available at: https://www.washingtonpost.com/nation/2021/07/27/tennessee-pastor-greg-locke-masks/. Accessed: December 17, 2022.

159 Suliman, A. and Villegas, P. (2021) Conservative radio host and vaccine critic dies of Covid-19 complications *Washington Post*. Available at: https://www.washingtonpost.com/nation/2021/08/09/dick-farrel-dies-covid19/. Accessed: December 17, 2022.

160 AP. (2021) Tennessee won't incentivize Covid shots – but pays to vax cows. *Politico*. Available at: https://www.politico.com/news/2021/08/03/tennessee-covid-shots-vax-cows-502249?utm_campaign=KHN%3A%20First%20Edition&utm_medium=-email&_hsmi=146424670&_hsenc=p2ANqtz-8G95ka-OvVmdwpN7Yvjddr BV9Oszy-EAMRp6bce8k6IUjdnXoWuZfW2yE7NuHzcMMABD25oNHty VPfhpJPL_VSrDSe5Q&utm_content=146424670&utm_source=hs_email. Accessed: December 17, 2022.

161 Stucka, M. (2021) Booming U.S. cases account for one-fifth the world total. *Los Angeles Daily Tribune/ USA Today*. Available at: https://losangelesdailytribune.com/booming-us-cases-account-for-one-fifth-the-world-total-nih-to-decide-whether-to-offer-booster-shots-this-fall-live-covid-updates-usa-today/. Accessed: December 17, 2022.

162 Pettus, EW. (2021) Mississippi breaks its one-day hospitalization record. *AP News*. Available at: https://apnews.com/article/health-education-coronavirus-pandemic-mississippi-6fa32e24bacaf6d8f59ee74beabbffdb?utm_campaign=KHN%3A%20 First%2Edition&utm_medium=email&_hsmi=149111670&_hsenc=p2ANqtz-8nN ZHub2O3E3yTHuwuqz0EiyWpGYwdf-eBrqeuOpsTte1fop9GEQzneG ZATJEMCBAQ9XgvgFoHQ0BMVj8kqXIUwvbfMg&utm_content=149111670&utm_source=hs_email. Accessed: December 17, 2022.

163 Wen, L. (2021) The pandemic has become more dangerous for children. Here's how to help keep them safe. *Washington Post*. Available at: https://www.washingtonpost.com/opinions/2021/08/11/pandemic-has-become-more-dangerous-children-heres-how-help-keep-them-safe/?utm_campaign=wp_week_in_ideas&utm_medium=email&utm_source=newsletter&wpisrc=nl_ideas. Accessed: December 17, 2022.

164 Kumar Raghav, and P, Mohanty S. (2020) Are graphene and graphene-derived products capable of preventing COVID-19 infection? *Med Hypotheses*. 144: 110031. 10.1016/j.mehy.2020.110031. Epub 2020 Jun 24. PMID: 33254479; PMCID:

PMC7313523. Available at: https://pubmed.ncbi.nlm.nih.gov/33254479/. Accessed: December 17, 2022.

165 Slotnik, D. and Weiland, N. (2021) The prospect of booster shots is igniting a global health debate *New York Times.* Available at: https://www.nytimes.com/2021/08/16/world/booster-shots-debate.html?campaign_id=185&emc=edit_yct_20210816&instance_id=38030&nl=coronavirus-tracker&regi_id=10879457&segment_id=66363&te=1&user_id=5c81c9183ba5aa9fd6 82e58291889859. Accessed: December 17, 2022.

166 Holcombe, M. (2021) U.S. Covid cases among children are surging. Experts warm it may get worse. *CNN Health.* Available at: https://www.cnn.com/2021/08/25/health/us-coronavirus-wednesday/index.html?utm_campaign=KHN%3A%20First%20Edition&utm_medium=email&_hsmi=152650396&_hsenc=p2AN qtz-_qZ4zG_O4zS080Iui3-uSVE8BcaojvBnVBloaBVkpHpKb02k1vqjtV4JIhu FOoGxfU2AY5UTi3eGTNq4P1IMqgi_GweQ&utm_content=152650396&utm_source=hs_email. Accessed: December 17, 2022.

167 Powell, TB. (2021) Louisiana reports record number of Covid deaths. *CBS News.* Available at: https://www.cbsnews.com/news/louisiana-covid-19-deaths-highest-daily-total-pandemic/. Accessed: December 17, 2022.

168 Barrabi, T. (2021) South Florida doctors stage walkout amid surge of unvaccinated Covid-19 patients. *Fox News.* Available at: https://www.foxnews.com/us/south-florida-doctors-walkout-unvaccinated-covid-19-patients. Accessed: December 17, 2022.

169 Imbler, S and Anthes, A. (2021) How the Delta variants infiltrated an elementary school classroom. *New York Times.* Available at: https://www.nytimes.com/2021/08/28/health/coronavirus-schools-children.html?searchResultPosition=1&action=click& module=RelatedLinks&pgtype=Article. Accessed: December 17, 2022.

170 Huang, L., Yao, Q., Gu, X., Wang, Q. et al. (2021) 1-year outcomes in hospital survivors with COVID-19: a longitudinal cohort study. *The Lancet.* 2021 Aug 28;398: 10302: 747–58. 10.1016/S0140-6736(21)01755-4. Erratum in: Lancet. 399:10337 p:1778. PMID: 34454673; PMCID: PMC8389999. Available at: https://www. thelancet.com/journals/lancet/article/PIIS0140-6736(21)01755-4/fulltext. Accessed: December 17, 2022.

171 Vogel G. (2021) Unethical? Unnecessary? The booster debate intensifies. *Science.* 373: 6558: 949–50. 10.1126/science.373.6558.949. PMID: 34446586. Available at: https://www.science.org/content/article/unethical-unnecessary-covid-19-vaccine-booster-debate-intensifies. Accessed: December 17, 2022.

172 Hallerman, T. and Teegardin, C. (2021) Atlanta docs plead with public to get shots as Kemp bans Covid mandates by cities. *Atlanta Journal-Constitution.* Available at: https://www.ajc.com/news/atlanta-news/atlanta-hospitals-say-covid-cases-pushing-ers-to-the-brink/SC3ZJWQBY5AF5JJ26PFE4EUBIY/. Accessed: December 17, 2022.

173 Sun, L and Achenbach, J (2021) Unvaccinated people were 11 times more likely to die of Covid-19, CDC reports finds. *Washington Post.* Available at: https://www.washingtonpost.com/health/2021/09/10/moderna-most-effective-covid-vaccine-studies/. Accessed: December 17, 2022.

174 Kavi, A. (2021) Biden's vaccine push: What you need to know. *New York Times.* Available at: https://www.nytimes.com/2021/09/09/us/politics/biden-vaccine-plan-highlights. html?utm_campaign=KHN%3A%20First%20Edition&utm_medium=email&_hsmi=157948700&_hsenc=p2ANqtz-_T507uAvv7COmrGh09jQEAJjxLK2 CVi2VjIgstom06PoyPVsr4GPVsu8gHN4QGE8DIn07fNGKdLRSGb7ioMk5J

bvlu3Q&utm_content=157948700&utm_source=hs_email. Accessed: December 17, 2022.

175 Jha, A. (2021) What the Sturgis rally shows us about the Delta variant. *Washington Post*. Available at: https://www.washingtonpost.com/outlook/2021/09/07/sturgis-covid-delta-variant/. Accessed: December 17, 2022.

176 Sonmez, F., Sotomayor, M., and Alfaro, M. GOP condemnation of Biden Coronavirus mandate fuels concern other vaccine requirements could be targeted. *Washington Post*. Available at: https://www.washingtonpost.com/politics/republicans-vaccines-mandate-covid/2021/09/13/751c7bde-14a3-11ec-9589-31ac3173c2e5_story.html. Accessed: December 17, 2022.

177 Bartoloni, G. (2021) Il grande flop della protesta No-Vax. Ma la Lega vota contro il Green-Pass. *La Repubblica*. Available at: https://www.repubblica.it/politica/2021/09/01/news/contro_green_pass_lega_flop_manifestazioni-316162719/?ref=nl-rep-a-bgr. Accessed: December 17, 2022.

178 Parker-Pope, T. (2021) Worried about breakthrough infections? Here's how to navigate this phase of the pandemic. *New York Times*. Available at: https://www.nytimes.com/article/breakthrough-infections-covid-19-coronavirus.html. Accessed: December 17, 2022.

179 Antonelli, M., Penfold, RS., Merino, J., and Sudre, CH. (2021) Risk factors and disease profile of post-vaccination SARS-CoV-2 infection in UK users of the COVID Symptom Study app: a prospective, community-based, nested, case-control study. *Lancet Infect Dis* 22: 1: 43–55. doi: 10.1016/S1473-3099(21)00460-6. Epub 2021 Sep 1. PMID: 34480857; PMCID: PMC8409907. Available at: https://www.thelancet.com/action/showPdf?pii=S1473-3099%2821%2900460-6. Accessed; December 17, 2022.

180 Sullivan, S., Sotomayor, M., Pager, T., and Stein, J. (2021) Democrats sort through painful sacrifices as social bill enters final stretch. *Washington Post*. Available at: https://www.washingtonpost.com/politics/democrats-sorting-through-painful-sacrifices-as-social-bill-enters-final-stretch/2021/09/11/49c4106c-122f-11ec-bc8a-8d9a5b534194_story.html. Accessed: December 17, 2022.

181 Owens, C. (2021) Democrats' historic compromise on prescription drug prices. *Axios*. Available at: https://www.axios.com/2021/07/15/democrats-health-care-congress-prescription-drugs-insurance. Accessed: December 17, 2022.

182 Fuchs, H., Ollstein, A., and Wilson, M. (2021) Drug industry banks on its Covid clout to halt Dems' push on prices. *Politico*. Available at: https://www.politico.com/news/2021/09/02/drug-prices-democrats-lobbying-508127. Accessed: December 17, 2022.

183 Otterman, S. and Goldstein, J. (2021) NY hospitals face possible mass firings as workers spurn vaccines. *New York Times*. Available at: https://www.nytimes.com/2021/09/24/nyregion/coronavirus-hospitals-vaccines.html?action=click&module=Well&pgtype=Homepage&section=New%20York. Accessed: December 17, 2022.

184 Abelson, R. (2021) Many health workers at big hospital chains with vaccine mandates are getting shots. *New York Times*. Available at: https://www.nytimes.com/2021/09/29/health/us-hospital-workers-vaccine.html?campaign_id=185&emc=edit_yct_20210929&instance_id=41567&nl=coronavirus-tracker&regi_id=10879457&segment_id=70168&te=1&user_id=5c81c9183ba5aa9fd682e58291889859. Accessed: December 17, 2022.

185 Blake, A. (2021) The evidence is building: Vaccine mandates work – and well. *Washington Post*. Available at: https://www.washingtonpost.com/politics/2021/09/29/evidence-is-building-vaccine-mandates-work-well/. Accessed: December 17, 2022.

186 Pandey, E. (2021) The rise of hiring (and firing) based on vaccination status. *Axios.* Available at: https://www.axios.com/2021/09/29/vaccine-mandates-business-job-postings?utm_source=newsletter&utm_medium=email&utm_campaign=newsletter_axioswhatsnext&stream=science. Accessed: December 17, 2022.

187 Knight, V. and Appleby, J. (2021) Biden releases a new plan to combat Covid, but experts say there's still a way to go. *Kaiser Health News.* Available at: https://khn.org/news/article/biden-promise-tracker-vaccination-progress-plan-to-get-covid-under-control/. Accessed: December 17, 2022.

188 Assistant Secretary for Planning and Evaluation (ASPE) (2021) Unvaccinated for Covid-19 but willing: Demographic factors, geographic patterns and changes over time. *ASPE Issue Brief.* Available at: https://aspe.hhs.gov/sites/default/files/2021-08/unvaccinated-but-willing-ib.pdf. Accessed: December 17, 2022.

189 Weber, L. and Barry-Jester, A. (2021) One half of states have rolled back public health powers in pandemic. *Kaiser Health News.* Available at: https://khn.org/news/article/over-half-of-states-have-rolled-back-public-health-powers-in-pandemic/?utm_campaign=KHN%3A%20First%20Edition&utm_medium=email&_hsmi=159714944&_hsenc=p2ANqtz-_BLjbTwjJZKUFzbMdGYpvxSeELQ9mLoRScd_ZxnPmU42DTQhW7LSYWannAv6wS-UFLOHyk67JorpfrBYNo3N_WujhZGQ&utm_content=159714944&utm_source=hs_email. Accessed: December 17, 2022.

190 Caputo, M. and Fineout, G. (2021) DeSantis flirts with the anti-vaccine crowd. *Politico.* Available at: https://www.politico.com/states/florida/story/2021/09/15/desantis-flirts-with-the-anti-vaccine-crowd-1391038. Accessed: December 17, 2022.

191 Archibald, R. (2021) Alabama saw more deaths in 2020 than any year in history. *Alabama.* Available at: https://www.al.com/news/2021/09/alabama-saw-more-deaths-in-2020-than-any-year-in-history.html?utm_source=newsletter&utm_medium=email&utm_campaign=newsletter_axiosam&stream=top. Accessed: December 17, 2022.

192 Gomez, AM. (2021) Ask KHN PolitiFact: Is my cloth mask good enough to face the Delta variant. *Kaiser Health News.* Available at: https://khn.org/news/article/ask-khn-politifact-is-my-cloth-mask-good-enough-to-face-the-delta-variant/?utm_campaign=KHN%3A%20First%20Edition&utm_medium=email&_hsmi=161506999&_hsenc=p2ANqtz-gGx49_MNRUtr1uxBWXj2u5k9jN8o2zF0ZFRc8mD6BeqBGXwXJQvHNMccK2x7fdneigHhCV_BRnRzPl3D6B35tgskdMQ&utm_content=161506999&utm_source=hs_email. Accessed: December 17, 2022.

193 Centers for Disease Control (CDC). (2021) How to know and tuck your mask to improve fit. *CDC.* Available at: https://www.youtube.com/watch?v=GzTAZDsNBe0. Accessed: December 17, 2022.

194 CDC. (2021) Improve the fit and filtration of your mask to reduce the spread of Covid-19. *CDC.* Available at: https://public4.pagefreezer.com/browse/CDC%20Covid%20Pages/11-05-2022T12:30/; https://www.cdc.gov/coronavirus/2019-ncov/prevent-getting-sick/mask-fit-and-filtration.html. Accessed: December 17, 2022.

195 Stone, W. (2021) I got a 'mild' breakthrough case. Here is what I wish I had known. *Kaiser Health News.* Available at: https://khn.org/news/article/first-person-perspective-breakthrough-covid-case-health-reporter-hindsight-advice/?utm_campaign=KHN%3A%20First%20Edition&utm_medium=email&_hsmi=161506999&_hsenc=p2ANqtz-967nviVNbamBWNDfeAZhYbDsC0cJzeP-B-KfLaWJmepZvuBC4fOIXxMwKkIE6x-DyanPwOf8lqwUt

NHz33C6W3FHEjGA&utm_content=161506999&utm_source=hs_email. Accessed: December 17, 2022.

196 Baker, S. (2021) Covid deaths are finally falling. *Axios.* Available at: https://www. axios.com/2021/10/07/covid-cases-deaths-vaccines-winter?utm_source=newsletter &utm_medium=email&utm_campaign=newsletter_axiosvitals&stream=top. Accessed: December 17, 2022.

197 Wells, G., Horwitz, J., and Seetharaman, D. (2021) Facebook knows that Instagram is toxic for teen girls, documents show. *Wall St Journal.* Available at: https://www.wsj. com/articles/facebook-knows-instagram-is-toxic-for-teen-girls-company-documents-show-11631620739?utm_source=newsletter&utm_medium=email&utm_campaign=newsletter_axiosvitals&stream=top. Accessed: December 17, 2022.

198 Wells, G., Horwitz, J., and Seetharaman, D. (2021) Facebook knows that Instagram is toxic for teen girls, documents show. *Wall St Journal.* Available at: https://www.wsj. com/articles/facebook-knows-instagram-is-toxic-for-teen-girls-company-documents-show-11631620739?utm_source=newsletter&utm_medium=email&utm_campaign=newsletter_axiosvitals&stream=top. Accessed: December 17, 2022.

199 National Academies of Sciences, Engineering, and Medicine. (2020) *Encouraging Protective COVID-19 Behaviors among College Students.* Washington, DC: The National Academies Press. https://doi.org/10.17226/26004. Available at: https://nap.nationalacademies.org/download/26004. Accessed: December 17, 2022.

200 Johnson, CY. (2021) A scientific hunch. Then silence. Until the world needed a life-saving vaccine. *Washington Post.* Available at: https://www.washingtonpost.com/science/2021/10/01/drew-weissman-mrna-vaccine/. Accessed: December 17, 2022.

201 Sah, P., Moghadas, SM., Vilches, TN., Shoukat, A. et al. (2021) Implications of suboptimal COVID-19 vaccination coverage in Florida and Texas. *Lancet Infect Dis.* 21: 11: 1493–94. doi: 10.1016/S1473-3099(21)00620-4. Epub 2021 Oct 7. PMID: 34627498; PMCID: PMC8497018. Available at: https://www.thelancet.com/action/showPdf?pii=S1473-3099%2821%2900620-4. Accessed: December 17, 2022.

202 Achenbach, J. and Abutaleb, Y. (2021) Messy, incomplete U.S. data hobbles pandemic response. *Washington Post.* Available at: https://www.washingtonpost. com/health/2021/09/30/inadequate-us-data-pandemic-response/?utm_campaign=KHN%3A%20First%20Edition&utm_medium=email&_hsmi=165766208&_hsenc=p2ANqtz-93J346py2YQZNFkOVuWf-vZpFkepOcBTAy gzZnnYG8yTsW-ZaY5Dq0QXYWb7LwckMjFwucvN0pBRXmXso9mMkpovZDL w&utm_content=165766208&utm_source=hs_email. Accessed:December 17, 2022.

203 Economist (2021) In many rich countries Covid-19 has slashed life expectancy to below 2015 levels. *Economist.* Available at: https://www.economist.com/graphic-detail/2021/09/29/in-many-rich-countries-covid-19-has-slashed-life-expectancy-to-below-2015-levels?utm_campaign=coronavirus-special-edition&utm_medium=newsletter&utm_source=salesforce-marketing-cloud. Accessed: December 17, 2022.

204 Frankel, TC. (2021) The biggest employers are successfully enacting vaccine mandates. Many smaller employers need help. *Washington Post.* Available at: https://www.washingtonpost.com/business/2021/10/05/corporate-vaccine-push/?utm_campaign=wp_to_your_health&utm_medium=email&utm_source=newsletter&wpisrc=nl_tyh&wpmk=1&pwapi_token=eyJ0eXAiOiJKV1QiLCJhbGciO iJIUzI1NiJ9.eyJjb29raWVuYW1lIjoid3BfY3J0aWQiLCJpc3MiOiJDYXJ0YSIsIm Nvb2tpZXZhbHVlIjoiNTk2YjYxNTNhZGU0ZTI0MTE5YjI4MmIzIiwidG FnIjoiNjE1ZTA0MzM5ZDJmZGE5ZDQxMDA3YTgyIiwidXJsIjoiaHR0cH

M6Ly93d3cud2FzaGluZ3RvbnBvc3QuY29tL2J1c2luZXNzLzIwMjEvM
TAvMDUvY29ycG9yYXRlLXZhY2NpbmUtcHVzaC8_dXRtX2NhbXBhaWduPX
dwX3RvX3lvdXJfaGVhbHRoJnV0bV9tZWRpdW09ZW1haWwWwmdXRtX3N
vdXJjZT1uZXdzbGV0dGVyJndwaXNyYz1ubF90eWgmd3Btaz0xIn0.3MLunN
Rwh_ZLXTbOfRbrRQaHwuZl BKBMgkBI 7FfDhY Accessed: December 17, 2022.

205 Barret, P., Hendrix, J., and Sims, G. (2021) How tech platforms fuel U.S. political
polarization and what government can do about it. *Brookings*. Available at: https://www.
brookings.edu/blog/techtank/2021/09/27/how-tech-platforms-fuel-u-s-political-po-
larization-and-what-government-can-do-about-it/?utm_campaign=Brookings%20
Brief&utm_medium=email&utm_content=164358241&utm_source=hs_email.
Accessed: December 17, 2022.

206 Thomas, T., Ming, L., Rainey, T., and Gardner, G. (2021) Where Biden's vaccine mandate
will hit and miss. *Politico*. Available at: https://www.politico.com/news/2021/10/07/
biden-vaccine-mandate-counties-515337?utm_campaign=KHN%3A%20First%20
Edition&utm_medium=email&_hsmi=168409879&_hsenc=p2ANqtz-_4Ksm
4Krii_anAOkHgTBIQjs_K3wvMbHHTS4izzlK4IY5gc-A0u2y3FRvhstOgpXaK
inX6b5FuJGMFIbt2K8uN33usKg&utm_content=168409879&utm_source=hs_
email. Accessed: December 17, 2022.

207 Sarkissian, A. (2021) How a doctor who questioned vaccine safety became De Santis'
surgeon general pick. *Politico*. Available at: https://www.politico.com/states/florida/
story/2021/09/29/how-a-doctor-who-questioned-vaccine-safety-became-desantis-
surgeon-general-pick-1391488. Accessed: December 17, 2022.

208 Sokol, S. (2021) Jewish GOP candidate blames Soros and 'deep state' for Covid-
19. *Haaretz*. Available at: https://www.haaretz.com/us-news/2021-10-11/ty-article/.
highlight/jewish-gop-senate-candidate-blames-soros-and-deep-state-for-covid-
19/0000017f-ef03-d4a6-af7f-ffc71ac00000. Accessed: December 17, 2022.

209 Galston, WA. (2021) For Covid-19 vaccinations, party affiliation matters more than race and
ethnicity. *Brookings*. Available at: https://www.brookings.edu/blog/fixgov/2021/10/01/
for-covid-19-vaccinations-party-affiliation-matters-more-than-race-and-ethnic-
ity/?utm_campaign=Brookings%20Brief&utm_medium=email&utm_con-
tent=165955443&utm_source=hs_cmail. Accessed: December 17, 2022.

210 Carbajal, E. (2021) Covid-19 moving toward endemic in New York City, health
officials say. *Becker's Hospital Review*. Available at: https://www.beckershospital
review.com/public-health/covid-19-transitioning-to-endemic-in-new-york-city-
health-officials-say.html. Accessed: December 17, 2022.

211 Talev, M. (2021) Convincing the unvaccinated. *Axios*. Available at: https://www.
axios.com/2021/07/20/coronavirus-unvaccinated-refuse-shot-axios-ipsos-poll.
Accessed: January 14, 2023.

212 Edwards, J. (2021) Georgia's medical board mum as doctors spread Covid-19 misinformation. *Atlanta Journal-Constitution*. Available at: https://www.ajc.com/news/coro-
navirus/georgias-medical-board-mum-as-doctors-spread-covid-19-misinformation/
CRWP7IZFBBEBPFSAVIW7AGD7CM/?utm_source=Iterable&utm_medium=
email&utm_campaign=campaign_3110932. Accessed: December 17, 2022.

213 Smith, JA. (2021) Six reasons why humans wear masks. *Greater Good Magazine*.
Available at: https://greatergood.berkeley.edu/article/item/six_reasons_why_humans_
wear_masks?utm_source=Greater+Good+Science+Center&utm_cam
paign=180037573c-EMAIL_CAMPAIGN_GG_Newsletter_Octo
ber_28_2021&utm_medium=email&utm_term=0_5ae73e326e-1800375
73c-74759204. Accessed: December 17, 2022.

214 Goldfield, N. (2021) The challenges and opportunities of Peace through Health in a Covid era. *Baystate Medical Center Grand Rounds.* Available at: https://www.youtube.com/watch?v=lccWYHiWzA0. Accessed: December 17, 2022.

215 Macaya, M., Matani, M., Wagner, M., and Rocha, V. (2021) Colin Powell dies. *CNN.* Available at: https://www.cnn.com/politics/live-news/colin-powell-dies-10-18-21/index.html. Accessed: December 17, 2022.

216 Mandavilli, A. (2021) Omicron prompts swift reconsideration of boosters among scientists *New York Times.* Available at: https://www.nytimes.com/2021/12/01/health/covid-omicron-booster-shots.html?utm_campaign=KHN%3A%20First%20Edition&utm_medium=email&_hsmi=190183580&_hsenc=p2ANqtz–XfuN89LP0VdunYhKScCv5hniFgzhhpzckcrNoD8pP6zG5OyRpoEp8IQOrlzR5Tr44cvn70BA7PXzIEzAXx6QhMmaCUA&utm_content=190183580&utm_source=hs_email. Accessed: December 17, 2022.

217 Voltz, M. (2021) Hospitals refused to give Ivermectin to patients. Lockdowns and political pressure followed. *Kaiser Health News.* Available at: https://khn.org/news/article/ivermectin-covid-treatment-hospital-threats-political-pressure/?utm_campaign=KHN%3A%20First%20Edition&utm_medium=email&_hsmi=190183580&_hsenc=p2ANqtz-8b0-EOYtLd8Qpt10RTFm4bnEEDXw3-BI9w2FuH-Je82i2yIWo2hN4IbWkYoC2FlPdRLN7Q6SBnH-ArGADJX49lne3oTQ&utm_content=190183580&utm_source=hs_email. Accessed: December 17, 2022.

218 Yong, E. (2021) Why health care workers are quitting in droves. *The Atlantic.* Available at: https://www.theatlantic.com/health/archive/2021/11/the-mass-exodus-of-americas-health-care-workers/620713/?utm_source=newsletter&utm_medium=email&utm_campaign=atlantic-daily-newsletter&utm_content=20211123&silverid=%25%25RECIPIENT_ID%25%25&utm_term=The%20Atlantic%20Daily. Accessed: December 17, 2022.

219 Boorstein, M. (2021) Marcus Lamb, head of Daystar, a large Christian network that discouraged vaccines, dies after getting Covid-19. *Washington Post.* Available at: https://www.washingtonpost.com/religion/2021/11/30/marcus-lamb-daystar-covid-vaccine-medical-freedom/. Accessed: December 17, 2022.
Weisman, J. (2021) G.O.P. fights Covid mandates. Then blames Biden as cases rise. *New York Times.* Available at: https://www.nytimes.com/2021/11/24/us/politics/republicans-biden-coronavirus.html. Accessed: December 17, 2022.

220 Papenfuss, M. (2021) White House doctor who raved about Trump's health now says Omicron is election ruse. *Yahoo News.* Available at: https://news.yahoo.com/white-house-doctor-raved-trumps-024430725.html?fr=sycsrp_catchall. Accessed: December 17, 2022.

221 Government Accounting Office (GAO). (2021) Behavioral health and Covid-19. *GAO.* Available at: https://www.gao.gov/assets/720/717988.pdf. Accessed: December 17, 2022.

222 Dawn. (2021) 115,000 health workers have died from Covid, says WHO. *Dawn.* Available at: https://www.dawn.com/news/1625500. Accessed: December 17, 2022.

223 McPhilips, D. and Cole, D. (2021) Outgoing NIH director says Trump and other Republicans pressured him to endorse unproven Covid-19 remedies and to fire Fauci. *CNN.* Available at: https://www.cnn.com/2021/12/19/politics/francis-collins-trump-political-pressure-republicans/index.html?utm_campaign=KHN%3A%20First%20Edition&utm_medium=email&_hsmi=197756001&_hsenc=p2ANqtz-_FcyK8uItAp_D3I3XvUoWsx1dSmjxL_QzzgbrkGQBbp6dYGPfbbdKx-2wfIp_Y_5NU

24V1d3fbYVDLilUBcdLSitkXrg&utm_content=197756001&utm_source=hs_
email. Accessed: December 17, 2022.

224 McCardle, M. (2021) Harsher and harsher punishments are not the way to convince the
unvaccinated. *Washington Post.* Available at: https://www.washingtonpost.com/opin-
ions/2021/12/15/targeting-vaccine-resistance-lets-leave-punishment-aside/?utm_
campaign=wp_week_in_ideas&utm_medium=email&utm_source=newsletter&w
pisrc=nl_ideas. Accessed: December 17, 2022.

225 Gerson, M. (2021) How is the GOP's coronavirus recklessness compatible with pro-life.
Washington Post. Available at: https://www.washingtonpost.com/health/2021/12/09/
ron-johnson-mouthwash-covid/. Accessed: December 17, 2022.

226 Sun, LH. (2021) Two years into this pandemic, the world is dangerously unprepared for the next one, report says. *Washington Post.* Available at: https://www.
washingtonpost.com/health/2021/12/08/next-pandemic-global-health-secu-
rity-index/?utm_campaign=wp_politics_am&utm_medium=email&utm_
source=newsletter&wpisrc=nl_politics&carta-url=https%3A%2F%2Fs2.
washingtonpost.com%2Fcar-ln-tr%2F3578d59%2F61b0a3259d2fdab56bbab
fa2%2F596b6153ade4e24119b282b3%2F10%2F60%2F61b0a3259d2fdab56b
babfa2. Accessed: December 17, 2022.

227 Knight, V. (2021) The vaccine rollout was a success. But events within and beyond
Biden's control stymied progress. *Kaiser Health News.* Available at: https://khn.org/
news/article/biden-covid-vaccine-2021/?utm_campaign=KHN%3A%20First%20
Edition&utm_medium=email&_hsmi=197756001&_hsenc=p2ANqtz-oAJKp
GUEE6TNROBViLOORNwozr452mMGB9rAvgeWzggChWYwLJtmdeCvGui
MFZ0JhYkRRaiuRFA2w_cyzvLV8wzViVw&utm_content=197756001&utm_
source=hs_email. Accessed: December 17, 2022.

228 Banco, E. (2021) 'It is embarrassing': The CDC struggles to track Covid cases as
Omicron looms. *Politico.* Available at: https://www.politico.com/news/2021/12/20/
cdc-covid-omicron-delta-tracking-525621?utm_campaign=KHN%3A%20First%20
Edition&utm_medium=email&_hsmi=198219700&_hsenc=p2ANqtz-_T-ccmt
C7u7p3vdB9varhgL-aAkDmybBVN2R2RVfT6S2NVKQB92PETVbaw2uwi
UOWXYp5HJuWfywO46QFIP3VXgfsC9A&utm_content=198219700&utm_
source=hs_email. Accessed: December 17, 2022.

229 United Nations News and Features. (2021) How can we end covid? The UN's global
vaccine… *United Nations Web TV.* Available at: https://media.un.org/en/asset/k1x/
k1xtz75djz. Accessed: December 17, 2022.

230 Johnson, CK. (2021) One year of vaccines: Many lives saved, many needlessly lost. *AP.*
Available at: https://apnews.com/article/coronavirus-pandemic-science-health-fran
cis-collins-57ab6ae016acec5ee5ca268cc682879c?utm_campaign=KHN%3A%20
First%20Edition&utm_medium=email&_hsmi=195201705&_hsenc=p2ANqtz-
8juvMujkiBvXN0XBx-Saep6TBxWnLCRPJG_d4RCjIyX4I_g9SmV5xOV1Qdzcl
JBvU-XhyCy_mWkZmyaSFbbOln3WKDLA&utm_content=195201705&utm_
source=hs_email. Accessed: December 17, 2022.

231 Sanger-Katz, M. (2021) On more generous terms, Obamacare proves newly popular. *New York Times.* Available at: https://www.nytimes.com/2021/12/22/upshot/
on-more-generous-terms-obamacare-proves-newly-popular.html. Accessed: December
17, 2022.

232 Milbank, D. (2021) Sarah Palin's anti-vax talk shows Republicans have become a death
cult. *Washington Post.* Available at: https://www.washingtonpost.com/opinions/2021/
12/20/sarah-palin-anti-vax-tpusa-tconference/. Accessed: December 17, 2022.

233 Shpigel, J. (2021) Netanyahu party lawmaker likens Israel's Covid restrictions to 'concentration camps' Haaretz. Available at: https://www.haaretz.com/israel-news/2021-12-26/ty-article/.premium/likud-lawmaker-calls-covid-restrictions-to-concentration-camps/0000017f-dbff-d856-a37f-ffffb3450000. Accessed: December 16, 2022.

234 Grynbaum, MM. (2021) Fox News host's incendiary Fauci comments follows a network pattern. *New York Times*. Available at: https://www.nytimes.com/2021/12/23/business/media/fox-anthony-fauci-jesse-watters.html. Accessed: December 17, 2022.

235 Boorstein, M. (2021) Marcus Lamb died of Covid-19 after his network discouraged vaccines. But some Christian leaders don't want to talk about it. *Washington Post*. Available at: https://www.washingtonpost.com/religion/2021/12/03/marcus-lamb-daystar-vaccine-televangelist-graham/.

236 Kimball, S. (2021) Business groups ask White House to delay Biden Covid vaccine mandate till after the holidays. *CNBC*. Available at: https://www.cnbc.com/2021/10/25/businesses-ask-white-house-to-delay-biden-covid-vaccine-mandate-until-after-holidays.html. Accessed: December 17, 2022.

237 Banco, E., Cancryn, A., and Overmohle, S. Biden officials now fear booster programs will limit global vaccine supply. *Politico*. Available at: https://www.politico.com/news/2021/12/31/biden-novavax-production-covid-omicron-526283. Accessed: December 17, 2022.

238 Jackson, C. (2022) Most Americans not worried about Covid going into 2022 holidays. *Ipsos*. Available at: https://www.ipsos.com/en-us/news-polls/axios-ipsos-coronavirus-index?utm_source=newsletter&utm_medium=email&utm_campaign=newsletter_axiosvitals&stream=top. Accessed: January 1, 2023.

239 Levy, R. (2022) Health care workers are panicked as desperate hospitals ask infected staff to return. *Politico*. Available at: https://www.politico.com/news/2022/01/10/doctors-covid-staff-shortage-526842. Accessed: December 11, 2022.

240 AP (2022) Arizona provider OK's virus-positive hospital workers. *AP*. Available at: https://apnews.com/article/coronavirus-pandemic-health-arizona-pandemics-dd7cec1fca4f9aeb9f535fd29fd1ce0f?utm_campaign=KHN%3A%20First%20Edition&utm_medium=email&_hsmi=200392340&_hsenc=p2ANqtz-1HTi0KDJNdWIbQAqP5TkT_tsoyXRdyR-QfYDVHuOD134s2_qyfsy1EV9thQEmkKa3hznMmU4aGHqIknd_TKcQEGO17A&utm_content=200392340&utm_source=hs_email. Accessed: December 11, 2022.

241 Nuzzo, JB. and Gostin, LO. (2022) The First 2 Years of COVID-19: Lessons to Improve Preparedness for the Next Pandemic. *JAMA*. Jan 18;327: 3: 217–18. 10.1001/jama.2021.24394. PMID: 34989763. Available at: https://jamanetwork.com/journals/jama/fullarticle/2787943. Accessed: December 11, 2022.

242 Borio, LL., Bright, RA., and Emanuel, EJ. (2022) A National Strategy for COVID-19 Medical Countermeasures: Vaccines and Therapeutics. *JAMA*. 327: 3: 215–16. 10.1001/jama.2021.24165. Available at: https://jamanetwork.com/journals/jama/fullarticle/2787946. Accessed: December 11, 2022.

243 Adashi, EY. and Cohen, IG. (2022) The pandemic preparedness program: Reimagining public health. *JAMA*. 327: 3: 219–20. 10.1001/jama.2021.23656. PMID: 34989800. Available at: https://jamanetwork.com/journals/jama/article-abstract/2787947. Accessed: December 11, 2022.

244 Stolberg, SG. (2022) Former Biden advisers urge a pandemic strategy for the 'new normal'. *New York Times*. Available at: https://www.nytimes.com/2022/01/06/us/politics/former-biden-advisers-pandemic-strategy.html. Accessed: December 11, 2022.

245 Feldman, J. (2022) A year in how has Biden done in his response. *JM Feldman.* Available at: https://jmfeldman.medium.com/a-year-in-how-has-biden-done-on-pandemic-response-88452c696f2. Accessed: December 17, 2022.

246 Tartof SY, Slezak JM, Fischer H, Hong V, et al. (2021) Effectiveness of mRNA BNT162b2 COVID-19 vaccine up to 6 months in a large integrated health system in the USA: a retrospective cohort study. *Lancet* 16: 398: 1407–16. 10.1016/S0140-6736(21)02183-8. Epub 2021 Oct 4. PMID: 34619098; PMCID: PMC8489881. Available at: https://www.thelancet.com/journals/lancet/article/PIIS0140-6736(21)02183-8/fulltext. Accessed: December 11, 2022.

247 Firozi, P. and Chiu, A. (2022) How often can you safely re-use your N-95 or KN-95 mask. *Washington Post.* Available at: https://www.washingtonpost.com/health/2022/01/13/kn95-n95-mask-reuse-omicron/. Accessed: December 11, 2022.

248 Lempert, R (2022) The vaccine mandate cases, polarization and jurisprudential norms. *Brookings.* Available at: https://www.brookings.edu/blog/fixgov/2022/01/15/the-vaccine-mandate-cases-polarization-and-jurisprudential-norms/?utm_campaign=Brookings%20Brief&utm_medium=email&utm_content=201257255&utm_source=hs_email. Accessed: December 11, 2022.

249 Bella, T. (2022) Florida health official on leave after encouraging employees to get vaccinated. *Washington Post.* Available at: https://www.washingtonpost.com/health/2022/01/19/florida-raul-pino-vaccinated-leave-desantis/. Accessed: December 11, 2022.

250 Padamsee, TJ., Bond, RM., Dixon, GN., et al. (2022) Changes in COVID-19 vaccine hesitancy among black and white individuals in the US. *JAMA Netw Open.* 5: 1: e2144470. 10.1001/jamanetworkopen.2021.44470. Available at: https://jamanetwork.com/journals/jamanetworkopen/fullarticle/2788286?utm_source=STAT+Newsletters&utm_campaign=dfc960724a-MR_COPY_01&utm_medium=email&utm_term=0_8cab1d7961-dfc960724a-152403458. Accessed: December 11, 2022.

251 Heesakkers, H., van der Hoeven, JG., Corsten, S., et al. (2022) Clinical outcomes among patients with 1-year survival following intensive care unit treatment for COVID-19. *JAMA.* 327: 6: 559–65. 10.1001/jama.2022.0040. Available at: https://jamanetwork.com/journals/jama/fullarticle/2788504. Accessed: December 11, 2022.

252 Nolen, S. (2022) Rich countries lure health workers from low income countries to fight shortages. *New York Times.* Available at: https://www.nytimes.com/2022/01/24/health/covid-health-worker-immigration.html. Accessed: December 11, 2022.

253 Cha, AE. (2022) America's split-screen pandemic: Many families resume their lives even as hospitals are overwhelmed. *Washington Post.* Available at: https://www.washingtonpost.com/health/2022/01/28/texas-omicron-pandemic/?utm_campaign=wp_. Accessed: December 11, 2022.

254 U.S. Government Accounting Office Significant Improvements Are Needed for Overseeing Relief Funds and Leading Responses to Public Health Emergencies. *US Government Accounting Office.* https://files.gao.gov/reports/GAO-22-105291/index.html. Accessed: December 11, 2022.

255 Shear, M., Stolberg, S., LaFraniere, S., and Weiland, N. (2022) Biden's pandemic fight: Inside the setbacks of the first year *New York Times.* Available at: https://www.nytimes.com/2022/01/23/us/politics/biden-covid-strategy.html. Accessed: December 11, 2022.

256 Senator Lamar Alexander. (2020) Preparing for the next pandemic. *U.S. Senate.* Available at: https://www.help.senate.gov/imo/media/doc/Preparing%20for%20the%20Next%20Pandemic.pdf. Accessed: December 11, 2022.

257 Stern, J. and Wu, K. (2022) Endemicity is meaningless. *The Atlantic.* Available at: https://www.theatlantic.com/health/archive/2022/02/endemicity-means-noth ing/621423/?utm_source=newsletter&utm_medium=email&utm_campaign=atlan tic-daily-newsletter&utm_content=20220202&utm_term=The%20Atlantic%20 Daily. Accessed: December 11, 2022.

258 Wen, L. (2021) The vaccinated will make different choices about what they can do now. That's OK. *Washington Post.* Available at: https://www.washingtonpost.com/ opinions/2021/04/30/how-decide-what-activities-bring-back-once-youre-vacci nated/. Accessed: December 11, 2022.

259 Velasquez, D., Gondi, S., Lu, R., Pissaris, A. et al. (2021) GoTV Max: A novel mobile Covid-19 vaccine program. *NEJM Catalyst.* Available at: https://catalyst.nejm.org/ doi/full/10.1056/CAT.21.0174. Accessed: December 11, 2022.

260 McHugh, J. (2022) The 1918 flu didn't end in 1918. Here's what it's third year can teach us. *Washington Post.* Available at: https://www.washingtonpost.com/histo ry/2022/02/06/1918-flu-fourth-wave/. Accessed: December 11, 2022.

261 Goldfield, N. and Lerner, J. (2022) Ask Nurses and Doctors. *Robert Hubbell Podcast.* Available at: https://www.callin.com/episode/ask-nurses-and-doctors-SCRWxXN QLv. Accessed: November 27, 2022.

262 French, R. and Erb, R. (2022) Northern Michigan health director quits, cites anger over mask mandates. *Bridge Michigan.* Available at: https://www. bridgemi.com/michigan-health-watch/northern-michigan-health-director-quits-cites-anger-over-mask-mandates?utm_source=Bridge+Michigan&utm_cam paign=4521b1f272-Bridge+Newsletter+02%2F23%2F2022&utm_medium=e mail&utm_term=0_c64a28dd5a-4521b1f272-82373340. Accessed: December 11, 2022.

263 Ramachandran, V. (2022) As politics infects public health, private companies profit. *Kaiser Health News.* Available at: https://khn.org/news/article/as-politics-infects-pub lic-health-private-companies-profit/?utm_campaign=KHN%3A%20First%20 Edition&utm_medium=email&_hsmi=204219187&_hsenc=p2ANqtz–st-gUNX-9iEyaHDiXbb5ENXBDLsDQxVf9phTW9mTWe8cFP_cD_kCuZg3VTw7ByL-7F5A6XZJ6lKBEJRE8ul4gdCNBFVCA&utm_content=204219187&utm_ source=hs_email. Accessed: December 11, 2022.

264 Barry-Jester, AM. (2021) Hard lessons from a city that tried to privatize public health. *Kaiser Health News.* Available at: https://khn.org/news/article/detroit-hard-lessons-privatize-public-health/. Accessed: December 11, 2022.

265 Mazzei, P. (2022) The doctor giving De Santis' pandemic policies a seal of approval. *New York Times.* Available at: https://www.nytimes.com/2022/02/23/us/florida-sur geon-general-ladapo.html. Accessed: December 11, 2022.

266 Tufekci, Z. (2022) How many millions of lives might have been saved from Covid-19. *New York Times.* Available at: https://www.nytimes.com/2022/03/11/opinion/covid-health-pandemic.html. Accessed: November 27, 2022.

267 Alarcon, D. (2022) A pandemic tragedy in Guayaquil *The New Yorker.* Available at: https://www.newyorker.com/magazine/2022/03/14/a-pandemic-tragedy-in-guay aquil?utm_source=nl&utm_brand=tny&utm_mailing=TNY_Daily_Con trol_030722&utm_campaign=aud-dev&utm_medium=email&utm_term=tny_ daily_recirc&bxid=5bea06da24c17c6adf125b09&cndid=50856718&hasha= 5c81c9183ba5aa9fd682e58291889859&hashb=cebff94d072ef16164c89170f c47fd36337bb64d&hashc=8c6ed225fce9f934f5b1b6d643f99d2a761bd86aefbc7 f884c1cbe64c9dce77f&esrc=bounceX;. Accessed: November 27, 2022.

268 Mahtani, S. and Yu, T. (2022) Body bags, overflowing morgues and chaotic hospitals: Hong Kong's pandemic goes critical. *Washington Post.* Available at: https://www.washingtonpost.com/world/2022/03/09/hong-kong-covid-hospitals-morgues/. Accessed: November 27, 2022.

269 Hamblin, J. (2022) Can public health be saved, *New York Times.* Available at: https://www.nytimes.com/2022/03/12/opinion/public-health-trust.html. Accessed: November 27, 2022.

270 Ollstein, AM. (2022) Covid chaos fueled another public health crisis: STDs. *Politico.* Available at: https://www.politico.com/news/2022/03/12/covid-std-crisis-00015717. Accessed: November 27, 2022.

271 Llamas, D. (2022) Why do some people never get Covid. *New York Times.* Available at: https://www.nytimes.com/2022/03/08/opinion/people-never-get-covid.html?action=click&module=RelatedLinks&pgtype=Article. Accessed: November 27, 2022.

272 Spudich, S. and Nath, A. (2022) Nervous system consequences of Covid-19. *Science.* Available at: https://www.science.org/doi/10.1126/science.abm2052. Accessed: November 27, 2022.

273 Eulich, E and Lana, SM (2022) Two years income, pandemic resilience propels action. Available at: https://www.csmonitor.com/Daily/2022/20220310?cmpid=ema:ddp:20220310:1141128:read&sfmc_sub=61636896&id=1141128#1141128. Accessed: November 27, 2022.

274 Zamrini, E., Cheng, Y., Kokkinos, P. Faselis, C., et al. (2022) Cardiorespiratory Fitness Is Protective Against Alzheimer's and Related Disorders *Neurology* 98:18 Supplement: 1475. Available at: https://n.neurology.org/content/98/18_Supplement/1475. Accessed: November 27, 2022.

275 Ortis, J., Bacon, J., and Tebor, C. (2022) Boosted Americans 97 times less likely to die of virus than unvaccinated. *USA Today.* Available at: https://www.usatoday.com/story/news/health/2022/02/02/covid-cases-mandates-vaccines-deaths/9308759002/. Accessed: November 27, 2022.

276 Larsen, B., Hetherington, M., Greene, S., Ryan, T. et al. (2022) Counter-stereotypical messaging and partisan cues: Moving the needle on vaccines in a polarized U.S. *National Bureau of Economics Research.* Available at: https://www.nber.org/papers/w29896. Accessed: November 27, 2022.

277 Goldstein, J. and Otterman, S. (2022) What New York got wrong about the pandemic, and what it got right. *New York Times.* Available at: https://www.nytimes.com/2022/03/17/nyregion/new-york-pandemic-lessons.html?action=click&module=RelatedLinks&pgtype=Article. Accessed: November 27, 2022.

278 Brusselaers, N., Steadson, D., Bjorklund, K., Breland, S., et al. (2022) Evaluation of science advice during the COVID-19 pandemic in Sweden. *Humanit Soc Sci Commun.* 9: 1: 239. Available at: https://www.nature.com/articles/s41599-022-01097-5. Accessed: November 27, 2022.

279 Rizzo, S. (2022) Local health officials report threats, harassment and vandalism during the pandemic, study finds. *Washington Post.* Available at: https://www.washingtonpost.com/health/2022/03/17/public-health-official-harassment/. Accessed: December 11, 2022.

280 Woolf, SH., Masters, RK., and Aron, LY. (2022) Changes in Life Expectancy Between 2019 and 2020 in the US and 21 Peer Countries. *JAMA Netw Open.* 5: 4: e227067. 10.1001/jamanetworkopen.2022.7067. PMID: 35416991; PMCID: PMC9008499. Available at: https://jamanetwork.com/journals/jamanetworkopen/fullarticle/2791004. Accessed: November 27, 2022.

281 Stobbe. M (2022) Covid-19, overdoses pushed US to highest death toll ever. *AP.* Available at: https://apnews.com/article/covid-science-health-centers-for-disease-control-and-prevention-robert-anderson-ff2f01e401abce778bea8ac2e9c6e53e?utm_campaign=KHN%3A%20First%20Edition&utm_medium=email&_hsmi=209891651&_hsenc=p2ANqtz-9IATQN2pTGnf9DuEmAgtQ3fRYPMQg jLKM2-EcCqkNt1SdS_oLqAGVdA-Mlqq_FY68XrASclwKUxq_1WO6JIIZaKZ kKyw&utm_content=209891651&utm_source=hs_email. Accessed: November 27, 2022.

282 Tully, T. and Schorr, S. (2022) Why this coastal county has the highest death toll in its state. *New York Times.* Available at: https://www.nytimes.com/2022/04/10/nyregion/ocean-county-new-jersey-covid.html?utm_campaign=KHN%3A%20First%20Edition&utm_medium=email&_hsmi=209623319&_hsenc=p2ANqtz-_OIiHaBUsd 3FXorZ0g2jVq–ARa24Qcj5byIhsNMRP2yFlO-dwhIDtm9XzG8dDZZZ2Tqt JadMFFgS_qv-Nt8YOG–vTw&utm_content=209623319&utm_source=hs_email. Accessed: November 27, 2022.

283 Sullivan, A., Irving, S., Treston, J., Lerner, J. et al. (2022) Nurses and physicians as diplomats in the Covid culture wars. *American Nurse.* Available at: https://www.myamericannurse.com/nurses-and-doctors-as-diplomats-in-the-covid-culture-wars/. Accessed: November 27, 2022.

284 Panchal, N., Kamal, R., Cox, C., and Garfield, R. (2022) The implications of Covid-19 for mental health and substance abuse. *Kaiser Family Foundation.* Available at: https://www.kff.org/report-section/the-implications-of-covid-19-for-mental-health-and-substance-use-issue-brief/. Accessed: November 27, 2022.

285 Shi, D., Whitaker, M., Marks, K., Anglin, O. et al. (2022) Hospitalizations of children aged 5-11 with laboratory confirmed Covid-19. *Centers for Disease Control.* Available at: https://www.cdc.gov/mmwr/volumes/71/wr/mm7116e1.htm?s_cid= mm7116e1_w. Accessed: November 27, 2022.

286 Office of Governor Gavin Newson. (2021) Governor Newsom signs into law first-in-the-nation expansion of Medi-CAL to undocumented Californians 50 and over, bold initiatives to advance more equitable and prevention-focused health are. *CA. Gov.* Available at: https://www.gov.ca.gov/2021/07/27/governor-newsom-signs-into-law-first-in-the-nation-expansion-of-medi-cal-to-undocumented-californians-age-50-and-over-bold-initiatives-to-advance-more-equitable-and-prevention-focused-health-care/. Accessed: November 27, 2022.

287 Weiland, T. (2022) Loss of pandemic aid stresses hospitals that treat the uninsured. *New York Times.* Available at: https://www.nytimes.com/2022/05/01/us/politics/covid-aid-hospitals-uninsured.html. Accessed: November 27, 2022.

288 Government Accounting Office. (2022) Scientific integrity: HHS Agencies need to develop procedures and train staff on reporting and addressing political interference. *Government Accounting Office.* Available at: https://www.gao.gov/assets/gao-22-105885.pdf. Accessed: November 27, 2022.

289 Huang, L., Li, X., Gu, X., Zhang, H., et al. (2022) Health outcomes in people 2 years after surviving hospitalisation with COVID-19: a longitudinal cohort study. *Lancet Respir Med.* 10: 9: 863–76. doi: 10.1016/S2213-2600(22)00126-6. Epub 2022 May 11. PMID: 35568052; PMCID: PMC9094732. Available at: https://www.thelancet.com/journals/lanres/article/PIIS2213-2600(22)00126-6/fulltext. Accessed: December 11, 2022.

290 Sharkey, SW., Lesser, JR., Menon, M., Parpart, M. et al. (2008) Spectrum and significance of electrocardiographic patterns, troponin levels, and thrombolysis in

myocardial infarction frame count in patients with stress (tako-tsubo) cardiomyopathy and comparison to those in patients with ST-elevation anterior wall myocardial infarction. *Am J Cardiol.* 101: 12: 1723–28. doi: 10.1016/j.amjcard.2008.02.062. Epub 2008 Apr 9. PMID: 18549847. Accessed: January 14, 2023.

291 Sampson, H. (2022) Cruise ships are smashing records despite Covid on board: "Life goes on". *Washington Post.* Available at: https://www.washingtonpost.com/ travel/2022/05/10/cruises-booking-covid-outbreaks/?utm_campaign=KHN%3A %20First%20Edition&utm_medium=email&_hsmi=2127452 85&_hsenc=p2ANqtz-9b-3BFuTP38Lm-NIuXv9h4kLyO2Pm7Z-o0tdI7_9kynvTAdeW1QlYhBttF3F23Xj8rWhX-JBRWHDEkq8Uw8vMaM PiVfQ&utm_content=212745285&utm_source=hs_email. Accessed: November 27, 2022.

292 Sullivan, A., Irving, S., Treston, J., Lerner, J. et al. (2022) Nurses and physicians as diplomats in the Covid culture wars. *American Nurse.* Available: https://www. myamericannurse.com/nurses-and-doctors-as-diplomats-in-the-covid-culture-wars/. Accessed: November 27, 2022.

293 University of Liverpool. (2022) Covid 19 Drug Interactions. *University of Liverpool.* Available at: https://www.covid19-druginteractions.org/checker. Accessed: September 4, 2022.

294 U.S. Food and Drug Administration (2022) FDA Updates on Paxlovid for Health Care Providers. *FDA.* Available at: https://www.fda.gov/drugs/news-events-human-drugs/fda-updates-paxlovid-health-care-providers. Accessed: September 4, 2022.

295 Velasquez-Manoff, M. (2022) The anti-vaccine movement's new frontier. *The New York Times.* Available at: https://www.nytimes.com/2022/05/25/magazine/anti-vaccine-movement.html. Accessed: November 27, 2022.

296 Gerson, M. (2022) Too many Americans are still in Covid denial. *Washington Post.* Available at: https://www.washingtonpost.com/opinions/2022/05/19/covid-million-americans-dead-complacency-ideology/. Accessed: December 11, 2022.

297 Warraich, H., Kumar, P., Nasir, K., Joynt Maddox, K., et al. (2022) Political environment and mortality rates in the United States, 2001-19: population based cross sectional analysis. *BMJ.* 377: e069308. 10.1136/bmj-2021-069308. PMID: 35672032; PMCID: PMC9171631. Available at: https://www.bmj.com/content/377/bmj-2021-069308. Accessed: August 28, 2022.

298 Violanti, J.M., Fekedulegn, D., McCanlies, E. and Andrew, M.E. (2022), "Proportionate mortality and national rate of death from COVID-19 among US law enforcement officers: 2020", *Policing: An International Journal.* 45:5: 881–91. https:// doi.org/10.1108/PIJPSM-02-2022-0022. Available at: https://www.emerald.com/ insight/content/doi/10.1108/PIJPSM-02-2022-0022/full/html. Accessed: August 28, 2022.

299 Gupta, A., Howell, S., Yannelis, C., and Gupta, A. (2021) Does private equity investment benefit patients? Evidence from nursing homes. *National Bureau of Economic Research.* https://www.nber.org/system/files/working_papers/w28474/w28474. pdf. Accessed: November 28, 2022.

300 Davis, HE., Assaf, GS., McCorkell, L., Wei, H., et al. (2021) Characterizing long COVID in an international cohort: 7 months of symptoms and their impact. *E Clinical Medicine.* 38: 101019. 10.1016/j.eclinm.2021.101019. Epub 2021 Jul 15. PMID: 34308300; PMCID: PMC8280690. Available at: https://www.thelancet.com/ journals/eclinm/article/PIIS2589-5370(21)00299-6/fulltext. Accessed: December 11, 2022.

301 Bhattaraj A. and Siegel R. (2022) Inflation is Making Homelessness Worse. *Washington Post*. Available at: https://www.washingtonpost.com/business/2022/07/03/inflation-homeless-rent-housing/. Accessed: August 28, 2022.

302 Cohen, R. (2022) Evictions are Life-Altering and Preventable. *Vox*. Available at: https://www.vox.com/23140987/evictions-housing-rent-assistance-erap-tenant. Accessed: August 28, 2022.

303 Yehuda, R. (2022) Trauma in the Family Tree *Scientific American* 327: 1: 50–55. doi:10.1038/scientificamerican0722-50. Available at: https://www.scientificamerican.com/article/how-parents-rsquo-trauma-leaves-biological-traces-in-children/. Accessed: August 28, 2022.

304 Levey, N. (2022). 100 Million People in America are Saddled with Health Care Debt. *Kaiser Health News*. Available at: https://khn.org/news/article/diagnosis-debt-investigation-100-million-americans-hidden-medical-debt/?utm_source=Sailthru&utm_medium=email&utm_campaign=VoxCare%2C%206/30/22&utm_term=VoxCare. Accessed August 28, 2022.

305 Instagram. (2022) Available at: https://www.instagram.com/p/CfcLk5pvmin/?igshid=MDJmNzVkMjY%3D. Accessed: August 28, 2022.

306 UNICEF. (2022) COVID-19 pandemic leads to major backsliding on childhood vaccinations, new WHO, UNICEF data shows. *UNICEF*. Available at: https://www.unicef.org/press-releases/covid-19-pandemic-leads-major-backsliding-childhood-vaccinations-new-who-unicef-data. Accessed August 23, 2022.

307 Weber, L. and Barry-Jester, AM. (2022) Conservative Blocs Unleash Litigation to Curb Public Health Powers. *Kaiser Health News*. Available at: https://khn.org/news/article/conservative-blocs-litigation-curb-public-health-powers/?utm_campaign=KHN%3A%20First%20Edition&utm_medium=email&_hsmi=219935716&_hsenc=p2ANqtz–D1Dv23WjSVeYsq5KdZHvwIGFT1GYfogb6YwlEfJAbYYsHoVOckVT-T643fJFO6L1uzLNZKGI4x7kd_TrpCNlQraIHTg&utm_content=219935716&utm_source=hs_email. Accessed August 23, 2022.

308 The White House. (2022). Fact Sheet: Biden Administration Outlines Strategy to Managed BA.5. *White House Briefing Room*. Available at: https://www.whitehouse.gov/briefing-room/statements-releases/2022/07/12/fact-sheet-biden-administration-outlines-strategy-to-manage-ba-5/. Accessed: August 23, 2022.

309 The Economist. (2022) Covid-19 Vaccines Saved an Estimated 20m Lives During the First Year. *The Economist*. Available at: https://www.economist.com/graphic-detail/2022/07/07/covid-19-vaccines-saved-an-estimated-20m-lives-during-their-first-year. Accessed: August 23, 2022.

310 Weixel, N. COVID-19 was third-leading US cause of death between March 2020 and October 2021. *The Hill*. Available at: https://thehill.com/policy/healthcare/3546647-covid-19-was-third-leading-u-s-cause-of-death-in-2020-and-2021/?utm_campaign=KHN%3A%20First%20Edition&utm_medium=email&_hsmi=218738910&_hsenc=p2ANqtz–QxCE_-lL5oEpBFguaiekN3F_sPqPRaKBfrLXVVuT-bSJnZAJG1wqYvjknUXlqfCvXx3_3oweyM_FebuhIIAA_b5xRKA&utm_content=218738910&utm_source=hs_email. Accessed August 23, 2022.

311 McCarthy, E. (2022) Meet the Covid Super-Chargers. *Washington Post*. Available at: https://www.washingtonpost.com/lifestyle/2022/07/21/no-covid-yet/. Accessed: August 22, 2022.

312 Weixel, N. (2022) GOP plots Fauci probe after midterms. *The Hill*. Available at: https://thehill.com/policy/healthcare/3571232-gop-plots-fauci-probe-after-mid

terms/?utm_campaign=KHN%3A%20First%20Edition&utm_medium=email&_hsmi=220673640&_hsenc=p2ANqtz-8PUL2E-8iTVmCm49sZvbQVBfW-xDjXEs-064GMpLUqS2QAwU78M3C9yELKDW6YnLfeR4a0ZkJy_9CoDVH2vln5ONX-9ifQ&utm_content=220673640&utm_source=hs_email. Accessed: August 22, 2022.

313 Ibid.

314 Browne, E., (2022) Joe Biden's Critics Use Covid News to Mislead People about Vaccines *Newsweek*. Available at: https://www.newsweek.com/joe-biden-positive-covid-vaccine-infections-claim-effective-1727075?utm_campaign=KHN%3A%20First%20Edition&utm_medium=email&_hsmi=220673640&_hsenc=p2ANqtz-_cvsKEAJT3RZpCqHD0q7efmO-. Accessed: August 22, 2022.

315 Doherty, E. (2022) Schools Look to Get Back on Track after 2 Terrible Years. *Axios*. Available at: https://www.axios.com/2022/08/01/schools-pandemic-students-learning-loss?utm_source=newsletter&utm_medium=email&utm_campaign=newsletter_axiosam&stream=top. Accessed: August 22, 2022.

316 Kuhfelt, M. and Lewis, K. (2022) Student Achievement in 2021-2022. *NWEA Research*. Available at: https://www.nwea.org/content/uploads/2022/07/Student-Achievement-in-2021-22-Cause-for-hope-and-concern.researchbrief-1.pdf. Accessed: August 22, 2022.

317 Topazian, RJ., McGinty, E., Han, H., et al. (2022) US Adults' Belief about Harassing or Threatening Public Health Officials during the Covid-19 Pandemic. *JAMA*. 5:7. Available at: https://jamanetwork.com/journals/jamanetworkopen/fullarticle/2794789?utm_source=newsletter&utm_medium=email&utm_campaign=newsletter_axiosvitals&stream=top. Accessed: August 22, 2022.

318 Bettelheim, A. (2022) 1 in 5 Americans Okay with Threatening Health Officials. *Axios*. Available at: https://www.axios.com/2022/08/01/1-in-5-americans-ok-with-threatening-health-officials?utm_source=newsletter&utm_medium=email&utm_campaign=newsletter_axiosvitals&stream=top. Accessed: August 22, 2022.

319 Goldfield, N. *Testimonial*. Available at: https://drive.google.com/file/d/1unzl7thd6c-7MkLunkXDyJP9qFBFKQI0s/view. Accessed August 22, 2022.

320 Francesca, P., Parlapiano, A., Sanger-Katz, M., and Washington, E. (2022) A Detailed Picture of What's in the Democrats' Climate and Health Bill. *New York Times*. Available at: https://www.nytimes.com/interactive/2022/08/13/upshot/whats-in-the-democrats-climate-health-bill.html?utm_campaign=KHN%3A%20First%20Edition&utm_medium=email&_hsmi=222804950&_hsenc=p2ANqt-8lEAi3kakV3PziM_SJTqaXbj1tPk65rrvuUm5g_TjdDrjZEtSn6mvNXQOFTg1rSHKFfoHwE32mcRMSrKf6ZfU0W44cYg&utm_content=222804950&utm_source=hs_email. Accessed: August 21, 2022.

321 Owens, C. (2022) The Coming Public-Private Drug-Pricing Divides. *Axios*. Available at https://www.axios.com/2022/08/15/prescription-drug-prices-medicare-employers?utm_source=newsletter&utm_medium=email&utm_campaign=newsletter_axiosvitals&stream=top. Accessed: August 21, 2022.

322 Allen, A. (2022) Big Pharma Went All In to Kill Drug Pricing Negotiations. *Kaiser Health News*. Available at: https://khn.org/news/article/big-pharma-oppose-drug-pricing-negotiations-history/. Accessed: August 21, 2022.

323 Achenbach, A. and Sun, L. (2022) Covid forecast: Major fall surge unlikely but variants are a wild card. *Washington Post*. Available https://www.washingtonpost.com/health/2022/09/03/fall-covid-surge-booster-2022/. Accessed: September 5, 2022.

324 Lapin, A., Minn. (2022) GOP Nominee for Governor Says Comparing Covid Policies to the Holocaust is 'Legitimate'. *Jewish Telegraphic Agency*. Available at: https://

www.jta.org/2022/08/24/politics/minn-gops-nominee-for-governor-says-comparing-covid-policies-to-the-holocaust-is-legitimate?utm_source=JTA_Maropost&utm_campaign=JTA_DB&utm_medium=email&mpweb=1161-47463-28280; Accessed: September 5, 2022.

325 Reardon, S. (2022) First U.S. polio case in nearly a decade highlights the importance of vaccination. *Scientific American.* Available at: https://www.scientificamerican.com/article/first-u-s-polio-case-in-nearly-a-decade-highlights-the-importance-of-vaccination/?utm_source=newsletter&utm_medium=email&utm_campaign=health&utm_content=link&utm_term=2022-08-22_featured-this-week&spMailingID=71989175&spUserID=NTg0MzIwNjc0ODg0S0&spJobID=2251932421&spReportId=MjI1MTkzMjQyMQS2. Accessed: September 5, 2022.

326 Ellington, S. and Olson, CK. (2022) Safety of COVID-19 mRNA vaccines in pregnancy. *The Lancet.* Available at: https://www.thelancet.com/action/showPdf?pii=S1473-3099%2822%2900443-1. Accessed: September 5, 2022.

327 Rabin, RC. (2022) U.S. Life expectancy fall again in 'Historic' setback. *New York Times.* Available at: https://www.nytimes.com/2022/08/31/health/life-expectancy-covid-pandemic.html. Accessed: September 5, 2022.

328 McFarling, UL. (2022) So much more to do': A hospital system's campaign to confront racism — and resistance to change — makes early strides. *Stat.* Available at: https://www.statnews.com/2022/08/25/mass-general-brigham-campaign-confront-racism-early-progress/?utm_source=STAT+Newsletters&utm_campaign=03eed60886-MR_COPY_01&utm_medium=email&utm_term=0_8cab1d7961-03eed60886-152403458. Accessed: September 5, 2022.

329 Romero, S., Rabin, RC., and Walker, M. How the pandemic shortened life expectancy in native American Communities. (2022) *New York Times.* Available at: https://www.nytimes.com/2022/08/31/health/life-expectancy-covid-native-americans-alaskans.html. Accessed: September 5, 2022.

330 https://www.cnbc.com/2022/09/01/us-health-officials-brace-for-another-fall-covid-surge-but-with-fewer-deaths.html

331 Kuodi, P., Gorelik, Y., Zayyad, H. Wertheim, O. et al. (2022) Association between BNT162b2 vaccination and reported incidence of post-COVID-19 symptoms: cross-sectional study 2020-21, Israel. *npj Vaccines* 7: 101 Available at: https://doi.org/10.1038/s41541-022-00526-5. Accessed: November 26, 2022.

332 Hillis, S., N'konzi, JN., Msemburi, W., Cluver, N. et al. (2022) Orphanhood and Caregiver Loss Among Children Based on New Global Excess COVID-19 Death Estimates. *JAMA Pediatr.* 176: 1145–48. Available at: doi:10.1001/jamapediatrics.2022.3157. Accessed: November 26, 2022.

333 Hart, A. (2022) He stood his ground: California state senator will leave office as champion of tough vaccine laws. *Kaiser Health News.* Available at: https://khn.org/news/article/california-senator-richard-pan-champion-tough-vaccine-laws/?utm_campaign=KHN%3A%20First%20Edition&utm_medium=email&_hsmi=225106212&_hsenc=p2ANqtz-8DsuitmYFMeJa6_TFZPagd1_fU7-UGTp36Hld0-5sqzrr8PEy66Cgtu8vde5N_SvQ2SuEXqzQPZ2p7AGHjEigjS9mxOA&utm_content=225106212&utm_source=hs_email. Accessed: November 26, 2022.

334 Hillis, S., N'konzi, JN., Msemburi, W., Cluver, N. et al. (2022) Orphanhood and Caregiver Loss Among Children Based on New Global Excess COVID-19 Death Estimates. *JAMA Pediatr.* 176: 1145–48. Available at: doi:10.1001/jamapediatrics.2022.3157. Accessed: November 26, 2022.

335 Oshin, O. (2022) Fauci fears "anti-vaxxer" attitudes could cause outbreaks of non-Covid disease. *The Hill.* Available at: https://thehill.com/policy/health-care/3649593-fauci-fears-anti-vaxxer-attitude-could-cause-outbreaks-of-non-covid-diseases/?utm_campaign=KHN%3A%20First%20Edition&utm_medium=email&_hsmi=226460475&_hsenc=p2ANqtz-9yfsmFYvd6g8esVICzLrcWnLTRRaf8sfJKyWan5vbBIMvOKYrDYWBKfn3njgSUTMX12XDtADVqNjzYHYxFQXkMMSqNDQ&utm_content=226460475&utm_source=hs_email. Accessed: November 26, 2022.

336 AP News. (2022) Thousands of striking nurses return to work in Minnesota. *AP News.* Available at: https://apnews.com/article/health-covid-duluth-strikes-bd9e5d5d2205d63b989c4a2f08cbe316?utm_campaign=KHN%3A%20First%20Edition&utm_medium=email&_hsmi=226268508&_hsenc=p2AN-qtz-_D2pLCJE3kFsr3i6TsnR-CN3b7cPGOkWIJilZXdjoeU00rEJiuNlAra87Z-dPO3lC7ADWf-kuELilFvtPPiNK8JPZAePg&utm_content=226268508&utm_source=hs_email. Accessed: November 26, 2022.

337 Government Accounting Office. (2022) Covid-19 in Nursing Homes *U.S. Government Accounting Office.* Available at: https://www.gao.gov/assets/gao-22-105133.pdf. Accessed: November 26, 2022.

338 Alvarez, D. and Mullen. (2022) For the Underinsured: A combination eye-and-psych exam. *The New Yorker.* Available at: https://www.newyorker.com/humor/daily-shouts/for-the-underinsured-a-combination-eye-and-psych-exam. Accessed: November 26, 2022.

339 Pitel, P. (2022) Don't be fooled by medical experts. *Jacksonville Sun* Available at: https://mcusercontent.com/4b1ae8f547095b3561188d2c6/files/f4c3edde-8380-5cb3-af0d-d85d91b6335d/Dont_be_Fooled_.pdf. Accessed: December 11, 2022.

340 Goldfield, N., Kaminski, M., and Lerner, J. (2022) Voting for the common health of Pennsylvania. *Trib Live.* Available at: https://triblive.com/opinion/dr-norbert-gold-field-dr-mitch-kaminski-and-jeffrey-c-lerner-voting-for-the-common-health-of-pa/. Accessed: January 14, 2023.

341 Bowser, M., Dr Oz says uninsured Americans have no 'right to health' in resurfaced clip *Yahoo Life.* Available at: https://www.yahoo.com/lifestyle/dr-oz-says-uninsured-americans-180511104.html?guccounter=1. Accessed: December 11, 2022.

342 Karlamangla, S. (2022) Once known for vaccine skeptics, Marin tells now them "you're not welcome." *New York Times.* Available at: https://www.nytimes.com/2022/10/02/us/covid-vaccine-marin-california.html. Accessed: November 26, 2022.

343 Hoffman, J. (2022) Half of adults have heard little or nothing about new Covid boosters, study finds. *New York Times.* Available at: https://www.nytimes.com/2022/09/30/health/omicron-booster-covid.html. Accessed: December 11, 2022.

344 Young, E. (2022) The pandemics legacy is already clear. All of this will happen again. *The Atlantic.* Available: https://www.theatlantic.com/health/archive/2022/09/covid-pandemic-exposes-americas-failing-systems-future-epidemics/671608/?utm_source=newsletter&utm_medium=email&utm_campaign=atlantic-daily-newsletter&utm_content=20220930&utm_term=The%20Atlantic%20Daily. Accessed: November 26, 2022.

345 Mahr, K. and Banco, E. (2022) No quick fixes: Walensky's push for change at CDC meets reality. *Politico.* Available at: https://www.politico.com/news/2022/10/21/rochelle-walensky-change-cdc-00062874. Accessed: November 24, 2022.

346 Mahr, K., (2022) CDC Director orders agency overhaul, admits flawed COVID-19 response. *Politico* Available at: https://www.politico.com/news/2022/08/17/cdc-agency-overhaul-covid-19-response-00052384. Accessed: November 24, 2022.

347 Montez, JK., Mehri, S., Monnat, NM., Beckfield, J. et al. (2022) US state policy contexts and mortality of working-age adults. *PLOS One.* 17: 10: e0275466. Available at: https://doi.org/10.1371/journal.pone.0275466 Accessed: November 26, 2022.

348 Wallace, J., Goldsmith-Pinkham, P., and Schwartz, J. (2022) Excess death rates for Republicans and Democrats during the Covid-19 pandemic. *NBER Working Papers.* 30512. Available at: https://www.nber.org/papers/w30512. Accessed: November 26, 2022.

349 Goldfield, N., Lerner, J., and Kaminski, M. Who is better suited to fight addiction crisis? Fetterman or Oz? Doctors weigh in. *GoErie, PA* Available: https://www.goerie.com/story/opinion/columns/2022/10/21/experts-say-fetterman-would-strengthen-addiction-overdose-fight-in-pa-by-supporting-health-insurance/69580309007/. Accessed: November 26, 2022.

350 Garfinkel, P. Val Demings has demonstrated her support for containing health care costs. (2022) *West Volusia Beacon* Available at: https://beacononlinenews.com/2022/10/25/val-demings-has-demonstrated-her-support-for-containing-health-care-costs/. Accessed: November 26, 2022.

351 Israelsen-Hartley, S. (2022) A rural doctor and the fight against Covid. *The Assembly* Available at: https://www.theassemblync.com/health/rural-doctors-covid-vaccines/?utm_campaign=wp_to_your_health&utm_medium=email&utm_source=newsletter&wpisrc=nl_tyh. Accessed: January 14, 2023.

352 Kimball, S. (2022) Less than 50% of nursing home residents have received Omicron booster ahead of expected winter Covid wave *CNBC* Available at: https://www.cnbc.com/2022/12/15/covid-most-nursing-home-residents-have-not-received-omicron-booster.html?utm_campaign=KHN%3A%20First%20Edition&utm_medium=email&_hsmi=238217488&_hsenc=p2ANqtz-9ZeM6blaCLKPYeKf0pKQv0vFP-V51OFNX8WSI-gnwllAQIraEhDxdX3qjpo5i7MTyzGryaeBYPQHAWXfXSUE2I8-dSzQ&utm_content=238217488&utm_source=hs_email. Accessed: January 14, 2023.

353 Mueller, B. (2022) New Covid booster shots cut risk of hospitalization by half, CDC reports *New York Times* Available at: https://www.nytimes.com/2022/12/16/health/covid-boosters.html. Accessed: January 14, 2023.

354 Otterman, S. and Piccoli, S. (2023) Nurses do on strike at 2 New York City hospitals *New York Times* Available at: https://www.nytimes.com/2023/01/09/nyregion/nurses-strike-nyc-hospitals.html. Accessed January 14, 2023.

355 Robbins, R., Thomas, K., and Silver-Greenberg, J. (2022) How a sprawling hospital chain ignited its own staffing crisis. *New York Times.* Available at: https://www.nytimes.com/2022/12/15/business/hospital-staffing-ascension.html. Accessed January 14, 2023.

356 Lin, S., Deng, X., Ryan, I., Zhang, K., et al. (2022) COVID-19 Symptoms and Deaths among Healthcare Workers, United States. *Emerg Infect Dis.* 28: 8: 1624–41. 10.3201/eid2808.212200. Epub 2022 Jul 7. PMID: 35798004; PMCID: PMC9328912. Available at: https://www.ncbi.nlm.nih.gov/pmc/articles/PMC9328912/pdf/21-2200.pdf. Accessed: January 14, 2023.

357 Topol, E. (2023) The Coronavirus is speaking to us. It's saying it's not done with us *Washington Post.* Available at: https://www.washingtonpost.com/opinions/2023/01/08/xbb-covid-variant-immune-evasive-pandemic/. Accessed: January 14, 2023.

358 Editorial Board (2023) Congress has not stepped up to fight Covid-19 – or the next pandemic. *Washington Post.* Available at: https://www.washingtonpost.com/

opinions/2023/01/08/covid-19-pandemic-congress-funding/. Accessed January 14, 2023.

359 Kohrs, R. (2023) Will America's public health reckoning ever come? *Stat* Available at: https://www.statnews.com/2023/01/11/will-americas-public-health-reckoning-ever-come/?utm_source=STAT+Newsletters&utm_campaign=5fc4f3805c-MR_COPY_01&utm_medium=email&utm_term=0_8cab1d7961-54c4f3805c-152403458. Accessed: January 14, 2023.

360 Hsu, T. (2022) As Covid-19 continues to spread, so does misinformation about it *New York Times* Available at: https://www.nytimes.com/2022/12/28/technology/covid-misinformation-online.html. Accessed January 14, 2023

361 Gounder, C. (2023) Grant Wahl was a loving husband. I will always protect his legacy *New York Times* Available at: https://www.nytimes.com/2023/01/08/opinion/grant-wahl-celine-gounder-vaccine.html. Accessed January 14, 2023.

362 Stripling, J. (2023) Florida Surgeon General used 'flawed' science, faculty peers say *Washington Post* Available at: https://www.washingtonpost.com/education/2023/01/04/ladapo-surgoen-general-university-florida/. Accessed January 14, 2023.

363 Arnsdorf, I. (2022) DeSantis reverses himself on coronavirus vaccines, moving to right of Trump *Washington Post* Available at: https://www.washingtonpost.com/politics/2022/12/17/desantis-vaccine-reversal/. Accessed January 14, 2023.

364 Office of the Florida Governor. (2022) Governor Ron DeSantis Petitions Florida Supreme Court for Statewide Grand Jury on COVID-19 Vaccines and Announces Creation of the Public Health Integrity Committee. *Office of the Florida Governor* Available at: https://www.flgov.com/2022/12/13/governor-ron-desantis-petitions-florida-supreme-court-for-statewide-grand-jury-on-covid-19-vaccines-and-announces-creation-of-the-public-health-integrity-committee/. Accessed January 14, 2023.

365 Johnson, A. (2022) Can politics kill you? Research says increasingly the answer is yes *Washington Post* https://www.washingtonpost.com/health/2022/12/16/politics-health-relationship/?utm_campaign=KHN%3A%20First%20Edition&utm_medium=email&_hsmi=238504070&_hsenc=p2ANqtz-_LNnLdFiWaD5e9WvSjQVHd1sip7N_zNhN9u0spb1X8VGGt09w0TQYxZJ_IwQ-XneEiRyUX9DRqZgM_nNAgd7rrSnU-6g&utm_content=238504070&utm_source=hs_email. Accessed January 14, 2023.

366 Dress, B. (2022) GOP governor challenges DeSantis on vaccines: 'We shouldn't undermine science' *The Hill* https://thehill.com/homenews/sunday-talk-shows/3779764-gop-governor-challenges-desantis-on-vaccines-we-shouldnt-undermine-science/

367 Mazzei, P. (2023) Obamacare is everywhere in the unlikeliest of places: Miami *New York Times* Available at: https://www.nytimes.com/2023/01/11/us/obamacare-aca-miami-fl.html. Accessed: January 14, 2023.

368 Xu, S., Huang, R., S., L., Hong, V., et al. (2023) A safety study evaluating non-COVID-19 mortality risk following COVID-19 vaccination. *Vaccine.* 16;41: 3: 844–54. 10.1016/j.vaccine.2022.12.036. Epub 2022 Dec 20. PMID: 36564276; PMCID: PMC9763207. Available at: https://www.sciencedirect.com/science/article/pii/S0264410X22015614. Accessed: February 13, 2023.

369 Dixon, M. (2023) DeSantis pushes to make Covid-19 changes permanent. *Politico* Available at: https://www.politico.com/news/2023/01/17/desantis-covid-19-changes-anti-vax-00078192. Accessed: February 13, 2023.

370 Rovner, J. (2023) Au revoir, Public Health Emergency. *Kaiser Health News* Available at: https://khn.org/news/podcast/podcast-khn-what-the-health-283-covid-public-health-emergency-finale-medicaid-unwinding-february-2-2022/?utm_campaign=KHN%3A%20First%20Edition&utm_medium=email&_hsmi=244454881&_hsenc=p2ANqtz-_7VOUKwdrvTPH728Rkc83inoGq4ijpJTskTHRRaYivc26hiaaZ7fF99Cdyxg8I77tRhUJKhLDWVQmmq39enQ4FlhiSaA&utm_content=244454881&utm_source=hs_email. Accessed: February 13, 2023.

371 Belluck, P. (2023) Long Covid is keeping significant numbers of people out of work, study finds. *New York Times* Available at: https://www.nytimes.com/2023/01/24/health/long-covid-work.html?utm_campaign=KHN%3A%20First%20Edition&utm_medium=email&_hsmi=243119539&_hsenc=p2ANqtz-8rnMx6mhhRmEn53bwfGUayHAlFYu8_Bs4_GDxl1099l5wfLLRcHoL-_-XlGlbDWLQI46cbdMy01ikpfOqJqMfyVoU3qQ&utm_content=243119539&utm_source=hs_email. Accessed: February 13, 2023.

372 Solis, S. (2023) Massachusetts data shows drain of family doctors. *Axios* Available at: https://www.axios.com/local/boston/2023/01/25/massachusetts-doctos-family-drain?utm_source=newsletter&utm_medium=email&utm_campaign=newsletter_axioslocal_boston&stream=top. Accessed: February 13, 2023.

373 Reinhart, E. (2023) Doctors aren't burned out from overwork. We're demoralized by our health system. *New York Times*. Available at: https://www.nytimes.com/2023/02/05/opinion/doctors-universal-health-care.html

374 Gurley, L. (2023) Why nurses say they are striking and quitting in droves. Washington Post Available at: https://www.washingtonpost.com/business/2023/01/14/nurses-strike-staffing-unions/?utm_campaign=KHN%3A%20First%20Edition&utm_medium=email&_hsmi=241981500&_hsenc=p2ANqtz-_yFKvDoPcQHoo95SJBc9lm19heeHGDotw6zDK25Fk1PhEcAgZ2WhZIUsNuZmCSVX3TdApqkSRSA8cX_hV0T2nPdn4lZw&utm_content=241981500&utm_source=hs_email. Accessed: February 13, 2023.

Chapter 4

American Fragility during and after the COVID Pandemic

The Role to Date of Health Professionals and Health Professional Associations

Introduction

All political sides agree the United States is increasingly fragile and conflict-prone. Here, "conflict" implies at least a constitutional crisis at a national level which the historian Robert Kagan believes has already arrived.[1] Conflict could devolve into ongoing violence of the kind that broke out on January 6, 2021. In addition, on a national level, a large percentage of Americans, particularly many self-identified Republicans, do not view the American government as legitimate.[2] But what do fragility and legitimacy mean?

This chapter will define these terms, very briefly summarize the overall political "fragility landscape" in terms of Republicans versus Democrats, and then discuss how health professionals both at the individual and organizational level have unfortunately contributed to increased American fragility and decreased legitimacy. Health professionals have, for example, contributed to the saga over the inappropriate use of Hydroxychloroquine to treat COVID. This chapter also highlights the role that health professional organizations, such as American Medical Association (AMA), have played in the ongoing battle against COVID misinformation.

DOI: 10.4324/9781003426257-5

Lastly, this chapter highlights the role that individual physicians such as Simone Gold have had in propagating COVID misinformation.

Two bottom lines emerge from this chapter. While we might hope or expect that all health professionals would believe in science, the reality is that, given human nature, some of my cohort don't believe in science. As extensively discussed by Brian Klaas in his book *Corruptible: Who Gets Power and How It Changes Us*,[3] there are health professionals for whom political power "trumps" science. Secondly, I agree with Klaas's perspective that "those who control—not those being controlled—are the ones we need to worry about." For physicians, it is organized medicine and, in particular, the American Medical Association (AMA) and the Federation of State Medical Boards that are the "controllers." As this chapter will document, there are opportunities for improvement.

One Definition of Fragility and Legitimacy

> "States are fragile when state structures lack political will and/or capacity to provide the basic functions needed for poverty reduction, development and to safeguard the security and human rights of their populations."[4]

> "'Legitimacy' is a term increasingly used to denote that a state is acceptable to most of its people and population groups."[5] "State legitimacy can derive from a range of sources, including the effectiveness of public institutions in their performance of various functions, such as service delivery; and their degree of representation and accountability. Legitimacy does not derive solely from effectively functioning institutions, however. Such institutions must resonate with societies in order for them to be considered legitimate."[6]

I have already highlighted the fact that the performance of the United States during this pandemic is far worse than that of any other industrialized country. Again, the United States suffered ten times the death rate as Australia. This is one clear indication of the country's fragility.

Yet the words "fragility" and "legitimacy" have different meanings for all elements of the political spectrum. Both Republicans and Democrats agree that our government is increasingly fragile, if not outright illegitimate. What are the implications of different political points of view for health care responses to the pandemic? As we will see, the Republican and Democratic (R and D) labels still have relevance. But from a political point of view, the R and D labels have many flavors.

The R and D Labels with the Understanding That I Am Oversimplifying—But Only Somewhat

The Republican Party has under its umbrella members and people in positions of power who support traditional capitalism, ranging from minimal taxation to federal support for businesses as advocated by, for example, the Chamber of Commerce to small "g" government at a state level; government suffused with a Christian religious perspective; and single-issue advocates, such as those against abortion, in favor of gun rights or oil drilling. A segment of the Republican party, particularly that part aligned with Donald Trump, supports authoritarianism, including white supremacy and fascism.[7]

The Democratic Party has under its umbrella members who promote national or federal authority over issues such as abortion rights, universal health insurance, consumer protection, and gun control. Like Republicans, Democrats support traditional capitalism, albeit with federal assistance and/or rules for engagement. A majority of Democrats, or at least those who wield power at all levels of the federal government, uphold our traditional privately run health system. As of this writing, Democratic lawmakers who advocate a single-payer system—or other government domination of an economic sector (socialism)—are in a distinct minority within the Democratic party.

Challenging as it may be to accept, there are facts pertaining to the COVID pandemic. Vaccines save lives.[8] Many Republicans either deny that fact or state that it is an infringement on individual rights for government/society to demand that all eligible people be vaccinated, even in sectors of the economy such as health care or education, where, for example, a small number of unvaccinated people can impact the entire population, especially the most vulnerable.

Misinformation abounds about vaccines and COVID in general.[9] Republicans are much more likely to articulate scientifically inaccurate statements about the pandemic. With 99% (849 out of 853) of all the links to her scientific and general pronouncements rated as unreliable, Sarah Palin exemplifies this predicament.[10] And society or government has had to make judgments using scientific facts, such as whether or not and how to keep schools open for face-to-face instruction. Unfortunately, as some Republicans are not relying on facts to make their judgments, it is difficult to have an honest conversation examining the pros and cons of a particular decision.

Importantly, Republicans are also more likely to make ad hominem attacks on public scientists.

> "We are not going to be like (Dr. Anthony) Fauci in the '80s, claiming that families could get AIDS by sitting and watching TV together," DeSantis said at a press conference in Rockledge, where he and state health officials were addressing opioid treatment. After asking the Governor's Office for clarification of DeSantis' reference, they sent a link to a long-form 1983 interview with Fauci where he said the "full extent of transmissibility" of the disease was not known.[11]

Republicans have regularly attacked our already weak public health system to the point that there is an eroding public trust in our public health professionals.

The Tragic Case of Hydroxychloroquine: Physicians Enabling Republican Party Misinformation; Connection between Political Parties, Politicians, Celebrities, and Physicians

In part because it is mostly (but not at all exclusively) physicians who are able to prescribe medication, I will focus this section on the medical profession. At the start of the pandemic, Donald Trump promoted hydroxychloroquine. It is important to highlight the timeline for that endorsement, the importance of the endorsement of individual physicians, and the lack of pushback from organized medicine. What I find most fascinating is the change in the physician prescribing pattern in response to politician endorsement of a medication. The political affiliation of physicians who prescribed hydroxychloroquine should also be noted.

Brief timeline of the rise and fall of hydroxychloroquine as summarized from an article in the *Washington Post*;[12] I *highlight* in bold the names of physicians:

> *March 16*: Tesla CEO Elon Musk tweets a link to a March 13 paper suggesting that the antimalarial drug chloroquine might be effective at treating COVID-19.
>
> A few hours earlier, the drug gets its first mention on Fox Business network, from Fox contributor *Marc Siegel, a doctor*. "In terms of treatments, remdesivir"—an antiviral—"looks very promising. I will tell you something you don't know: the South Koreans have tried chloroquine, that's for malaria," Siegel says. "Hydroxychloroquine is something we use for arthritis. Those look very promising." That evening, Gregory Rigano, one of the authors of the paper Musk linked to, appears on Laura Ingraham's Fox News show. He says that hydroxychloroquine can "just get rid of [the virus] completely." Rigano is an attorney, not a doctor. He'd written the paper with the help of *James Todaro, an ophthalmologist and tech investor*.
>
> *Mid-March*: Trump speaks with Oracle chairman Larry Ellison, who in February hosted a major fund-raising event for President Trump in California. Ellison suggests that the government establish a system (based on Oracle's database tools) to track the use of chloroquine and hydroxychloroquine as possible treatments for COVID-19, the disease caused by the new coronavirus. Others raise the idea in the same period, including Mehmet Oz (*Dr. Oz*), a regular on Fox News who the *New York Times* reports had contacted Trump advisers.
>
> *March 17*: *A French doctor named Didier Raoult* is part of a group of researchers who publish a paper suggesting that a combination of hydroxychloroquine and the antibacterial medication azithromycin (which is often sold under the brand name Z-Pak) could be effective against the disease. The study later draws significant scrutiny, including from the journal where it was published.

Anthony S. Fauci, a leading member of the White House coronavirus task force, appears on Ingraham's Fox News program that evening. "We have to be careful, Laura, that we don't assume something works based on an anecdotal report that's not controlled," he said. "And I refer specifically to hydroxychloroquine. There's a lot of buzz out there on the Internet, on the social media about that. We need to look at it in a scientific way."

March 18: Rigano appears on Tucker Carlson's Fox News show. Ingraham touts the Raoult study.

March 19: Trump for the first time mentions the drug during a daily briefing on the pandemic.

March 21: Trump promotes the unproven combination of hydroxychloroquine and azithromycin on Twitter. It could be "one of the biggest game changers in the history of medicine," he speculates:

> HYDROXYCHLOROQUINE & AZITHROMYCIN, taken together, have a real chance to be one of the biggest game changers in the history of medicine. The FDA has moved mountains— Thank You! Hopefully they will BOTH (H works better with A, International Journal of Antimicrobial Agents)....
> —Donald J. Trump (@realDonaldTrump)
> March 21, 2020

Later that day, he retweets this tweet. He also retweets a tech investor's citation of the Raoult study. By the end of March 21, Fox News and Fox Business have mentioned chloroquine or hydroxychloroquine 176 times.

March 27: Asked about the drug, Trump explicitly rejects *Fauci's* view.

March 28: The FDA provides emergency-use authorization for hydroxychloroquine and chloroquine to treat COVID-19.

March 29: Speaking during a briefing in the Rose Garden, Trump says that the hydroxychloroquine and Z-Pak combination is being tested with patients in New York. He thanks the FDA for approving its use.

April 21: Guidelines published by the National Institutes of Health (NIH) recommend against the hydroxychloroquine-azithromycin combination "because of the potential for toxicities." The NIH offers no recommendation about the use of hydroxychloroquine alone.

April 22: Rick Bright, the former director of the Biomedical Advanced Research and Development Authority, alleges that he was demoted because he objected to the administration's promotion of chloroquine and hydroxychloroquine.

April 23: Trump is asked during the daily coronavirus briefing why he has stopped promoting the drugs. "I haven't at all. I haven't at all. What are you say—we'll see what happens," Trump replies. "We've had a lot of very good results and we had some results that perhaps aren't so good. I don't know. I just read about one, but I also read many times good. So I haven't at all.

And it's a—it's a great—for malaria, for lupus, for other things. And we'll see what it is."

April 24: The FDA formally warns against taking the medicines Trump has promoted due to "serious heart rhythm problems."

By the end of the day on April 22, the most recent day for which data are available, Fox News and Fox Business had mentioned those two drugs 1,375 times.

It goes without a saying that a patient cannot take hydroxychloroquine without a prescription from a licensed health professional. The overall estimated number of hydroxychloroquine or chloroquine prescriptions dispensed in March and April 2020 increased from 819,906 in 2019 to 1,312,859 in 2020.[13] A recent study provides a fascinating picture of what parts of the country had the highest increase:

> Increases in hydroxychloroquine prescriptions were higher in areas of the country with greater support for Trump in the 2016 and 2020 elections. Our results suggest a 2% increase in weekly hydroxychloroquine prescription rates for every percentage point increase in DMA-level vote share for Trump. We find evidence of this disproportionate increase among high-Trump-supportive areas when accounting for DMA sociodemographic characteristics and health system capacity.... The robustness of the results when using Republican House of Representatives votes instead of Trump votes also underscores the notion that partisan identification, rather than solely Trump support, drives our observed effects. This robustness check reflects the broader partisan divide over hydroxychloroquine among politicians and pundits rallying for or against Trump's endorsement.[14]

Were patients driving the demand, or did political affiliations and preferences of physicians play a role? While both liberal and conservative physicians responded to Donald Trump's endorsement, we know that physicians who identified themselves as politically conservative responded significantly more.[15]

Physicians Working against Vaccines and in Favor of COVID Misinformation; the Role of Organized Medicine

Organized medicine can be divided into two broad categories: organizations, such as the American Medical Association (AMA), which represent the economic and professional interests of, in this case, all physicians, and licensing boards, which have the power to grant and take away medical licenses.

The AMA has taken official policy positions against, for example, vaccine disinformation[16]:

> While disinformation has run rampant during the COVID-19 pandemic, we know unscientific claims are being made about other health conditions and other public health initiatives are being undermined. We are committed to doing everything we can to stop the spread of disinformation and providing accurate, evidence-based information—the lives of our patients and the public depend on it.[17]

Unfortunately, the AMA, like all other medical professional associations, has done little beyond these public service announcements to combat misinformation. Chapters 8–11 specify options that the AMA and other professional medical associations could pursue.

Each state has the power to license medical professionals. I am licensed to practice in the state of Massachusetts and cannot practice anywhere else without applying for licensure in the state I wish to practice. According to the website of the Federation of State Medical Boards (FSMB), "to protect the public from the unprofessional, improper, unlawful or incompetent practice of medicine, each of the states and territories making up the United States of America defines the practice of medicine within their borders and delegates the authority to enforce the law to a regulatory board."[18] The FSMB was just over one hundred years old in 2022.[19] The origin of the state medical boards goes back to the American War of Independence, with the idea of states' rights in any regulation of the medical profession always preeminent over federal rights. State legislatures have the power to license health professionals. They decide whether or not and under what rules to empower a state licensure board to, in turn, take charge of the licensing process.

In July 2021, the FSMB issued a "formal statement warning that spreading COVID-19 vaccine misinformation could put physicians' licenses at risk." What has happened after the FSMB issued this formal warning? To my knowledge, only one physician has lost his license. Licensing specialty boards such as the American Board of Internal Medicine (ABIM) have been very careful in emphasizing political polarization without highlighting the fact that it is Republicans that are politicizing COVID.[20] The reason for this political weakness is in part the justified fear that Republican-dominated legislatures will, as some already have, limited the ability of state licensing boards to address COVID misinformation. Policy options will be discussed more fully in Chapters 8–11.

Each state licensure board has power vested in it from state legislatures. Currently, more than half of the states have either passed or proposed legislation either restricting board authority or explicitly allowing the off-label treatment of COVID-19, or both.[21] All of these are states dominated by Republicans. Unfortunately, Republican lawmakers in some states protect health professionals who peddle COVID disinformation.[22] At least one state, North Dakota, has passed legislation allowing physicians to prescribe Ivermectin.[23]

With respect to medical professional organizations tasked with issuing licenses to physicians, Carl Coleman has recently reviewed the legal issues surrounding disciplining doctors accused of misinformation.[24] He concluded: "disciplinary actions against physicians who disseminate medical misinformation can be justified in only one set of circumstances: when physicians disseminate misinformation with knowledge that it is false or with reckless disregard of whether it is true." At least one physician, Steven LaTulippe in Oregon, lost his medical license after continuing to insist that his patients not wear masks.[25] As of February 2022, state licensure boards have disciplined eight physicians for spreading COVID misinformation.[26]

Other than Steven LaTulippe, no one else to my knowledge has lost their medical license for spreading COVID misinformation. Joseph Ladapo, the Florida surgeon general and director of the Florida Department of Health, has not lost his license, nor has the Florida Department of Health Medical Quality Assurance Program (the state licensure board) undertaken any investigation despite the many false statements he has made about COVID vaccines and the efficacy of face masks.[27] In response to inquiries about the lack of a more forceful response, the FASB president stated:

> "People assume that licensing boards are on the lookout, they're on the internet," says Dr Humayun Chaudry, president of the Federation of State Medical Boards. "They actually don't have the resources—neither the money nor the manpower—to monitor what happens on the internet or social media."[28]

In another article, Carl Coleman concludes:

> In most cases the medical profession should emphasize alternative strategies for responding to misinformation that raise fewer constitutional concerns. For example, private hospitals and other health care organizations could revoke physicians' privileges or terminate their employment for spreading false or misleading information about medical matters. Medical specialty boards (which, unlike licensing boards, are nongovernmental entities) could treat disseminating medical falsehoods as grounds for revoking certifications. Professional associations can also play an important role in calling out misinformation when they see it and disseminating the truth.[29]

The FASB, AMA, and other health professional organizations have largely restricted their fight against COVID to public pronouncements.

Physicians Working against Vaccines and in Favor of COVID Misinformation; the Role of Individual Physicians and the Case of Simone Gold

The following provides just a sampling of what the Center for Countering Digital Hate (CCDH) calls the "Dirty Dozen,"[30] a number of whom are physicians:

> Dr. Rashid Buttar posted on twitter that COVID-19 "was a planned operation" and shared an article alleging that most people who got vaccinated against the coronavirus would be dead by 2025. His tweets are a recent addition to a steady stream of spurious claims about the COVID-19 vaccines and treatments. Another example is Dr. Sherri Jane Tenpenny's June testimony, before Ohio state legislators, that the vaccine could cause people to become magnetized. Clips from the hearing went viral on the internet. Earlier in the pandemic, on April 9, 2020, Dr. Joseph Mercola posted a video about whether hydrogen peroxide could treat the coronavirus; it was shared more than 4,600 times. In the video, Mercola said that inhaling hydrogen peroxide through a nebulizer could prevent or cure COVID-19.

Focusing on one health professional—and I will highlight Simone Gold—illustrates both the challenges in disciplining physicians spreading COVID misinformation and, as important (or possibly even more so), the connection between physicians seeking the limelight and politicians and celebrities only too willing to welcome such physicians to their fold.

From the website of a right-wing Republican member of the House of Representatives, dated September 9, 2022:

> Rep. Louie Gohmert (TX-01) joined Dr. Simone Gold today as she was released from federal prison after she was unjustly prosecuted by the Biden Administration's Department of Justice. He also presented her with a flag which was flown over the U.S. Capitol to celebrate her invaluable work and contributions to public health, medical freedom and our God-given constitutional rights.

The congressman released the following statement:

> Dr. Gold is a patriot and an American hero. In the early days of the COVID-19 pandemic, she exposed the world to life-saving early treatment options that undoubtedly saved many lives. Tragically, her sound medical advice was viciously attacked and suppressed by a corrupt media captured by pharmaceutical companies with a clear financial agenda.

After having her name and reputation shamefully dragged through the mud, the Biden administration's DOJ threw her in prison for peacefully walking into the U.S. Capitol on January 6 and delivering a speech. Dr. Gold is the definition of what a political prisoner looks like—something I never thought I'd see here in the United States of America.

God Bless Dr. Gold. History will not look kindly upon those who persecuted—and prosecuted—doctors who spoke out against the COVID lockdown, mask and vaccine mandates.[31]

What did Simone Gold do to deserve federal prison? How did she come to that point where she was sentenced to six months in prison? Is Simone Gold still able to practice medicine? What did she do to deserve the praise of a Republican member of Congress who is, himself, under investigation for his role in the January 6, 2021, insurrection?

Simone Gold was the only physician caught, tried, and convicted for taking part in the January 6 insurrection. At her sentencing, Gold asked for leniency. "I made a mistake. I have consistently said so. I deeply regret going inside the Capitol."[32]

Yet in August 2022, Simone Gold moved from, in her words, "the communist state" of California to Florida. The Florida Department of Health Services issued her a license to practice medicine, and she established a medical practice (according to her website) while she was in federal prison. It is worth quoting extensively from her website, GoldCare Health and Wellness. Under the tab "Who We Are" are the following statements:

We founded the civil liberties organization, America's Frontline Doctors

2020 revealed an irreparable system that has been gaining power for many years in America. Centuries ago, Founding Father Benjamin Rush stated:

Unless we put medical freedom into the Constitution, the time will come when medicine will organize into an undercover dictatorship to restrict the art of healing to one class of Men and deny equal privileges to others; the Constitution of the Republic should make a special privilege for medical freedoms as well as religious freedom.

President Ronald Reagan also recognized the need for medical freedom in 1961, when he said:

One of the traditional methods of imposing statism or socialism on a people has been by way of medicine. It's very easy to disguise a medical program as a humanitarian project.

Many have cautioned this government overreach through the guise of medical safety. The propaganda surrounding COVID-19 inflicted intense fear in many Americans. Believing we were keeping our loved ones safe, we allowed ourselves to be controlled and consequently lost our freedoms.

A movement—a resistance—took action to help the American people no longer be manipulated and controlled. GoldCare™ is built on those same philosophies of freedom, honesty and resistance to provide a safe harbor for people seeking the truth!

We welcome all like-minded individuals into a new method of health care—regardless of where you've been on your healthcare journey. We'll meet you where you're at now and show you a new path to medical freedom.

In addition, under the FAQ tab, the question "Is ivermectin or hydroxychloroquine available?" was answered: "Clinicians practice medicine based on your unique needs, including writing any prescription that's in your best interest. And we will help you find 'freedom pharmacies' that honor these prescriptions, but we'll never receive incentives for any referrals."[33]

Concluding Comments

A December 2021 poll documented that most Americans feel that physicians do not have the right to spread false information about the COVID pandemic.[34] More specifically:

- 91% of adults said doctors don't have the right to intentionally spread misinformation or false health information.
- 83% said a physician's responsibility to share credible information with their patients and the public outweighs their protected right to speech.
- 78% said medical doctors who intentionally spread misinformation about COVID-19 should be disciplined in some way and expressed varying levels of support for actions such as warnings, fines, or license suspension or revocation.

Furthermore, according to the poll, the public had strong feelings about the consequences of physicians spreading COVID misinformation:

Doctors who intentionally spread misinformation about COVID-19 should...

- *78%*: Receive a warning
- *89%*: Have to pay a fine
- *80%*: Have their license temporarily suspended
- *58%*: Have their license permanently revoked

The public's perception is significant because recent polling has demonstrated that the public believes that public health is important to the health of the United States and supports increased funding but today lacks a high level of trust in public health institutions.[35]

The Florida medical licensure board has not disciplined Dr. Ladapo using any of these penalties that the American public recommends. Self-identifying as a Republican predicts both lack of vaccination and even death. This and many other personal tragedies of the COVID pandemic highlight the importance of individual health professionals and health professional organizations taking a stronger stance in favor of science. See Chapters 8–11 for options that health professional organizations should consider to protect the public from health professionals who spread scientifically inaccurate information.

Notes

1 Leonhardt, D. (2022) A "crisis coming": Twin threats to American democracy. *New York Times.* Available at: https://www.nytimes.com/2022/09/17/us/american-democracy-threats.html. Accessed: November 20, 2022.

2 Stokes, B. (2021) Polls shows Americans do not believe in "American democracy". *German Marshall Fund.* Available at: https://www.gmfus.org/news/poll-shows-americans-dont-believe-american-democracy Accessed: November 20, 2022.

3 Klaas, B. (2021) Corruptible: Who Gets Power and How it Changes Us. New York: Scribner

4 OECD (2007). *Principles for Good International Engagement in Fragile States and Situations.* Paris: OECD. Available at: https://www.oecd.org/dac/conflict-fragility-resilience/docs/38368714.pdf. Accessed November 20, 2022.

5 OECD (2010). *The State's Legitimacy in Fragile Situations: Unpacking Complexity.* Paris: OECD. Available at: https://www.oecd.org/dac/conflict-fragility-resilience/docs/the%20States%20legitmacy%20in%20FS.pdf. Accessed: November 20, 2022.

6 Haider, H. (2010). *State-Society Relations and Citizenship in Situations of Conflict and Fragility.* GSDRC Topic Guide Supplement. Available at: https://gsdrc.org/wp-content/uploads/2015/07/CON88.pdf. Accessed: November 20, 2022.

7 Nichols, T. (2022) Fear of fascism. *The Atlantic.* Available at: https://www.theatlantic.com/newsletters/archive/2022/08/fear-of-fascism/671289/ Accessed: November 19, 2022.

8 Wappes, J. (2022) Covid vaccines saved an estimated 20 million in 1 year. *CIDRAP.* Available at: https://www.cidrap.umn.edu/news-perspective/2022/06/covid-19-vaccines-saved-estimated-20-million-lives-1-year Accessed: November 20, 2022.

9 Hsu, T. (2022) As Covid-19 continues to spread, so does misinformation about it. *New York Times.* Available at: https://www.nytimes.com/2022/12/28/technology/covid-misinformation-online.html. Accessed: December 28, 2022.

10 Macdonald, M. and Brown, M. (2022) Republicans are increasingly sharing misinformation, research finds. *Washington Post.* Available at: https://www.washingtonpost.com/politics/2022/08/29/republicans-democrats-misinformation-falsehoods/ Accessed: November 20, 2022.

11 Gankarski, AG (2022) Governor DeSantis blasts Anthony Fauci AIDS policy in Monkeypox comments. *Florida Politics.* Available at: https://floridapolitics.com/archives/543778-desantis-monkeypox/ Accessed: November 20, 2022.

12 Bump, P. (2022) The rise and fall of Trump's obsession with Hydroxychloroquine. *Washington Post.* Available at: https://www.washingtonpost.com/politics/2020/04/24/rise-fall-trumps-obsession-with-hydroxychloroquine/ Accessed: November 20, 2022.

13 Bull-Otterson, L., Gray, EB., Budnitz et al. (2020) Hydroxychloroquine and Chloroquine Prescribing Patterns by Provider Specialty Following Initial Reports of Potential Benefit for COVID-19 Treatment — United States, January–June 2020. *MMR Morbidity and Mortality Report.* Available at: https://www.ncbi.nlm.nih.gov/pmc/articles/PMC7470458/ Accessed: October 1, 2022.

14 Madanay, F., McDevitt, RC., Ubel, PA. (2022) Hydroxychloroquine for COVID-19: Variation in Regional Political Preferences Predicted New Prescriptions after President Trump's Endorsement. *J Health Polit Policy Law.* 47: 4: 429–51. Available at: https://read.dukeupress.edu/jhppl/article/47/4/429/293751/Hydroxychloroquine-for-COVID-19-Variation-in. Accessed: October 1, 2022.

15 Ibid.

16 American Medical Association. AMA adopts policy to combat disinformation by health professionals. Available at: https://www.ama-assn.org/press-center/press-releases/ama-adopts-policy-combat-disinformation-health-care-professionals. Accessed: November 20, 2022.

17 Ibid.

18 Federation of State Medical Boards. *Annual Report 2022.* Available at: https://www.fsmb.org/siteassets/advocacy/publications/fsmb-current-annual-report.pdf. Accessed: November 20, 2022.

19 For a history of the Federation of State Medical Boards, see: Johnson, DA. and Chaudhry, HJ. (2012) Medical licensing and discipline in America. New York: Lexington.

20 Baron, RJ. and Ejnes, YD. (2022) Physicians spreading misinformation on social media - Do right and wrong answers still exist in medicine? *N Engl J Med.* 387: 1: 1–3. doi: 10.1056/NEJMp2204813. Epub 2022 May 18. PMID: 35584154. Available at: https://www.nejm.org/doi/10.1056/NEJMp2204813?url_ver=Z39.88-2003&rfr_id=ori:rid:crossref.org&rfr_dat=cr_pub%20%200pubmed. Accessed: December 24, 2022.

21 State action on Coronavirus. *National Conference on State Legislatures.* Available at: https://www.ncsl.org/research/health/state-action-on-coronavirus-covid-19.aspx Accessed: November 20, 2022.

22 Ollove, M. (2022) States Weigh Shielding Doctors' Misinformation, Covid Remedies. *PEW Stateline.* Available at: https://www.pewtrusts.org/en/research-and-analysis/blogs/stateline/2022/04/06/states-weigh-shielding-doctors-covid-misinformation-unproven-remedies. Accessed: September 19, 2022.

23 Ibid. Accessed: October 1, 2022.

24 Coleman, CH. (2022) Physicians Who Disseminate Medical Misinformation: Testing the Constitutional Limits of Professional Disciplinary Action 20 First Amend. L. Rev. 113, *Seton Hall Public Law Research Paper.* Available at: SSRN: https://ssrn.com/abstract=3925250. Accessed: September 19, 2022.

25 Clark, C. (2022) Oregon doc loses license for not wearing mask, spreading misinformation. *MedPage Today.* Available at: https://www.medpagetoday.com/special-reports/exclusives/94593. Accessed: November 20, 2022.

26 Tahir, D. (2022) Medical boards get pushback as they try to punish doctors for Covid misinformation. *Politico*. Available at: https://www.politico.com/news/2022/02/01/covid-misinfo-docs-vaccines-00003383. Accessed: September 19, 2022.

27 Rubin, R. (2022) When physicians spread unscientific information about Covid-19. *Journal of the American Medical Association*. Available at: https://jamanetwork.com/journals/jama/fullarticle/2789369. Accessed: October 1, 2022.

28 Brumfiel, G. (2021) This Doctor Spread False Information About COVID. She Still Kept Her Medical License. *National Public Radio*. Available at: https://www.npr.org/sections/health-shots/2021/09/14/1035915598/doctors-covid-misinformation-medical-license. Accessed: October 1, 2022.

29 Coleman, C. (2022) License revocation as a response to physician misinformation: Proceed with caution. *Health Affairs Forefront*. Available at: https://www.healthaffairs.org/do/10.1377/forefront.20211227.966736/. Accessed: December 28, 2022.

30 Center for Countering Digital Hate. (2022) *The Disinformation Dozen*. Available at: https://counterhate.com/wp-content/uploads/2022/05/210324-The-Disinformation-Dozen.pdf. Accessed: November 20, 2022.

31 Press Release. (2022). Representative Gohmert Greets Dr Simone Gold as She is Released from Federal Prison. Available at: https://gohmert.house.gov/news/documentsingle.aspx?DocumentID=399995. Accessed: October 1, 2022.

32 Gentry, C. (2022) The anti-Covid-Vax founder of America's frontline doctors has a license to practice in Florida. *Health News Florida*. Available at: https://health.wusf.usf.edu/health-news-florida/2022-08-18/the-anti-covid-vax-founder-of-americas-frontline-doctors-has-a-license-to-practice-in-florida. Accessed: December 24, 2022.

33 Gold Health Care and Wellness (2022) Available at: https://goldcare.com. Accessed: November 20, 2022.

34 De Beaumont Foundation (2022) 9 in 10 Americans: Hold doctors accountable for spreading Covid misinformation. Available at: https://debeaumont.org/news/2021/disinformation-doctors-poll/. Accessed: November 20, 2022.

35 Robert Wood Johnson Foundation/ Harvard School of Public Health (2021) *The Publics Perspective of the United States' Public Health System*. Available at: https://www.rwjf.org/en/library/research/2021/05/the-publics-perspective-on-the-united-states-public-health-system.html: Accessed: October 1, 2022.

INCREASING PUBLIC TRUST IN THE UNITED STATES; THE CRITICAL ROLE OF HEALTH PROFESSIONALS IN REBUILDING THE PUBLIC HEALTH SYSTEM AND DECREASING FRAGILITY

II

Chapter 5

COVID-19 and the Mental Health and Substance Abuse Crisis

Tragedy, Positive Changes, and Resilience

Newspaper headlines from the past two years of the pandemic provide a sense of the impact that the COVID-19 pandemic has had on the mental health and substance abuse of Americans:

> *Many Teens Report Emotional and Physical Abuse by Parents during Lockdown*[1]
>
> *"'What's the Point?' Young People's Despair Deepens as Covid-19 Crisis Drags On—*
>
> *COVID-19, Overdoses Pushed US to Highest Death Total Ever*[2]
>
> *How Loneliness Is Damaging Our Health: Even before the Pandemic, There Was an "Epidemic of Loneliness," and It Was Affecting Physical Health and Life Expectancy*[3]
>
> *Hundreds of Suicidal Teens Sleep in Emergency Rooms. Every Night. With Inpatient Psychiatric Services in Short Supply, Adolescents Are Spending Days, Even Weeks, in Hospital Emergency Departments Awaiting the Help They Desperately Need*[4]

DOI: 10.4324/9781003426257-7

Lost on the Frontline: Thousands of US Healthcare Workers Died Fighting Covid-19 in the First Year of the Pandemic; We Counted Them and Investigated Why[5]

The Foundational Skills for Learning Need to be Retaught[6]

This report from Wuhan, China, highlights the emotional toll exacted where COVID-19 started[7]:

> Another woman had spent days begging for an ambulance—at that time private cars were also barred from Wuhan's streets—for her father, but once it came, she could not get him a hospital bed. She brought him home, where he lay on the first floor because she didn't have the strength to carry him up the stairs. "He passed away there in front of her. She was making congee for him," Xu said. "She didn't get to say good bye." To ease such trauma may take years. It is easier for many of Wuhan's residents to block memories of the darkest days. There is also a shortage of good psychologists.

And this excerpt of a recent report highlights the global mental health challenges we face:

> The COVID-19 pandemic has increased the incidence of factors that adversely affect mental health (eg, family disputes, social isolation, fear of contagion, uncertainty, chronic stress, hopelessness, feelings of entrapment and burdensomeness, substance misuse, loneliness, domestic violence, child neglect or abuse, unemployment, and economic difficulties), while concurrently reducing access to mental health services.... policy makers are focused on efforts to mitigate the pandemic's devastating economic and social impacts, and the long-term consequences on mental health are being overlooked.

Is this quote from an author working in the United States? Europe? No—it is about Iran.[8]

Introduction

Throughout this pandemic, Americans and the media have been quite open about the mental health and substance abuse (MHSA) consequences of this tragedy. The sad fact is that despite all our knowledge about evidence-based optimal MHSA practices, we have barely scratched the surface of systematically addressing the ongoing MHSA crisis, which COVID-19 has only exacerbated. As Darrell Steinberg, mayor of Sacramento, California, and mental health advocate has stated: "Providing mental healthcare to people who need it the most is a voluntary act of government, and it shouldn't be. It should be a legal requirement."[9]

This chapter will summarize the data of the impact of COVID-19 on MHSA with a particular, but not exclusive focus on the United States, point out some of the challenges we faced in our responses, and then specify what is being done and what should be done. I discuss some of the positive changes to our health system. I then highlight family, community, and societal responses to the MHSA Crisis.

I conclude the chapter by emphasizing that we need to be aspirational. This includes strengthening resilience, and the chapter will close with comments on how the vast majority of us, who choose to continue to live, must and do develop mechanisms of resilience as we confront the horrors of this pandemic. I bring out the role of healthcare professionals and their impact on the resilience of individuals and society during the pandemic. I also highlight the impact of the pandemic on health professional resilience.

An excellent report[10] from the U.S. Government Accounting Office highlights the dramatic mental health consequences of the COVID-19 pandemic and calls attention to six groups of people who have suffered the most during this pandemic. They are:

- healthcare workers,
- people of color,
- people with preexisting behavioral health conditions, including substance abuse,
- young adults,
- children and adolescents, and
- people facing financial distress.

The Data

MHSA disorders increased across the board during the pandemic.[11] Among the key takeaways from recent surveys:

- in January 2021, 41% of adults reported symptoms of anxiety and/or depressive disorder;
- from June 2020, 13% of adults reported new or increased substance use due to coronavirus-related stress, and 11% of adults reported thoughts of suicide in the past 30 days.[12]

Variation in state-level suicide rates is largely driven by rates of suicide by firearm. Suicides involving firearms vary from the lowest rate of 1.8 per 100,000 in New

Jersey and Massachusetts to a high of 20.9 per 100,000 in Wyoming. More than twice as many suicides by firearm occur in states with the fewest gun laws relative to states with the most laws.

Young adults have experienced several pandemic-related consequences, such as closures of universities and loss of income, that may contribute to poor mental health. During the pandemic, a larger than average share of young adults (ages 18–24) have reported symptoms of anxiety and/or depressive disorder (56%). Compared to all adults, young adults are more likely to report substance use (25% versus 13%) and suicidal thoughts (26% versus 11%).

Research from prior economic downturns shows that job loss is associated with increased depression, anxiety, distress, and low self-esteem and may lead to higher rates of substance-use disorder and suicide. During the pandemic, adults in households with job loss or low incomes have reported higher rates of symptoms of mental illness than those without job or income loss (53% versus 32%). Research during the pandemic points to concerns around poor mental health and well-being for children and their parents, particularly mothers, as many experienced challenges with school closures and lack of child care. Women with children were more likely to report symptoms of anxiety and/or depressive disorder than men with children (49% versus 40%). In general, both before and during the pandemic, women have reported higher rates of anxiety and depression than men.

The pandemic has disproportionately affected the health of communities of color. Non-Hispanic black adults (48%) and Hispanic or Latinx adults (46%) are more likely to report symptoms of anxiety and/or depressive disorder than non-Hispanic white adults (41%). Historically, these communities of color have faced challenges accessing mental health care.

Many essential workers continue to face challenges, including a greater risk of contracting the coronavirus than other workers. Compared with nonessential workers, essential workers are more likely to report symptoms of anxiety or depressive disorder (42% versus 30%), starting or increasing substance use (25% versus 11%), and suicidal thoughts (22% versus 0.8%) during the pandemic.[13]

With respect to children and adolescents, key takeaways from a recent study include[14]:

■ Deaths due to drug overdose among adolescents nearly doubled from 2019 (282 deaths) to 2020 (546 deaths). In the same period, the largest increases in these deaths were among adolescent males (deaths more than doubled), as well as Black (deaths more than tripled) and Hispanic (deaths more than doubled) adolescents.

■ Suicides are the second-leading cause of death among adolescents. These deaths have increased since 2010 but slowed in recent years. It is possible that not all suicides have been captured, as they may have been misclassified as drug overdose deaths. In 2020, across racial and ethnic groups, suicide death rates were highest among American Indian and Alaska Native adolescents

(22.7 per 100,000), followed by white adolescents (4.5 per 100,000). Adolescent males had higher rates of suicide than their female peers (8.7 versus 3.9 per 100,000); however, rates of self-harm were higher (and increased faster) for females.

■ The share of adolescents experiencing anxiety and/or depression has increased by one-third since 2016 but held relatively steady from 2019 (15%) to 2020 (16%). In 2020, anxiety and/or depression was more pronounced among adolescent females than males. Anxiety and/or depression was higher among white and Hispanic adolescents and lower among black adolescents.

■ In 2021, many adolescents reported adverse experiences such as emotional abuse (55%), parental job loss (29%), hunger (24%), and physical abuse (11%). Some of these experiences were more pronounced among female and lesbian, gay, or bisexual (LGB) adolescents. Research shows that gun violence, including but not limited to school shootings, has continued to rise in recent years and may be linked to poor mental health outcomes among youth.

■ Access to mental health care may have worsened during the pandemic, with declines in the utilization of care among both Medicaid and private insurance pediatric beneficiaries. Before the pandemic, the rate of mental health treatment was low and varied across demographics. Reasons for not receiving care included cost and a lack of providers.

■ Gun violence continues to rise and may lead to negative mental health impacts among children and adolescents. An increasing number of children and adolescents have been exposed to gun violence in recent years. There were forty-two school shootings across the United States in 2021[15] – the highest on record for a single year—and in 2020 firearms became the leading cause of death among children aged 19 and younger.[16] Research suggests that children and adolescents may experience negative mental health impacts,[17] including symptoms of anxiety, in response to school shootings and gun-related deaths in their communities.[18] Other research[19] found that youth antidepressant use increased following exposures to fatal school shootings.

A remarkable COVID-19 statistic: in the six months between April and October 2021, the number of children experiencing the death of a parent or primary caregiver as a result of COVID-19 nearly doubled, to more than 5.2 million globally, surpassing the total number of reported COVID-19 deaths worldwide.[20] The impact of mental health and substance abuse issues on people's lives is staggering. Just as I am writing this, I am working with a young mother using ten bags of heroin a day laced with fentanyl (she has a prescription for Narcan,® to counteract an overdose) who is now in withdrawal, and we are trying to convince her to switch to Suboxone,® a well-known treatment for heroin addiction.

Finally, health care workers have suffered tremendously. Let us not forget the health professionals who have lost their lives to the pandemic.[21] And aside from physical attacks on health care workers,[22] they have been afflicted by serious mental health issues. Many have quit.[23] A recent study by the Physicians Foundation, as quoted by Richard Mollica and colleagues, found that doctors were severely affected by the COVID-19 pandemic: 61% reported often experiencing feelings of burn-out[24]; 57% had experienced inappropriate feelings of anger, tearfulness, or anxiety; 46% had isolated themselves from others; and more than 55% know of a physician who has either considered, attempted, or died by suicide. I continue to keep in mind the tragic story of the emergency room physician who committed suicide early on during the pandemic.[25] Despite the high incidence of mental health symptoms, only 14% of doctors sought medical attention.

Compounding Social Factors That Are Worsening the MHSA Crisis

Homelessness
Loss of Schooling
The Lack of Integrated Primary and MHSA Services
Racism and the MHSA Crisis

Homelessness, Suicide, Drug Overdoses

These factors are all interlinked. Simply put, no home means no health, no stability in life. Veronica, a patient of mine—she is almost seventy—sleeps in her car in a Walmart parking lot. Frank carries around a mattress to the home of different friends. Because of his unstable housing, he can't use his sleep apnea machine, thus worsening his high blood pressure and asthma.

Overdoses during the pandemic increased nationally by 30% to 92,000, while suicides actually dropped by about 10% to 44,000. Why, when these two tragedies typically go in tandem? The supply of fentanyl has actually gone up during the pandemic.[26] Increased isolation is also in part to blame for increased overdoses. But even though a great deal has been written about this divergence, we don't understand the reasons. Suicides and overdoses represent another tragedy that the United States has not effectively dealt with.

Loss of Schooling

"Something that we continuously come back to is that our ninth graders were sixth graders the last time they had a normative, uninterrupted school year," said Jennifer Fine, a high school counselor in Chicago. "Developmentally, our students have skipped over crucial years of social and emotional development."[27] In 2022, reading and math scores went down, the first time this has occurred since a national association started tracking data in the 1970s.[28]

The Lack of Integrated Primary and MHSA Services

You would think that with all the publicity about the abysmal state of MHSA services, we as a country could pull together on this issue and provide adequately paid mental health services to those who need them. But the insurance industry and many employer lobbyists, among other groups, are against such an approach.[29] For example, according to a recent report, health insurers "covered nutritional counseling for medical conditions like diabetes, but not for mental health conditions such as anorexia nervosa, bulimia nervosa, and binge-eating disorder." And, of course, navigating the system for effective mental health services is daunting, if not impossible.[30] Chapter 8 presents my suggestions on how to integrate primary and MHSA services.

Racism and the MHSA Crisis

COVID-19 continues to decimate the Black community. As reported by Dylan Scott in his excellent column for *Vox* in 2020, we saw the collision of two public health crises—police violence and the coronavirus.[31] Scott believes that COVID illustrates:

> the nation's structural racism, in two important ways. First, police violence is a public health risk. In almost any way you measure it, the US criminal justice system is prejudiced against black Americans, and black people are much more likely to be subjected to state-sanctioned violence in the US compared to white Americans.... Black men, by far the most at-risk group, face one in 1,000 odds of being killed by the police over the course of their lives.

Blacks are significantly overrepresented in the American penal system. Suicide in prison accounts for 34% of all deaths; suicide rates for prisoners are four times the rate of the general public.[32] Even more disturbing, most of those who committed suicide were never convicted of any crime.[33] Beyond the high rate of suicide, the overall COVID-19 care in prisons constitutes another stain on our national conscience.[34]

Auspicious Trends, My Hopes Concerning MHSA Services, and the Inevitable Human Response of Resilience

From "COVID-19 Notes," February 15, 2021:

> For myself, I have a constant sense of dread hanging over me; this pandemic gnaws. One of my patients last week who was still under quarantine was hospitalized with COVID pneumonia. I encouraged her, in a positive but firm tone of voice (I've known her for years), that

she needed to be in quarantine for 5 more days. She told me that she just couldn't take it mentally any more and had already gone to the store—even though she was highly infectious. Who knows how many people she might have infected by going out? If you "have" to go out we know now the importance of not only double masking out also how to put them on to minimize discomfort (important for me, as I have a deformed ear from a prior accident).

And then 18 months later, July 25, 2022:

As I work on this chapter of the book on this day, I have the same feeling—a sense of dread about the future. How can I not feel the same sense of dread that I felt two years ago when I see data documenting that death and hospitalization rates for COVID have increased 38% and 15% respectively in the past two weeks?

And as can be seen from the same date as my diary note immediately above, hospitals and healthcare workers continue to suffer, get sick, and die:

Hospitals across the country are grappling with widespread staffing shortages, complicating preparations for a potential Covid-19 surge as the BA.5 subvariant drives up cases, hospital admissions and deaths. Long-standing problems, worker burnout and staff turnover have grown worse as Covid-19 waves have hit health care workers again and again— and as more employees fall sick with Covid-19 themselves.

Despite the overall tragedy of the COVID-19 pandemic, there are positive trends in three areas related to MHSA services, though these trends are very tenuous at best:

- Systemic changes to our health system impacting MHSA services.
- Family, community, and societal responses to the MHSA crisis.
- The "inevitable" human response—the individual will to live or resilience in the face of crisis; recovery versus resilience.

Systemic Changes to Our Health System Impacting MHSA Services

The most dramatic change to our delivery system that had a positive impact on MHSA is telehealth. Without the almost ubiquitous presence of telehealth, untold more individuals would have died, including health professionals who would have been exposed to, for example, depressed and anxious patients with COVID-19. A caveat, however. The vast majority of my patients could access only the telephonic, not the video version of telehealth. I am not sure why this occurred. But through this pandemic, I learned a valuable lesson. Possibly in part because I've been in practice for more than forty-five years, I found that the vast majority of ambulatory care encounters could be dealt with on the phone.

Tele MHSA visits were and continue to be a game changer in the overall delivery of MHSA services. Telehealth made possible the efficient, rapid, and effective connection between patients and therapists without putting the therapist at risk and allowing the patient to have the interaction from home. At the height of the pandemic, 40% of mental health encounters took place via telehealth, and the most recent data indicates that it has decreased only slightly, down to 35%. Contrast this with just over 10% of outpatient visits occurring via telehealth.[35] Importantly, individuals living in rural health areas, those at high risk for suicide and/or overdose, among other conditions, were more likely to access telehealth as compared with those living in urban areas (55% versus 35%). In addition, "Telehealth availability increased by 77% from 2020 to 2021 for mental health treatment facilities and by 143% for substance use disorder treatment facilities. By January 2021, 68% of outpatient mental health facilities and 57% of substance use disorder treatment facilities in the sample were offering telehealth."[36]

Paying for telehealth is necessary but hardly sufficient if we are to adequately respond to pandemic crises and rising socioeconomic disparities. Chapter 8 provides my suggested response.

Family, Community, and Societal Responses to the MHSA Crisis

Christian Science Monitor (CSM) reporters met five people across five countries twice—the first time one year after the World Health Organization declaration of the COVID pandemic. CSM reporters went back again one year later to see how they were doing.

> During that first year, a surprising resilience emerged amid a global crisis with no end in sight.... And while reflecting on the loss of loved ones, regretting polarization within families and society, and suffering a dulling weariness, many also speak of a new sense of agency, whether through opportunities or through changing perspectives.
>
> Steven Taylor, a psychologist at the University of British Columbia who wrote a book on the psychology of pandemics, conducted research about how Americans and Canadians perceive they are doing now. His team found that about 77% of participants reported moderate to high improvement in at least one respect, like valuing friends and family, gratitude for each day, or a greater feeling of self-reliance.[37]

Valuing friends and family, gratitude for each day, and/or a feeling of self-reliance are all attitudes that can emerge and dominate one's outlook on life, especially if two additional factors are in play: trust in society's ability to care for your basic needs and, crucially, COVID-19's physical impact on one's family. Communities represent "a way station" between families and societies. Families, communities, and societies can under the best of circumstances embody differing aspects of resilience. Health professionals can make an impact at each of these levels. In turn, each of these levels affects the resilience of health professionals.

Here are two family scenarios:

> I've already alluded to my situation: Both of my adult children came "home" at the start of the pandemic and lived next door. They could have stayed as long as they wished. Our son and his wife, in fact, decided to remain in the town we live in. They were able to continue to work remotely.

Contrast my situation with this one:

> Carol Schumacher, 56, who was raised in the remote community of Chilchinbeto in the Navajo Nation, has lost 42 family members to Covid-19 over the last two years. The dead included two brothers aged 55 and 54, and cousins as young as 18 and 19.... The nearest hospital was a long drive away on dirt roads, she said, "and there's no guarantee about the quality of care there even if you make it in time. Some families don't even have transportation or running water. Imagine dealing with that."[38]

Imagine the impact on those individuals who survive when they've lost so many members of their family. The situation is even more challenging for the millions of children who have, as highlighted in the beginning of this chapter, lost one or both parents.

With respect to family, community, or social resilience, researchers generally agree that social capital is key. Ichiro Kawachi defines social capital as "those features of social relationships—such as levels of interpersonal trust and norms of reciprocity and mutual aid—that facilitate collective action for mutual benefit."[39] Social capital taps into a "collective dimension of society external to the individual."[40] Several articles have documented the positive relationship between social capital and decreased COVID-19 mortality and morbidity.[41] Another study documented the relationship between social capital, public health interventions, and COVID-19 outcomes:

> Using data for over 2,700 US counties, we investigate how social capital explains the level and growth rate of infections. We find that moving a county from the 25th to the 75th percentile of the distribution of social capital would lead to a 18% and 5.7% decline in the cumulative number of infections and deaths, as well as suggestive evidence of a lower spread of the virus. Our results are robust to many demographic characteristics, controls, and alternative measures of social capital ... public health interventions cannot be disconnected from the social forces that are present

at a local level. Moreover, stable and vibrant communities are not luxuries, but rather important priorities for managing emergencies. Investing in social capital and interpersonal relationships helps us manage negative shocks and retain levels of interconnectedness and well-being.[42]

The "Inevitable" Human Response—the Individual Will to Live or Resilience in the Face of Crisis: Recovery Versus Resilience

One can examine resilience through different lenses: social, mental, and physical health; health system, economic, ecological, governance, and individual.[43] This chapter focuses on resilience as it pertains to individual and health professional social and mental health; and the mental health aspects of the health system. Chapter 8 focuses on other aspects of resilience in particular the overall health system and governance.

First, one must examine the terms *recovery* and *resilience*. Recovery is not the same as resilience. A significant minority of my COVID-19 patients have not recovered. That is, they have not returned to their baseline of either emotional or physical functioning or both. As discussed in my diary in Chapter 3, Alice was intubated for several weeks during the initial phases of the pandemic. More than a year later she quickly becomes short of breath after walking a few steps. Her emotional state is fragile. Yet on some fundamental level, she is resilient; she has told me that if nothing else, she wants to be there for her kids. Sergei, hospitalized with COVID-19 pneumonia at the same time as his daughter, who also had COVID-19, continues to be short of breath after walking a few steps. If it wasn't for his children, Sergei tells me, he would have given up treating his diabetes, which requires taking insulin, a long time ago. He is illiterate and learning-disabled, which makes his diabetes difficult to control. So, Sergei and Alice have not recovered, yet they are resilient. Both Sergei and Alice enjoy life in their own ways.

I utilize Mollica's characterization of the word *resilience* at the individual level, which he states is a key element of self-care. According to Mollica, resilience is defined as "good adjustment across the mental, physical, and spiritual domains in the face of adversity." Resilience consists of five capacities:

- ability to experience reward and motivation in a positive and optimistic way,
- ability to work and be productive in spite of fear,
- adaptation of social behaviors to promote altruism, social bonding, and teamwork,
- use of cognitive skills to see negative experiences in a more "positive" light, and
- development of meaning and spiritual purpose in life.[44]

Not surprisingly, open communication is one of the most important predictors of resilience.[45]

While many have appropriately emphasized the mental health challenges that COVID-19 has brought on, this chapter concludes by accentuating human resilience in the face of the COVID-19 tragedy.[46] The research literature, in fact, documents that, in the words of one leading researcher, "decades of research have consistently shown that the most common outcome following potential trauma is a stable trajectory of health functioning or resilience." Continuing to quote from the CSM article that included interviews with five people over a period of two years:

> By most measures, Obdulia Montealegre Guzmán shouldn't be "okay."
>
> For the past 20 years, the taco vendor has joined the din of informal work in Mexico's bustling capital—organ grinders reaching out their hats for tips, vendors weaving through busy intersections hawking bubblegum, and cooks crowding sidewalks with their mobile food stalls.
>
> When the pandemic arrived, the streets went silent. And as clients holed up at home, informal workers like Ms. Montealegre had no source of income and little or no safety net. More than 40% of the Mexican population already lived in poverty pre-pandemic. COVID-19 landed informal workers in a "double situation of vulnerability," according to the United Nations.
>
> But inside a narrow market that spans three city blocks in a working-class neighborhood, where the snip-snip-snip of poultry shears competes with slow-tempo ranchero ballads from a distant boombox, Ms. Montealegre has re-imagined her makeshift stall selling prepared food and drinks at open-air markets with a slick, new business model.
>
> Today, her team of six dresses in matching face masks, aprons, and baseball caps. Each item is emblazoned with their new brand: a mustachioed man in a sombrero, holding a taco and giving an enthusiastic thumbs-up. And while she serves up steak *huaraches* smothered in cheese and crispy *flautas* to hungry shoppers, she's keeping track of orders coming in over a new WhatsApp ordering system, and advertising on Facebook.[47]

Ms Monteleagre has "re-imagined" her business model and herself. She is resilient in the face of the horrors of the pandemic.

The Impact of Health Professionals on the Resilience of Individuals and Society during the Pandemic: The Impact of the Pandemic on Health Professional Resilience

We have already discussed how public health is an integral part of social capital. Better public health services can lead to greater trust. At the health professional level, this chapter has also summarized what we know of the burnout and consequent early retirement of many health professionals. In some studies, the rate of burnout among health professionals has approached 60%.[48] Hospitals, in particular, have tried to respond with interventions recognizing that, as Mollica stated, health professionals are a "treasure." He and others have presented specific recommendations on how health care institutions can nurture this national treasure.[49]

Among the most disadvantaged people in the United States are the undocumented. They form a sizable percentage of my clinical practice, as our office serves the largest number of undocumented in western Massachusetts. We do not have firm empirical data documenting the impact of health professionals on the social capital of undocumented people. I will highlight just one example of the connection between health professionals and individual social capital.

Dr. Marty Nathan started La Cliniquita at our practice in the early 2000s. Its mission is to "provide medicines, medical supplies, needed specialty care and food to those with no other options."[50] We have collected innumerable anecdotal stories from La Cliniquita documenting its impact on the lives of the undocumented.

As I detail in my COVID Notes in Chapter 3, the undocumented suffered more than Americans already suffering from socioeconomic disparities as many undocumented had significant food insecurity. The COVID lockdown resulted in the loss of jobs with consequent loss of income. Just a week before I wrote this, I saw an undocumented patient found to be pregnant and food insecure. She was given a food voucher on the spot—via the Cliniquita program. Food insecurity is not uncommon, especially in the winter months.

The following is an "anecdotal story," a profound poem that one of the nurses working where I practice wrote as she reflected on the care that she, as a health care professional, tries to give to the undocumented. As the poem dramatically, to my mind, demonstrates, this health professional's care surely increases the resilience of any of the undocumented patients that she engages with to face this pandemic.

1,933 miles
(From Mexico to Massachusetts)
By Ahriel Burston

Walk a mile in someone else's shoes they say
But what about 1,933?
The distance traveled from village to clinic
In the shoes of this woman sitting right before me
With sun worn skin, child on your back and one deep in your womb
I pause when I realize I have never met anyone stronger than you
When you leave our visit I'm sobered to have met living, breathing sacrifice
The personification of the question, "how far would you go for a better life?"
Would you work jobs no one else would want for pay no one else would take?
Would you leave family and friends and all you've known? Is that a sacrifice you
 think you could make?

Would you risk your health for your pay, fearing to take a day off?
Faced with the reality you are dispensable and your family can't afford that loss.
I know I couldn't do what so many have already done.
So I do that little that I can to serve them each day when they come
Walk a mile in someone else's shoes they say
But what about 1,933?

The distance traveled from village to clinic in shoes of men and women braver
than any you may ever meet.[51]

I believe that the act of writing this poem was part of the resilience-strengthening process for this nurse.

Concluding Comments

While I've had a sense of dread throughout this pandemic, I hold other feelings at the same time. I don't feel optimistic—not after the abysmal performance of American leadership during this pandemic. But if I didn't also feel a strong sense of joy, I could not go on. My daughter, son, and his wife were with us for the first year of the pandemic. Partly because of this, my son and his wife decided to move to the town in which we live. They now live fifteen minutes away. My wife has told me countless times that the period of the pandemic was probably the happiest in her life. She was able to get a great deal of her own artwork done—she has had two books published during the pandemic—and appreciated the specialness of having our children live next door during this time.

Maybe it isn't joy. Maybe I've developed a greater sense of equanimity or acceptance of what comes my way. Is that part of the aging process? Or am I "using my cognitive skills to see my negative experience in a positive light"? For those of us lucky with resources—both physical and emotional—we can try to focus on the beauty of life that is all around us while pursuing efforts to make a difference in other people's lives. This may be the essence of resilience.

Notes

1 Barry, E. (2022) Many teens report emotional and physical abuse by parents during lockdown. *New York Times*. Available at: https://www.nytimes.com/2022/03/31/health/covid-mental-health-teens.html. Accessed: November 20, 2022.

2 Stobbe, M. (2022) Covid-19, overdoses pushed US to highest death total ever *AP News* Available at: https://apnews.com/article/covid-science-health-centers-for-disease-control-and-prevention-robert-anderson-ff2f01e401abce778bea8ac2e9c6e53e?utm_campaign=KHN%3A%20First%20Edition&utm_medium=email&_hsmi=209891651&_hsenc=p2ANqtz-9IATQN2pTGnf9DuEmAgtQ3fRYPMQgjLKM2-EcCqkNt1SdS_oLqAGVdA-Mlqq_FY68XrASclwKUxq_1WO6JIIZaKZkKyw&utm_content=209891651&utm_source=hs_email. Accessed: November 20, 2022.

3 Leland, J. (2022) How loneliness is damaging our health. *New York Times* Available at: https://www.nytimes.com/2022/04/20/nyregion/loneliness-epidemic.html. Accessed: November 20, 2022.

4 Richtel, M. (2022) Hundreds of suicidal teens sleep in emergency rooms every night. *New York Times* Available at: https://www.nytimes.com/2022/05/08/health/emergency-rooms-teen-mental-health.html?utm_campaign=KHN%3A%20 First%20Edition&utm_medium=email&_hsmi=212437486&_hsenc=p2AN qtz-96u_e5ZsxZWpAGqbEQCwgzI2eGa6CG5eUOMgBYlPslLx-wNrGlJWqDa J15LutjwKFsFLBsV1djdH_42unYsjgUErnR3g&utm_content=212437486&utm_ source=hs_email. Accessed November 20, 2022.

5 Manchester Guardian and Kaiser Health News. (2022) Lost on the frontline *Manchester Guardian* Available at: https://www.theguardian.com/us-news/ng-interactive/2020/ aug/11/lost-on-the-frontline-covid-19-coronavirus-us-healthcare-workers-deaths-database. Accessed: November 20, 2022.

6 Miller, CC. and Pallaro, B. (2022) 328 School counselors on the pandemics effect on children: Anxiety is filling our kids. *New York Times*. Available at: https://www. nytimes.com/interactive/2022/05/29/upshot/pandemic-school-counselors.html. Accessed November 20, 2022.

7 Su, A. (2021) A year after the Covid-19 pandemic began, Wuhan has become a city of forgetting. *Los Angeles Times*. Available at: https://www.latimes.com/world-nation/ story/2021-02-14/wuhan-becomes-a-city-of-forgetting. Accessed: November 20, 2022.

8 Doshmangir, L., Gholipour, K., and Gordeev, VS., (2022) *The Lancet*. Available at: https://www.thelancet.com/journals/lanpsy/article/PIIS2215-0366(22)00203-6/ fulltext. Accessed November 20, 2022.

9 See https://steinberginstitute.org/qa-darrell-steinbergs-longtime-focus-on-mental-health/ Accessed: December 24, 2022.

10 Government Accounting Office. (2021) Behavioral health and Covid-19. *Government Accounting Office*. Available at: https://www.gao.gov/assets/720/717988.pdf. Accessed November 20, 2022

11 Centers for Disease Control. (2022) Anxiety and depression. Household Pulse Survey. *National Center for Health Statistics* Available at: https://www.cdc.gov/nchs/covid19/ pulse/mental-health.htm. Accessed: November 20, 2022.

12 Morbidity and Mortality Weekly Report. (2022) Mental health, substance abuse, and suicidal ideation during the Covid-19 Pandemic. *Centers for Disease Control* Available at: https://www.cdc.gov/mmwr/volumes/69/wr/mm6932a1.htm?s_cid= mm6932a1_w. Accessed: November 20, 2022.

13 Panchal, N., Kamal, R., Cos, C., and Garfield, R. (2021) The implications of Covid-19 for menbtal health and substance abuse. *Kaiser Family Foundation* Available at: https://www.kff.org/coronavirus-covid-19/issue-brief/the-implications-of-covid-19-for-mental-health-and-substance-use/. Accessed: November 20, 2022.

14 Panchal, N., Rudowitz, R., and Cox, C. (2022) Recent trends in mental health and substance abuse concerns among adolescents. *Kaiser Family Foundation*. Available at: https://www.kff.org/coronavirus-covid-19/issue-brief/recent-trends-in-mental-health-and-substance-use-concerns-among-adolescents/. Accessed: November 20, 2022.

15 Cox, JW., Rich, S., Chiu, A., Thacker, H. et al. (2022) More than 320,000 students have experienced gun violence at school since Columbine. (2022) *Washington Post*. Available at: https://www.washingtonpost.com/graphics/2018/local/school-shootings-database/. Accessed: November 20, 2022. Riehm, KE., Mojtabai R., Adams, L.

et al. (2021) Adolescents concerns about school violence or shootings and association with depressive, anxiety and panic symptoms. *JAMA Network Open*. Available at: https://jamanetwork.com/journals/jamanetworkopen/fullarticle/2785658. Accessed November 20, 2022.

16 Goldstick, JE, Cunning, R., Cunningham, P. (2022) Common causes of death in children and adolescents in the United States. *New England Journal of Medicine*. 385: 1955–56. Available at https://www.nejm.org/doi/full/10.1056/NEJMc2201761 Accessed November 21, 2022.

17 Cimolai, V., Schmitz, J., and Sood, AB. (2021) Effects of mass shootings on the mental health of children and adolescents. *Curr Psychiatry Rep*. 23: 12. https://doi.org/10.1007/s11920-021-01222-2

18 Vasan, A., Mitchell, HK., Fein, JA., Buckler DG, et al. (2021) Association of neighborhood gun violence with mental health–related pediatric emergency department utilization. *JAMA Pediatr*. 175: 12: 1244–51. 10.1001/jamapediatrics.2021.3512. Available at: https://jamanetwork.com/journals/jamapediatrics/article-abstract/2784065. Accessed: November 21, 2022.

19 Rossin-Slater, M., Schnell, M., Schwandt, H., and Uniat, L. (2020) Local exposure to school shootings and youth antidepressant use. *PNAS* 117: 38: 23484–89. Available at: https://www.pnas.org/doi/full/10.1073/pnas.2000804117. Accessed: November 21, 2022.

20 Hillis, SD., Blenkinsop, A., Villaveces, A., Annor, FB. et al. (2021) COVID-19-associated orphanhood and caregiver death in the United States. *Pediatrics*. 148: 6: e2021053760. 10.1542/peds.2021-053760. Epub ahead of print. PMID: 34814177. Available at: https://publications.aap.org/pediatrics/article/148/6/e2021053760/183446/COVID-19-Associated-Orphanhood-and-Caregiver-Death?autologincheck=redirect ed?nfToken=00000000-0000-0000-0000-000000000000. Accessed: November 21, 2022.

21 Rezba, C. (2020) Nobody Accurately Tracks Health Care Workers Lost to COVID-19. So She Stays Up At Night Cataloging the Dead *Pro Publica*. Available at: https://www.propublica.org/article/nobody-accurately-tracks-health-care-workers-lost-to-covid-19-so-she-stays-up-at-night-cataloging-the-dead?utm_source=sailthru&utm_medium=email&utm_campaign=majorinvestigations&utm_content=feature. Accessed: December 24, 2022.

22 Larkin, H. (2021) Navigating attacks against health care workers in the COVID-19 era. *JAMA*. 325: 18: 1822–24. 10.1001/jama.2021.2701.

23 Wan, W. (2021) Burned out by the pandemic, 3 in 10 health care workers consider leaving the profession. *Washington Post*. Available at : https://www.washingtonpost.com/health/2021/04/22/health-workers-covid-quit/; Accessed: November 21, 2022.

24 Mollica, RF., Fricchione, GL. (2021) Mental and physical exhaustion of health-care practitioners. *Lancet*. 398: 10318: 2243–44. 10.1016/S0140-6736(21)02663-5. PMID: 34922665; PMCID: PMC8676692.

25 Watkins, A., Rothfeld, A., Rashbaum, WK., Rosenthal, BM. (2020) Top ER doc who treated virus patients dies by suicide. *New York Times* Available at: https://www.nytimes.com/2020/04/27/nyregion/new-york-city-doctor-suicide-coronavirus.html. Accessed: November 21, 2022.

26 Ghose, R., Forati, AM., and Mantsch, AM. (2022) Impact of the Covid-19 pandemic on opioid overdose deaths. *Journal of Urban Health*. 99: 316–27. Available at: https://www.ncbi.nlm.nih.gov/pmc/articles/PMC8856931/pdf/11524_2022_Article_610.pdf. Accesed: November 21, 2022.

27 Miller, CC. and Pallaro, B. (2022) 328 School counselors on the pandemics effect on children: Anxiety is filling our kids. *New York Times*. Available at: https://www.nytimes.com/interactive/2022/05/29/upshot/pandemic-school-counselors.html. Accessed November 20, 2022.

28 Mervosh, S. (2022) The pandemic erased two decades of progress in math and reading. *New York Times* Available at https://www.nytimes.com/2022/09/01/us/national-test-scores-math-reading-pandemic.html; Accessed September 3, 2022.

29 Ollstein, AM. and Wilson, M. (2022) Mental health push in Congress sparks Lobbying frenzy. *Politico* Available at: https://www.politico.com/news/2022/02/13/mental-health-pandemic-congress-lobbying-00008372. Accessed; November 21, 2022.

30 Levey, NN. (2022) This doctor thought she could navigate US health care. Then her autistic son needed help. *Kaiser Health News*. Available at: https://khn.org/news/article/this-doctor-thought-she-could-navigate-us-health-care-then-her-autistic-son-needed-help/?utm_campaign=KHN%3A%20First%20Edition&utm_medium=email&_hsmi=203952590&_hsenc=p2ANqtz-8iSNIhQjWOzB-QFUImlrTgmMDKjcLnM4wW7D6WqNddyHhSU3Yg04-OR48354U71XT1wVL5v1T7134QD8UCkgerOloSgQ&utm_content=203952590&utm_source=hs_email. Accessed: November 21, 2022.

31 Scott, D. (2020) Two public health crises have collided in the protests over George Ffloyd's death. *Vox* Available at: https://www.vox.com/2020/6/1/21276957/george-floyd-protests-coronavirus-police-brutality-racism. Accessed: November 21, 2022

32 The Conversation. (2018) How mass incarceration hurts US health, in 5 charts. *The Conversation*. Available at: https://theconversation.com/how-mass-incarceration-harms-u-s-health-in-5-charts-90674. Accessed: November 21, 2022.

33 Ibid.

34 Rubin, A., Golden, T., and Webster, RA. (2020) Inside the U.S.'s largest maximum security prison Covid-19 raged. *Pro Publica* Available at: https://www.propublica.org/article/inside-the-uss-largest-maximum-security-prison-covid-19-raged?utm. Accessed: November 21, 2022

35 Lo, J., Rae, M., Amin, K et al. (2022) Telehealth has played an outsized role meeting mental health needs during the Covid-19 pandemic. *KFF* Available at: https://www.kff.org/coronavirus-covid-19/issue-brief/telehealth-has-played-an-outsized-role-meeting-mental-health-needs-during-the-covid-19-pandemic/. Accessed: November 21, 2022

36 Cantor, J., McBain, RK., Kofner, A., Hanson, R. et al. (2022) Telehealth adoption by mental health and substance use disorder treatment facilities in the COVID-19 pandemic. *Psychiatr Serv*. 73: 4: 411–17. 10.1176/appi.ps.202100191. Epub 2021 Aug 19. PMID: 34407631.

37 Eulich, W., Lllana SM. (2022) Two years in: Pandemic resilience propels renewed action. *Christian Science Monitor*. Available at: https://www.csmonitor.com/World/2022/0310/Two-years-in-Pandemic-resilience-propels-renewed-action. Accessed: November 21, 2022

38 Romero, S., Rabin, RC., and Walker, M. (2022) How the pandemic shortened life expectancy in native American communities *New York Times*. Available at: https://www.nytimes.com/2022/08/31/health/life-expectancy-covid-native-americans-alaskans.html Accessed: September 5, 2022.

39 Kawachi, I. (1999) Social capital and community effects on population and individual health. *Ann N Y Acad Sci*. 896: 120–30. 10.1111/j.1749-6632.1999.tb08110.x.

PMID: 10681893. Available at: https://pubmed.ncbi.nlm.nih.gov/10681893/. Accessed: November 21, 2022.

40 Lochner, K., Kawachi, I., Kennedy, BP. (1999) Social capital: a guide to its measurement. *Health Place* 4: 259. 10.1016/s1353-8292(99)00016-7. PMID: 10984580.

41 Snel, E., Engbersen G., de Boom, J., and van Bochove, M. (2022) Social capital as protection against the mental health impact of the COVID-19 Pandemic. *Front Sociol* 7:728541. 10.3389/fsoc.2022.728541. PMID: 35516815; PMCID: PMC9063781.

42 Makridis, CA. and Wu, C. (2021) How social capital helps communities weather the COVID-19 pandemic. *PLoS One.* 16: 1: e0245135. 10.1371/journal.pone.0245135. Erratum in: *PLoS One.* 2021 Sep 23, 16: 9: e0258021. PMID: 33513146; PMCID: PMC7846018.

43 Wernli, D., Clausin, M., Antulov-Fantulin, N., Berezowski, J. et al. (2021) Building a multisystemic understanding of societal resilience to the COVID-19 pandemic. *BMJ Glob Health.* 6: 7: e006794. 10.1136/bmjgh-2021-006794. PMID: 34301677; PMCID: PMC8300552.

44 Mollica R, Augusterfer, E., Friccione, G., Graziano, S., et al. (2020) New Self Care Protcol p. 2 Available at https://hprtselfcare.org. Accessed: November 21, 2022

45 Sherblom, JC., Umphrey, LR., and Swiatkowski, P. (2022) Resilience, Identity Tension, Hope, Social Capital, and Psychological Stress During a Pandemic. *Advers Resil Sci.* 3: 1: 37–51. 10.1007/s42844-021-00049-3. Epub 2021 Oct 30. PMID: 34746800; PMCID: PMC8556146. Available at: Accessed: December 24, 2022

46 Eulich, W. and Liana SW. (2022) Two Years in, Pandemic Resilience Propels Action. *Christian Science Monitor* Available at: https://www.csmonitor.com/Daily/2022/20220310?cmpid=ema:ddp:20220310:1141128:read&sfmc_sub=61636896&id=1141128#1141128. Accessed: August 27, 2022.

47 Ibid.

48 Rosen, B., Preisman, M., Read, H. et al. (2022) Providers' perspectives on implementing resilience coaching for healthcare workers during the COVID-19 pandemic. *BMC Health Serv Res* 22: 780 Available at: https://doi.org/10.1186/s12913-022-08131-x Accessed: January 15, 2023

49 Park, ER., Sylvia, LG., Streck, JM., and Luberto, CM. (2021) Launching a resiliency group program to assist frontline clinicians in meeting the challenges of the COVID-19 pandemic: Results of a hospital-based systems trial. *Gen Hosp Psychiatry.* 68: 111–12. 10.1016/j.genhosppsych.2020.10.005. Epub 2020 Nov 2. PMID: 33229013; PMCID: PMC7605784.

For more on self-care for health-care practitioners see also https://hprtselfcare.org/

50 For more information, see La Cliniquita Available at: https://www.lacliniquita.com. Accessed: November 21, 2022.

51 Burston, A (2021) 1,933 Available at: https://www.lacliniquita.com/casa/; Accessed: September 11, 2022. Reprinted with permission.

Chapter 6

COVID-19 Crisis Creates Opportunities for Community Health Resilience Plan

Community Health Workers at the Center

Norbert Goldfield, Robert Crittenden, Durrell Fox, John McDonough, Len Nichols, and Elizabeth Lee Rosenthal

This paper was written in April 2020, a scant two and a half years ago, but in pandemic time reckoning it was at the beginning of "COVID time." We knew so little; so little had yet happened. It is important to reprint this paper here (it was first published in the *Journal of Ambulatory Care* Management, 43, no. 3, in July–September 2020, under the title "Community-Centered Population Health"), as it provides more detail on the role of Community Health Workers (CHWs) in the proposed Community Health Resilience Plan (CHRP) which I discuss in detail in chapter 8. It is also worth reprinting just to see how far we have come in terms of treatment and how the situation has deteriorated in terms of the overall political situation in the United States. The version of the paper below contains a number of changes and adaptations for this book.

Introduction

Dealing with the COVID-19 coronavirus requires a coordinated transnational effort. As of early April, it has become apparent that the more medicalized and decentralized the society, the more widespread the virus. Still, the catastrophe is worldwide and exploding in the United States as we write these words attempting to draw meaning from it.[1]

The virus has exposed glaring weaknesses that cannot be unseen. The US healthcare system's embrace of patient-centered care is being tested. This has been the best that our US system has to offer, placing patients at the center of a clinical care team in a medical setting. By downplaying the importance of social and other structural determinants of health, including racial and ethnic inequities, we have worsened our current crisis. We have guaranteed that its burdens will be unequally borne by the most vulnerable among us, who, in turn, will ultimately impact the health of the whole community. By underfunding public health capacity for so long, and by downplaying early warning signs that pointed to the impending crisis, we have worsened the effects of the virus on us all and on our economy. Most tragically, we have lost sight of the individual at the center of care and, by extension, humanity as a whole. Patients come into care settings isolated from their family and caregivers, with some attended in hospital settings via telemedicine to ensure virus isolation. The patient often ends up alone, the sad epitome of individualism, and, in the absence of curative approaches, with only palliative care.

This outbreak is an intensive care and a public health challenge, as well as a humanitarian crisis. As Dr. Jim Yong Kim, former president of the World Bank and former director of Partners in Health, put it, "while governments around the world have been announcing massive, unprecedented stimulus packages to keep their economies from collapsing during the pandemic—efforts that are absolutely critical— what we are facing, fundamentally, is a public health crisis."[2]

In respect to the US healthcare system, we need to begin now to focus on a future system that embraces:

1. A community health resilience plan (CHRP) (defined below and in Chapter 8);
2. Pandemic solutions for the entire population; and
3. A long-term plan for the next pandemic, as discussed in the recent National Academy of Medicine report.[3]

We need a new paradigm, one that moves from a *patient-centered* care system to a *community-centered* health and social-care ecosystem. Unlike much of the current US medical care system, the community sector has lacked funding and development. Strong and consistent sources of support are needed to make this sector viable and keep it flourishing. After the passage of the Affordable Care Act (ACA) in 2010, Neal

Halfon and colleagues published an article entitled "Applying a 3.0 Transformation Framework to Guide Large-Scale Health System Reform."[4] Over that decade, no such fundamental transformation took place. This paper is intended to marshal the gaps and exposed shortcomings revealed by the COVID-19 coronavirus pandemic crisis and to integrate insights about upstream investments that have been made since the ACA to describe an aspirational but ultimately achievable concentration on population health. We believe this framework will not only better protect against future pandemics but also better serve individuals by centering on preserving and improving health in ways that address both health and social needs through focusing on serving people in the communities where they live.

In the near term, as there is no current and will be no coherent federal response to the COVID-19 pandemic, state and other local leaders have been implementing and will continue to implement different types of community-based efforts to control and suppress this pandemic. What will happen to all these initiatives, employing many people with varied backgrounds once the initial crisis passes? We suggest that these initiatives should evolve into a new health system with community health workers (CHWs) at its center. The remainder of this paper fleshes out the framework and the key unifying role that CHWs should play that would tie the different state/local initiatives dealing with this pandemic together into a focus on a community health resilience plan (CHRP).

A CHRP system with CHWs at its center will be resilient and robust enough to move us down the road toward recovery from COVID-19, and it can help prevent future pandemics, all within an evolving community-centered population health system. The remainder of this paper will specify

A. Short-term control and suppression pandemic solutions leading to CHRP

    1. The joint State of Massachusetts and Partners in Health Program

    2. The State of Washington initiatives

    3. A national response policy proposal

B. Middle-term development of the CHPR workforce team

In a separate companion article, "Fitting Community Health Resilience Plan (CHRP) into the Health Care Delivery Patchwork: The Politics of CHRP (Chapter 7 of this book),"[5] I examine political considerations necessary for evolving CHRP from the existing health care delivery patchwork.

Short-Term Control and Suppression Pandemic Solutions Leading to CHRP

Nonpharmaceutical interventions (NPIs) remain central for the management of COVID-19 because there are no licensed vaccines or coronavirus antivirals. States have taken the lead on this effort.[6] A good example of NPIs can be seen in the approach, as described below, taken by the State of Massachusetts in a public-private partnership between the State of Massachusetts and Partners in Health.[7] In addition, the State of Washington has partially implemented and is continuing to develop innovative uses of emergency response systems (EMS) often linked to local fire departments.[8] Other states are planning to follow suit. CHWs should and in some cases are assuming leadership roles, though not in a systematic manner.

Several critical components are needed in the short term. Foremost is a strong public health presence that is community focused. Having a number of capabilities is essential in order to accomplish what we know works early in an epidemic—testing, contact tracing, and isolation. CHWs represent the glue for such a strong community-focused public health presence. We propose a roadmap for moving a CHRP system forward, with CHWs playing an active leadership and partnership role at every turn.

First, *close monitoring of changes in epidemiology and of the effectiveness of public health strategies and their social acceptance.* This stage of control of the pandemic (which does not deal with the elimination of the virus) will be a long haul, as it involves not just immediate control but also long-term suppression. Along with some of the subsequent steps, this is exactly what, in theory, the April 3, 2020, announcement of the State of Massachusetts-led effort will accomplish.

Second, *continued evolution of enhanced communication strategies that provide general populations and vulnerable populations most at risk with actionable information for self-protection, including identification of symptoms and clear guidance for those seeking treatment.* As they are closest to the communities they are serving, CHW leadership and CHWs and other front-line staff will adapt these evolving communication strategies to best serve their local particular communities. CHWs have been part of a team of first responders for years; COVID-19 has helped people think differently about the term "first responders."

Third, *continued intensive source control, entailing the isolation of patients and persons testing positive for COVID-19, contact tracing and health monitoring, strict health-facility infection prevention and control, and use of other active public health control interventions with continued active surveillance and containment activities at all other sites, with regular reporting to the World Health Organization (WHO) and sharing of data.* CHWs will need to work with other specialized members of the community-based healthcare team in coordination with the hospital systems.

Keeping as many people as possible at home, via social distancing, is a critical component. From a concrete point of view, the Massachusetts Department of Public Health (DPH) recommendations are key:

> Scale up specially trained paramedics supported by physician telemedicine consultations, a 24/7 nurse call center, and remote laboratory and biometric monitoring can provide evaluation, testing, and clinical management and intervention for all aspects of care in the quarantine period for certain individuals with presumptive or confirmed Covid-19 infection.[9]

CHWs need to lead and be the focal point of this team, as they are best positioned to, for example, connect up and, as appropriate, work with paramedics in order to keep as many people at home as possible.

In addition, because a key COVID-19 complication is respiratory problems, another recommendation is to "modify and remotely support certain consumer continuous positive airway pressure (CPAP) devices and oxygen concentrators to support less-ill persons, thereby freeing up ICU beds. We are confident that with telemedicine and simple monitoring of blood oxygen saturation using widely available and low-cost consumer devices, many patients requiring supplemental oxygen can be safely cared for in their own homes."[10]

Fourth, *success in preventing and overcoming the challenges posed by the pandemic are dependent on intensified active surveillance, led by and implemented by CHWs.* This model should be followed for possible infections in all countries using the WHO-recommended surveillance case definition.

Fifth, *with widespread community transmission established and anticipated, the transition by the United States to include mitigation activities, especially if contact tracing becomes ineffective or overwhelming and an inefficient use of resources.* Examples of mitigation activities include social distancing, canceling public gatherings, school closure, remote working, home isolation, observation of the health of symptomatic individuals supported by telephone or online health consultation, and provision of essential life support such as oxygen supplies and mechanical ventilators, in both clinical and care settings. CHW leadership and action can be a key to the success of these endeavors among many communities, including those often left behind.

Sixth, *serological tests that can estimate current and previous infections in general populations need to be developed and then deployed.* CHWs can play an active role here in reaching marginalized populations to ensure that they have access to testing services and that any actionable results are reported to those impacted in a timely way with culturally appropriate messaging and needed support for action.

Seventh, *preparation to ensure the resilience of health systems in all countries.* Such preparation is already carried out for seasonal influenza, anticipating severe infections and the course of the disease in older people and other populations identified to be at risk of severe disease. State, national, and international agencies are needed to coordinate in a positive care coordination and supported referral feedback loop with CHWs and CHW-led local, state, and regional organizations.

Finally, *continued research and evaluation are important to understand the source of the outbreak and its impacts.* Collecting the evidence necessary for the prevention of future coronavirus outbreaks should begin with studies of animals and animal handlers in markets. As called for by Dr. Camara Jones, disaggregation of COVID-19 data to identify differential impacts of the virus on varied populations will be important.[11] CHWs can play a critical role in supporting this surveillance and assessment effort, building on their core skills in the area of individual and community assessment and in partnering in research and evaluation.[12] Evaluation of mitigation processes and system developments will also be key to learn from and improve future response capacity.

Case Examples of Population Health Response to the Pandemic: The Joint State of Massachusetts and Partners in Health Program; The State of Washington EMS/Fire Department Initiative

The responses implemented in the State of Washington and under development in Massachusetts exemplify the effort that needs to be replicated throughout the world. The State of Washington has a well-coordinated public health approach to COVID-19 with consistent leadership from the Governor and has implemented standard case identification, tracing, and isolation. In addition, the public EMS, part of local fire departments, has complemented this effort. Initially, the EMS leadership focused on testing and assisting in the management of first responder COVID contact. The initial goal was to ensure healthy people could return to work as soon as possible. That system included specified testing stations and a system to follow positives. This was put together rapidly partly because these same fire departments have developed community-focused case management systems for vulnerable people, people with behavioral health problems, and opiate use. They are currently working with their communities to develop better case management in more communities, including rural areas, and are developing systems focused on expanding their testing and tracing to the general population, complementing the work of the public health workers. They offer another model of CHRP and could potentially be partnered with CHWs to extend their reach more fully, allowing them to focus at practicing at the top of their scope.

In the Massachusetts partnership, the state has planned for, in tandem with three other partners, the training and deploying of hundreds of contact tracers (CTs), responsible for calling people who have been in close contact with confirmed COVID-19 patients. The CTs' work, combined with the state's response initiatives, will provide support to people in quarantine in order to contain the spread of COVID-19. CHWs will take on many of these roles, but other individuals with other types of backgrounds will certainly be engaged as well.

The Massachusetts Community Tracing Collaborative (CTC) is a partnership of four groups:

- MA COVID-19 Command Center: Provides overall direction and coordination;
- Commonwealth Health Insurance Connector Authority (CCA): Working with Accenture/Salesforce to enable a virtual support center and connectivity; and
- Massachusetts Department of Public Health (DPH): Maintains data, guides, and processes.
- Partners in Health (PIH): Hires and manages the workforce and contributes technical expertise from tuberculosis, HIV, cholera, and Ebola virus epidemics and decades of community-based interventions, many that include CHWs.

Finally, Scott Gottlieb, Mark McLellan (two health policymakers who have served under Republican administrations), and colleagues recently proposed a massive federal program that essentially outlines a federally funded national COVID-19 surveillance system.[13] In the current political climate in Washington, such efforts will not be easy to enact.

Middle-Term Development of the CHRP Workforce Team

The key element of the Community Health Resilience Plan (CHRP) system consists of a team that includes, at its center, frontline community-centered experts who will be empowered to:

a. implement neighborhood and home-centered care that includes case finding,
b. reinforce healthcare treatment plans, and
c. advance health promotion and preventive services.

That frontline professional is the community health worker (CHW). A nationally recognized definition adopted by the American Public Health Association (APHA) CHW section describes the CHW as a:

frontline public health worker who is a trusted member of and/or has an unusually close understanding of the community served. This trusting relationship enables the worker to serve as a liaison/link/intermediary between health/social services and the community to facilitate access to services and improve the quality and cultural competence of service delivery. A community health worker also builds individual and community capacity by increasing health knowledge and self-sufficiency through a range of activities such as outreach, community education, informal counseling, social support, and advocacy.[14]

To build this new CHRP system, we must create policy mechanisms to support it. Initial policy proposals include the following:

a. Support integration of CHWs through resources allocated to start and strengthen CHW services, including resources for capacity building and service implementation to ensure CHW-led workforce development.
b. Develop communications and connections between the CHWs, public health agencies, health care providers, behavioral health care, and social service providers, such as housing, food sources, and transportation.
c. Identify required skills for the CHW professional central to this reconfigured system. CHW's core roles and competencies[15] must be developed. Aspects of

lay-led Chronic and Infectious Disease Self-Management may be a critical added skill for CHWs.[16]

d. Encourage the development of state CHW standards through supporting CHW-driven professional guidelines and credentialing processes, including certification, as guided by the National Association of CHWs, established in 2019.

e. Promote a strategy of statewide pilots of CHRP that build on a number of successful and promising examples (such as the program instituted by Massachusetts). This will require congressional and Centers for Medicare and Medicaid Services action to support demonstrations of such programs that are from and for communities. States and their governors can lead by addressing issues that are specific to their communities and add to the national dialogue.

f. And, finally, remain mindful of longer-term population health strategies that will strengthen long-term health and social system resiliency and sustainability as immediate pandemic reactions are fashioned and long-term pandemic amelioration (not just viral suppression) strategies are developed.

Components of a CHW-Led Population Health Approach

Two overall types of skills are called for in a CHW-led population health approach. The first set of skills would be provided by CHWs. As they form the center of the population health approach, they should be familiar with the community. CHWs will be supported, at the center of the system (see Table 6.1 for the list of roles), by professionals trained in specialized care, who offer the second set of skills. Specialized care will consist of care that is appropriate for a pandemic (crucially, respiratory support) and is geared to the fact that much-specialized care is increasingly delivered

Table 6.1 Roadmap to Community Centered Population Health for Pandemic Control and Suppression with Community Health Workers at the Spoke

Integrated Community Health Workers to Support:

1. Ongoing Monitoring of Changes in Epidemiology and Impact of Mitigation Activities
2. Continued Evolution of Communication Strategies
3. Continued Intensive Source Control, Including Isolation
4. Intensified Active Surveillance
5. Timely Application of Mitigation Activities such as Social Distancing, Remote Working, and Home Isolation
6. Development and Deployment of Serological Testing
7. Preparation to Ensure the Resilience of Health Systems in All Communities and Countries
8. Ongoing Research and Evaluation on the Outbreak and on Responses Systems Processes

in the home (including, for example, infections needing intravenous antibiotics). Adequate, appropriate, and accessible mental health services are needed for both specialized care and pandemic response. The CHWs will require appropriate training to assess when and what type of specialized care to draw on for home visits and community gatherings.

Conclusions

What happens to the hundreds of Massachusetts-based CTs that Partners in Health has hired after the immediate pandemic is controlled and suppressed? What about the State of Washington EMS professionals who have expanded their professional expertise to include intimate knowledge of the communities that they work in? What if the federal program involving the US Public Health Service that Gottlieb et al. recommends comes to pass?[17] Are these federal employees temporary or permanent? The authors of this paper posit that such efforts should represent the next step in the evolution of our health system. Massachusetts, Washington, and other states could become laboratories highlighting both the challenges and opportunities that emerge from the work that is being implemented as we write to fight this pandemic. This could follow the pattern set by Massachusetts as the first state to enact what eventually became the Affordable Care Act (ACA). However, such an eventuality cannot happen unless political considerations are addressed and interest groups become involved, and at least a portion of them sign off, so that CHRP can begin. If CHRP is to become a reality and not just another aspirational document, we need to begin now to shape the outlines of this approach as specified in this paper and to start the political work necessary for its implementation. If the development of the CHW workforce is at the core of this, as we have proposed, then CHW leadership will need to be fully at the center of any planning activities impacting their workforce and the communities they serve. The next politically oriented companion paper details the opportunities and challenges to CHRP development and implementation.

Notes

1 Nacoti, M., Ciocca, A., Giupponi, A., Brambillasca, A. et al. (2020) At the epicenter of the Covid-19 pandemic and humanitarian crises in Italy March 20, 2020. *NEJM Catalyst.* Available at: https://catalyst.nejm.org/doi/pdf/10.1056/CAT.20.0080. Accessed: November 21, 2022.

2 Partners in Health. (2020) FAQs: Hiring, process behind PIH's efforts in MA Covid response. *Partners in Health.* Available at: https://www.pih.org/article/faqs-hiring-process-behind-pihs-efforts-ma-covid-response. Accessed: November 21, 2022.

3 Hick, Jl., Hanflink, D., Wynia, MK., and Pavia, AT. (2020) *Duty to plan: Health care, crisis standards of care, and novel coronavirus SARS-CoV-2.* Available at: https://nam.edu/duty-to-plan-health-care-crisis-standards-of-care-and-novel-coronavirus-sars-cov-2/.

Accessed: April 13, 2020. See also chapters 10 and 11 for summaries of additional, more recent National Academy of Medicine reports.

4 Halfon, N., Long, P., Chang, DI., Hester, J. et al. A. (2014) Applying a 3.0 transformation framework to guide large-scale health system reform. *Health Aff* (Millwood). 33: 11: 2003–11. 10.1377/hlthaff.2014.0485. PMID: 25367996.

5 Goldfield, N. (2020) Fitting community-centered population health (CCPH) into the existing health care delivery patchwork: The politics of CCPH. *J Ambul Care Manage.* 43: 3: 191–98. doi: 10.1097/JAC.0000000000000339. PMID: 32467432.

6 Heyman, D. and Shindo, N., (2020) WHO scientific and technical advisory group for infectious hazards Covid-19: What is next for public health? *Lancet* 395: 10224: 542–45. Available at: https://www.thelancet.com/journals/lancet/article/PIIS0140-6736(20)30374-3/fulltext. Accessed: December 25, 2022.

7 Partners in Health. (2020) PIH partners with Mass Governor's office on Covid-19 response. *Partners in Health.* Available at: https://www.pih.org/article/pih-partners-mass-governors-office-covid-19-response?fbclid=IwAR1oGTckFiBT7WxdWV6id Sc3d_L0ZbY-1Yg5ChJh85805-Td7XL0PSpN7oA. Accessed: December 14, 2022.

8 Washington State Dept of Health. (2020) Covid-19. *Washington State Dept of Health.* Available at: https://www.doh.wa.gov/Emergencies/Coronavirus. Accessed: December 14, 2022.

9 Master, R., Gottlieb, G., Margulies, D., and Kryder, K. (2020) The urgent need for a comprehensive and scalable care response to the COVID-19 pandemic in Massachusetts. *Boston Globe.* Available at: https://www.bostonglobe.com/2020/03/25/opinion/mass-needs-comprehensive-care-response-coronavirus/. Accessed: November 21, 2022.

10 Ibid.

11 Jones C. (2020) Coronavirus disease discriminates. Our health care doesn't have to. *Newsweek.* Available at: https://www.newsweek.com/2020/04/24/coronavirus-disease-discriminates-our-health-care-doesnt-have-opinion-1496405.html. Accessed: April 13, 2020.

12 See for more details Community Health Worker Core Consensus Project. Available at: https://www.c3project.org/. Accessed: November 21, 2022.

13 Gottlieb, S., Rivers, C., McClellan M., Silvis, L. et al (2020) National coronavirus response: A road map to reopening. *American Enterprise Institute.* Available at: https://www.aei.org/wp-content/uploads/2020/03/National-Coronavirus-Response-a-Road-Map-to-Recovering-2.pdf. Accessed November 21, 2022.

14 Community Health Worker Section, American Public Health Association. Available at: https://www.apha.org/apha-communities/member-sections/community-health-workers/. Accessed: November 21, 2022.

15 See for more details Community Health Worker Core Consensus Project. Available at: https://www.c3project.org/. Accessed: November 21, 2022.

16 Chronic Disease Self-Management For more information see: https://selfmanagementresource.com. Accessed: November 20, 2022.

17 Gottlieb, S., Rivers, C., McClellan, M., Silvis, L. et al. (2020) National Coronavirus Response A Road Map To Reopening. *American Enterprise Institute.* https://www.aei.org/wp-content/uploads/2020/03/National-Coronavirus-Response-a-Road-Map-to-Recovering-2.pdf. Accessed: December 25, 2022.

Chapter 7

Fitting Community Health Resilience Plan (CHRP) into the Existing Healthcare Delivery Patchwork

The Politics of CHRP

Prefatory note: This paper, written and published (in the *Journal of Ambulatory Care Management* 43, no. 3, in July–September 2020, under the title "Community-Centered Population Health") at the beginning of the pandemic in April 2020, retains its salience. The politics today around the proposed Community Health Resilience Plan (CHRP) described in Chapter 8 is the same as the politics in April 2020, with one major caveat. In that early period of the pandemic, I was aspirational and hoped that a restructuring of our health system could occur at a national level. The tragic reality is that there is no chance that the proposal described in Chapter 8 can come to pass at a national level— this even though any number of experts have published reports advocating on a national level many aspects of what I propose for statewide implementation in chapter 8. Toward the end of this chapter, I acknowledge back in 2020 that no national health program will occur and put my hopes into a statewide implementation.[1] While I don't detail the state-level political obstacles to what I propose in Chapter 8, the lamentable likelihood is that healthcare organizations, especially those serving our acute healthcare needs, will unfortunately be among those principally opposed. In contrast, employers could play a key role. Back in April 2020, I wrote about the economic cost of the pandemic.

DOI: 10.4324/9781003426257-9

At the time, I didn't appreciate the true unimaginably enormous economic, in addition to the tragic human, cost. It is thus employers, understandably focused on the bottom line, who could make the difference in making CHRP come to life.

This chapter will start with comparative comments on health systems in industrialized countries. I will then turn my focus to interest groups in the U.S. that determine the shape of the American health system. A focus on trust, discussed in the next section, is important as trust must underlie any consideration of substantial change in our very complex health system. Interest group engagement and the building up of trust are both critical if we are to consider the possibility of substantial health system change as described in more detail in Chapter 8. The version of the paper below contains a number of changes and adaptations for this book.

Introduction

The COVID-19 crisis has nakedly exposed the problems and huge holes in the healthcare system of the United States. Some European medical systems offer a contrast to the US system. Part of the reason that the United Kingdom has come together as a country is the population's faith and trust in its National Health Service.[2] Yet the United Kingdom has pursued an inconsistent response to the COVID-19 epidemic, resulting in many deaths. In contrast to the United Kingdom, Germany has a very popular universal health insurance system, together with an excellent public health infrastructure. These two features encouraged the forceful political leadership response that has resulted in massive testing and, thus far, many fewer deaths in Germany.[3]

The immediate challenge the United States faces in this and future pandemics is clear.

> In order to save lives, reduce COVID-19's burden on our healthcare system, ease strict social distancing measures, and confidently make progress toward returning to work and school, the United States must implement a robust and comprehensive system to identify all COVID-19 cases and trace all close contacts of each identified case. It is estimated that each infected person can, on average, infect 2 to 3 others. This means that if 1 person spreads the virus to 3 others, that first positive case can turn into more than 59,000 cases in 10 rounds of infections.[4]

While projections on deaths are inherently conjectural, scientists have factually determined that COVID-19 is highly transmissible. To address this hurdle, a recent report specifies:

> In order to trace all contacts, safely isolate the sick, and quarantine those exposed, we estimate that our public health workforce needs to add

approximately 100,000 (paid or volunteer) contact tracers to assist with this large-scale effort. This workforce could be strategically deployed to areas of greatest need and managed through state and local public health agencies that are on the front lines of COVID-19 response. To do this, we also estimate that Congress will need to appropriate approximately $3.6 billion in emergency funding to state and territorial health departments.[5]

It is unclear whether the executive branch will sign on to fund even 10,000 contact tracers (CTs), let alone the needed 100,000. At the same time, as of this writing, it is clear that a states-led effort with support from foundations and universities is emerging.[6] One could easily imagine a consortium that, for example, involves Northeastern states.[7] The critical question is whether a bipartisan group of states will work together. This will be especially important if, as seems likely, the federal executive branch remains on the sidelines. Yet, given the political polarization currently straining the country,[8] it is hard to imagine cooperation between states such as Florida and New York.

For today, we need to address the current pandemic from the point of view of both control and suppression. But such efforts could also provide insights into a post-pandemic restructuring of healthcare in this country. Take Massachusetts, which was the first state to pass legislation that eventually became the Affordable Care Act. What happens to the hundreds of CTs that Massachusetts is hiring to address this pandemic? This paper posits that the community health resilience plan (CHRP), as described in the companion paper (see Chapter 8), could represent the next step in the evolution of our health system. Massachusetts (among other states) could become a laboratory of a different order, demonstrating both the challenges and opportunities that emerge from the work that is being implemented to fight this pandemic. If CHRP is to become a reality and not just another aspirational document, political considerations must be addressed and interest groups become involved. However, while interest groups will ultimately determine the fate of CHRP, the key element in the theory of change is trust in government.[9] If one or several states succeed in addressing the COVID pandemic together with an associated, at least modest, economic resurgence, the population in those states could develop the trust in state leadership necessary to finally make fundamental changes in our healthcare system. Such change may be a once-in-a-lifetime or once-in-a-century opportunity. It is certain that the numbers of uninsured will skyrocket under the double pressures of illness and unemployment, and not just among the poor and young. The key question is whether this increase will lead to pent-up demand for significant change in our health system. This article argues yes, if there is sufficient trust in state leaders together with the mobilization of interest groups, discussed in the following section.

Interest Groups That Will Be Engaged in Any Implementation of CHRP

Major political actors will determine whether or not this country can finally evolve toward a system that truly focuses on community-centered population health. They include, in alphabetical order, with questions and/or brief comments appended:

Community Health Centers

Federally qualified health centers and others, many of them owned by hospitals, could play an important supportive role in shaping CHRP details. They have much to gain, as they have many community health workers already engaged in the community.

Consumer Groups

Consumers Union, Families USA, Protect Our Care, and Community Catalyst, among other consumer groups, could play *the* critical role in the implementation of the CHRP.

Employers

While initially employers might be opposed to CHRP, their engagement will be critical to any statewide CHRP implementation. This support is more likely to emerge if CHRP results in more productive/satisfied employees and, over time, lower healthcare costs. Will employers now realize that a CHRP approach offers a better outcome than the current patchwork? It is clear that employers, who largely see health insurance as a benefit requiring cost control, have been historically uninterested in the details of health system change. Might this pandemic open employers to considering alternatives, such as CHRP? Even if employers might become supportive, other interest groups in this list with a greater stake in the detailed functioning of our healthcare system will have to make the compelling argument. Employers might be supportive especially if they appreciate the severe economic cost of the pandemic.

Federal Government, Executive Branch

This sector of the government, in this (Trump) administration, would have to be dragged kicking and screaming into constructive action. The executive branch will have to be forced into covering the millions of newly uninsured.[10] So far, the executive branch has not and most likely will not exert leadership on issues such as a national shelter-in-place directive.[11] In completely missing virtually every opportunity to address the pandemic until it was too late, the executive branch has substituted not only primarily personal but also ideological grievances in its incompetent efforts to mount an effective national response.[12]

Federal Government, Congress

Together with state governments, this branch of government will be key to establishing CHRP. At this time, the House of Representatives (2020) is the only body that will be willing to consider legislation that could implement CHRP in a statewide demonstration-like initiative.

Federal Government, Judiciary

Though it will not come up until 2021, it is key that the Supreme Court does not rule against the constitutionality of the Affordable Care Act to ensure that as many people as possible have access to insurance and needed health services.

Health Insurers

The trade association America's Health Insurance Plans (AHIP) represents a formidable opponent and will have to be engaged, as it was for the passage of the Affordable Care Act (ACA) and for the defeat of the Clinton health reform effort. As proposed below, the only possibility to avoid all-out opposition is to start small, in one or a handful of states. The ideal situation is a state with one dominant private insurer in addition to the important typical domination of Medicaid.

AHIP also includes many managed care organizations (MCOs), both for-profit (e.g., United Health Care) and nonprofit (e.g., Kaiser). Logically, it is the MCOs that should be coordinating with and linking up with state departments of public health for CHRP. Although making it happen presents formidable organizational challenges, community health workers (CHWs), as discussed in the previous article (chapter 6), should act as the glue and form the center of CHRP. In such a system, they would be the link between MCOs and departments of public health. This organizational arrangement could encourage support from both MCOs and departments of public health. The challenge again will be payment. A regulatory approach similar to what is utilized in Germany could represent a framework for resolving the payment conundrum.

Health Professionals

Physicians, nurses, and all individual practitioners have their own professional associations that constitute important and powerful interest groups. These groups could be supportive of and will want to shape the contours of CHRP, provided that payment to professionals belonging to these groups continues (or increases) and that the implementation of CHRP does not lead to another bureaucracy. Overall payment to some categories of health professionals represents an unknown in the long term, as it is likely that the COVID-19 pandemic will lead to changes in health professional practice patterns in ways that we cannot foresee. That said, health professional associations might support CHW-centered CHRP as long as they could shape the details.

Hospital Associations

Will this pandemic force a political reckoning on the part of hospital executives that hospitals are not the appropriate center for population healthcare? Will this pandemic encourage the hospital industry to realize that it should focus on its core business, acute hospital care? Such an approach would constitute an off-loading of the pressure on hospitals for community outreach. This would, in turn, lead to the appropriate demise of accountable care organizations (ACOs), as hospitals will not be at the center of this CHRP system. At present, our American reality is that hospitals will still want to control the flow of money (via ACOs) or be guaranteed sufficient cash flow (as teaching hospitals). If we move to CHRP, hospitals will want to control the funds that will have to flow into these community entities. Despite this historical behavior, it is possible that hospitals could be induced to support CHTP that they do not control. Payment is the key to hospital support. Assuming that hospitals will insist on a continuation of the ACO movement, especially in states such as Massachusetts, where the ACO movement is strong, regulations will be needed that emphasize the CHW core of a true population health program.

Labor Unions

CHRP represents an important organizing opportunity—for the Service Employees International Union (SEIU), among others—for the hundreds of thousands of recently unemployed individuals. Labor unions could be critical to ensuring that these critical CTs or Community Health Workers (CHWs) obtain dignified payment and benefits. Unions such as SEIU have been at the forefront of efforts to promote CHWs, with hoped-for subsequent new union members to increase their ranks. In addition, labor unions such as the National Education Association, the United Auto Workers, and the Teamsters could see CHRP as a way to maintain employment for their own members.

Mayors and/or Local Public Health Departments, Together with Community Activists

The approach of empowering communities to build the health and social service ecosystem their residents actually need starts with elevating the voices and power of local government and community groups in a federalism of meaning. Local public health departments have to be far better funded and empowered. The coronavirus crisis has raised awareness of just how essential it is that local health departments cooperate with the local healthcare delivery and surveillance systems. Now is the time to provide sufficient funds for those functions, as well as others that can improve population health via the CHRP proposal (detailed in Chapter 8).

Pharmaceutical Companies and Device Manufacturers

The politics for these interest groups, especially pharma, will be tricky, considering that Americans are looking to "Big Pharma" for COVID-19 cures. New treatments and vaccines are all good for pharmaceutical and device manufacturers. However, their primary interest is to secure maximum prices for their products. Community health, which does not further this interest, would not be of concern to them. They are likely to be formidable opponents of any serious attempt to implement CHRP, and they are very well financed.

State Government

Together with Congress, this branch of government will be the key to any implementation of CHRP. States such as California, Massachusetts, New York, and Washington will likely lead the way. Before now, states have been at the forefront of many initiatives that have led to national implementation. If CHRP is to be put into effect, it will happen at a state level first, provided that its citizens have confidence and trust, as discussed below, in how the leadership has dealt with the COVID-19 pandemic.

The Importance of Trust

While Francis Fukuyama's book predicting the future success of liberal democracy[13] is arguably problematic at best, his book entitled *Trust: The Social Virtues and the Creation of Prosperity* has had longer staying power.[14] Most recently, Fukuyama highlighted two countries, South Korea and Germany, where there appears to be a high level of trust in government. What does trust mean? How does it relate to CHRP?

In his book, which weaves together trust and economics, Fukuyama emphasizes that standard economic theory does not apply to all human behavior. According to Fukuyama:

> The power of neoclassical (economic theory) rests on the fact that its model of humanity is accurate a good deal of the time: people can indeed be relied on to pursue their own selfish interests more often than they pursue some kind of common good.... the neoclassical premise is subject to significant qualification.... there are numerous occasions when people pursue goals other than utility.[15]

Fukuyama's conception of trust, adapted from others, "is the expectation that arises within a community of regular, honest, and cooperative behavior, based on commonly shared norms, on the part of other members of that community."[16] "Trust is built on two foundations. First, citizens must believe that their government has the expertise, technical knowledge, capacity, and impartiality to make the best available judgments…. The second foundation is trust in the top end of the political hierarchy."[17] Simply put, effectively implemented, CHRP could be a critical building block in reestablishing trust in government.

A Theory of Change

A public health crisis is unfolding, and the richest country in the world is struggling to effectively respond. Equipment, testing, and protective clothing are all in short supply. Most tragically, urgent messages about the importance of social distancing and the need for temporary shutdowns have been muddied by politics and poor leadership.[18] Could a strong public health system have averted this problem? Alas, in the United States, no such system exists. "In 2019, a consortium of public health organizations lobbied the federal government for $1 billion to help the nation's public health system modernize its data infrastructure. They were granted $50 million. In the wake of COVID-19, that sum has been increased to $500 million."[19]

Could this increase in funding be a sign that "the times they are a-changin'"? What would it take to not only rebuild our public health infrastructure but also imagine CHRP? State- or regionwide demonstrations, with stakeholders supported at first by foundations and over time by governmental programs, can mitigate the strength of the political forces that interest groups will inevitably marshal against such a major endeavor. The current Massachusetts effort could evolve into a statewide CHRP. Importantly, the Commonwealth Health Insurance Connector Authority (CCA), one of the four key organizations participating in the Massachusetts effort, could end up as a link between the structure administering the current Massachusetts system and a future CHRP. The CCA eventually developed into the health insurance exchanges that are such a critical part of the Affordable Care Act.

Politics will determine whether payment for the CHRP will consist of grafting a public health component on top of our traditional patient care system or whether a single CHRPP financial and administrative entity emerges—a form of a single-payer system. The latter may possibly make its debut as a response to this pandemic. Such a home-grown CHRP could bring together elements of the German health system (which allows for tightly regulated private insurers)[20] and the history of public health accomplishments of, among others, Partners in Health.[21] If the Massachusetts effort is successful, it is more likely that major employers in the Massachusetts-based high-tech industry and the dominant health insurer, Blue Cross Blue Shield, will be convinced to be supportive of CHRP.

The wealthy are particularly successful in blocking changes they don't like. The political scientists Martin Gilens of the University of California, Los Angeles, and Benjamin Page of Northwestern University have calculated that between 1981 and 2002, policies supported by at least 80 percent of affluent voters passed into law about 45 percent of the time, while policies opposed by at least 80 percent of those voters passed into law just 18 percent of the time. Importantly, the views of poor and middle-class voters had little influence.[22] Despite the fact that the poor are suffering disproportionately in the COVID-19 epidemic, many in the middle class are not just suffering economically but, more to the point, also losing their health insurance. Both the middle class and the poor will have to be a key political force in any push toward CHRP. This could very well happen if millions of newly uninsured emerge.

Above all, for CHRP legislation to pass, citizens will need to trust that governmental leadership—both public and private but led by public leaders—has the expertise to successfully implement CHRP. As a significant majority of American citizens will never exhibit this level of trust in the Trump administration,[23] for now, only the states will be able to implement CHRP. Before state leadership can win the trust of its citizens to make this happen, it must demonstrate its ability to control and suppress the pandemic and then begin at least a modest economic resurgence. With the support of senior public leadership, at least several of the interest groups described above should pose the question: What are states such as Massachusetts or Washington going to do with all the contact tracers (CTs) that they have hired and used so effectively to control and suppress this pandemic? How will we call on them with sufficient lead time before the next pandemic? In particular, citizen groups and unions will have to "connect the dots" and link CTs not just with an essential part of a strengthened public health system but one that could evolve into CHRP as defined in the previous paper.

Concluding Comments

The journalist and activist Masha Gessen wrote recently in the *New Yorker*, "In the Midst of the Coronavirus Crisis We Must Start Envisioning the Future Now."[24] She points to the impacts of this pandemic on our entire society: on us as human beings (for those of us that survive), our economic livelihoods, and our social fabric. These in turn will affect our political system.

To quote Gessen:

> Our political system, frayed as it was, is under extraordinary stress. The Supreme Court has delayed cases. The Justice Department is seeking extreme powers.[25] The Trump Administration is using the crisis as an opportunity to push through a more extreme version of its agenda. The President now lies to the nation daily not only on Twitter but also on live television, during briefings that he has turned into versions of his rallies. The election campaign is in a state of suspended animation. The borders are effectively closed. At the federal level, there is a real possibility that the coronavirus will paralyze the work of Congress, leaving the White House without check. At the local level, quarantine measures either have stopped or will stop all town councils, school boards, and community meetings. Local news media, an endangered species before the crisis, may have been dealt a final, fatal blow by the coronavirus.

Yes, it is true that we are polarized as a country even around the COVID-19 pandemic.[26] While many other countries are similarly polarized, Trump and his followers have singularly exacerbated polarization. Although it is unlikely that we, as Americans, can break through the societal logjam that Trump and his immediate circle have significantly increased (at least not until the November election), the COVID-19 pandemic provides us with a unique, once-in-a-century crisis and opportunity. Starting local, at the state level, is the American way. Trust and confidence, as described in this paper, in the implementation of the control and suppression of COVID-19 together with an at least modest economic resurgence could translate into support for local and/or statewide political leaders. These leaders could in turn work with interest groups to carry out major changes in our healthcare system.

Politics will ultimately determine how our current patient-centered acute care–focused healthcare system will change. The wealthy undoubtedly will continue to have an outsize influence on any legislation promoting CHRP. Despite this fact, we will at least think about becoming better in improving our response before the next pandemic hits. The question is whether the ongoing impact of this pandemic on our economic and social fabric will force states and Congress (the executive branch will continue to be MIA or, in fact, actively hostile) to flesh out different approaches to our next healthcare system, labeled as the Community Health Resilience Plan or CHRP. It is incumbent on all of us (policymakers, interest groups, and individuals) to contribute to this conversation and then act—now. While for the foreseeable future, CHRP will be impossible to build at a national level, CHRP can occur at a state level. It is fully described in the next chapter.

Notes

1 Wiseman, O. (2020) How Coronavirus Punctured the Brexit-Trump Parallels. *Politico.* Available at: https://www.politico.com/news/magazine/2020/04/11/coronavirus-uk-us-brexit-trump-177924. Accessed: November 21, 2022.

2 Ibid.

3 Tharoor, I. (2020) Where Germany had success in fighting coronavirus, Britain stumbled. *Washington Post.* Available at: https://www.washingtonpost.com/world/2020/04/13/where-germany-had-success-fighting-coronavirus-britain-failed/?utm_campaign=wp_todays_worldview&utm_medium=email&utm_source=newsletter&wpisrc=nl_todayworld. Accessed: April 13, 2020.

4 Watson, C., Cicero, A., Blumenstock, J. et al. (2020) *A national plan to enable comprehensive COVID-19 case finding and contact tracing in the US.* Baltimore, MD: Johns Hopkins University. Available at: https://www.centerforhealthsecurity.org/our-work/pubs_archive/pubs-pdfs/2020/a-national-plan-to-enable-comprehensive-COVID-19-case-finding-and-contact-tracing-in-the-US.pdf. Accessed: November 21, 2022.

5 Ibid.

6 Sun, L., William, W., Abutaleb, A. (2020) A plan to defeat coronavirus finally emerges, but it's not from the White House. *Washington Post.* Available at: https://www.washingtonpost. com/health/2020/04/10/contact-tracing-coronavirus- strategy. Accessed: November 21, 2022.

7 Craig, T. and Dennis, B. (2020) Governors form groups to explore lifting virus restrictions; Trump says he alone will decide. *Washington Post.* Available at: https://www.washington post.com/politics/governors-form-groups-to-explore- lifting-virus-restrictions-trump-says-he-alone-will- decide/2020/04/13/f04a401e-7d84-11ea-a3ee-13e1ae 0a3571_story.html. Accessed: November 21, 2022.

8 Gadarian, SK., Goodwin, SW., and Pepinsky, TB. (2021) *Partisanship, health behavior, and policy attitudes in the early stages of the COVID-19 pandemic. PLoS One.* 16: 4: e0249596. 10.1371/journal.pone.0249596. PMID: 33826646; PMCID: PMC8026027. Available at: https://journals.plos.org/plosone/article?id=10.1371/journal.pone.0249596. Accessed: December 25, 2022.

9 Fukuyama, F. (2020) The Thing That Determines a Country's Resistance to the Coronavirus. *The Atlantic.* Available at: https://www.theatlantic.com/ideas/archive/2020/03/thing-determines-how-well-countries-respond-coronavirus/609025/. Accessed: April 11, 2002.

10 Cancryn, A., Cook, N., and Luthi, S. (2020) How Trump surprised his own team by ruling out Obamacare. *Politico.* Available at: https://www.politico.com/news/2020/04/03/trump-obamacare-coronavirus-164285. Accessed: November 21, 2022.

11 Mahdani, A., Miller, Z., and Fram, A. (2020) Trump resists national shutdown, leaving it up to states. *AP News.* Available at: https://apnews.com/article/virus-outbreak-donald-trump-ap-top-news-politics-united-states-c90b24e60a4853c ebe96ec995b626f9b. Accessed: November 21, 2022.

12 Aytac, S., Rau, E., and Stokes, S. (2018) Beyond opportunity costs: Campaign messages, anger and turnout among the unemployed. *British Journal of Political Science.* Available at: https://www.cambridge.org/core/journals/british-journal-of-political-science/article/beyond-opportunity-costs-campaign-messages-anger-and-turnout-among-the-unemployed/444928192590BEE9B4FB47BB4B7507D9. Accessed: November 21, 2022.

13 Fukuyama, F. (1992) *The End of History and the Last Man.* New York: Free Press.

14 Fukuyama F. (1995) *Trust.* New York: Free Press.

15 Ibid. pp 18, 19.

16 Ibid. p. 19.

17 Fukuyama, F. (2020) The thing that determines a country's resistance to the coronavirus. *The Atlantic.* Available at: https://www.theatlantic.com/ideas/archive/2020/03/thing-determines-how-well-countries-respond-coronavirus/609025/. Accessed: November 22, 2022.

18 Interlandi, J. (2020) The U.S. approach to public health: Neglect, panic, repeat. *New York Times.* Available at: https://www.nytimes.com/2020/04/09/opinion/coronavirus-public-health-system-us.html. Accessed: Novemember 21, 2022.

19 Ibid.

20 Tikkanen, R., Osborn, R., Mossialos, E., Djordjevic, A. et al. (2020) *International health systems profile.* Germany Commonwealth Fund. Available at: https://www.commonwealthfund.org/international-health-policy-center/countries/germany. Accessed: November 22, 2022.

21 See https://www.pih.org

22 The Editorial Board. (2020) The America we need. *New York Times.* Available at: https://www.nytimes.com/2020/04/09/opinion/coronavirus-inequality-america.html?action=click&pgtype=Article&state=default&module=styln-opinion-inequality-series&variant=show&region=ABOVE_MAIN_CONTENT&context=opinion-inequality-promo. Accessed: November 21, 2022.

23 Boot, M. (2020) The second most dangerous contagion in America: Conservative Irrationality. *Washington Post*. Available at: https://www.washingtonpost.com/opinions/2020/04/12/second-most-dangerous-contagion-america-conservative-irrationality/. Accessed: November 22, 2022.

24 Gessen, M. (2020) In the midst of the Coronavirus crisis, we must start envisioning the future now. *The New Yorker*. Available at: https://www.newyorker.com/news/our-columnists/in-the-midst-of-the-coronavirus-crisis-we-must-start-envisioning-the-future-now?mbid=&utm_source=nl&utm_brand=tny&utm_mailing=TNY_CoronaVirus_040420&utm_campaign=aud-dev&utm_medium=email&bxid=5bea06da24c17c6adf125b09&cndid=50856718&hasha=5c81c9183ba5aa9f-d682e58291889859&hashb=cebff94d072ef16164c89170fc47fd36337bb64d&hashc=8c6ed225fce9f934f5b1b6d643f99d2a761bd86aefbc7f884c1cbe6 4c9dce77f&esrc=bounceX&utm_term=TNY_CoronaVirus. Accessed: November 22, 2022.

25 Swan, BW. (2020) DOJ seeks new emergency powers amid Coronavirus pandemic. *Politico*. Available at: https://www.politico.com/news/2020/03/21/doj-coronavirus-emergency-powers-140023?fbclid=IwAR08qgYEjLNmvRtFI9oOlUl8QJoTrIWj4U77elbeRBYAcz9_-JnBuyfHpQ. Accessed: December 25, 2022.

26 Gadarian, Goodwin, and Pepinksy op. cit.

Chapter 8

Building Trust in Public Health

Coordinating Our Public Health and Acute Care Systems

The healthcare system and the related entities that pay for care are often bystanders when it comes to the work and performance of the public health system. But their interdependence has rarely emerged as clearly as it has during the coronavirus pandemic.[1]

Introduction

During the COVID pandemic the population of the United States suffered to a much greater extent than people in other industrialized countries.[2] As already mentioned, the United States experienced ten times the death rate, adjusted for population, as compared to, for example, Australia. The key difference between the two countries is trust. Australians have a much greater trust in government than do Americans. After introductory comments that lay out the rationale for the Community Health Resilience Plan (CHRP), this chapter summarizes our national and state public health challenges. I then highlight the important role of community health workers (CHW) before detailing the details of the CHRP.

The roots of public distrust of government in the United States run deep and are multifaceted. But as it relates to the pandemic, a weak response characterized by poor communication between the health system and the public and between the public health system and medical care providers contributed to the problem.[3] To increase confidence in our public health system in a sustained manner, greater links between public health and communities and between the public health and acute care systems are essential.

We need a new paradigm, one that moves from a *patient-centered* care system (our traditional acute care, managed care, long-term care system) to a *community-centered* health and social care ecosystem also called CHRP. However, recognizing that a comprehensive national or federal public health initiative will be difficult if not impossible to implement in today's polarized climate, this chapter suggests a state-level approach, as in Massachusetts, the author's place of residence. In the United States, states have historically taken the lead on many important national issues. Of significance, both the legalization of gay marriage and the system of healthcare coverage advanced in the Affordable Care Act passed under President Barack Obama began in Massachusetts under a Republican governor. Thanks to bipartisan leadership, we can point to an effective statewide public health system with effective coordination between the public health and acute healthcare systems in Massachusetts that could be a model for the country.

These recommendations build on Massachusetts's history, already existing regulations, and recently passed and/or implemented initiatives, including the excellent report published in June 2022 by the Massachusetts Joint Committee on COVID-19 and Emergency Preparedness and Management (hereafter, the Joint Committee). The Massachusetts Joint Committee is an arm of the Massachusetts state legislature, the General Court of the Commonwealth of Massachusetts.[4]

This proposal addresses our pandemic public health needs today and for the future by

- coordinating our public health (PH) and patient care-centric systems (hereafter PCC). For the purposes of this chapter, PCC includes acute care, primary/specialty care, and long-term care, along with arrangements for managed care, including accountable care organizations (ACOs);
- using Community Health Workers (CHWs) to activate this engagement between PH and PCC health systems. Most importantly, CHWs represent the link between the two (PH and PCC) health systems.[5] While technology can provide a tremendous amount of information, a human interface, locally recognized in the community, can more effectively address the profound socioeconomic and simply human dimensions of any pandemic, including contact tracing. PH and PCC both already have CHWs, but they need to be better coordinated with each other. The CHW will be empowered to implement neighborhood- and home-centered care.
- adopting validated quality metrics tied to financial incentives to maximize quality outcomes;
- addressing the needs of the entire population with a focus on those most at risk; and

■ implementing this approach initially in several counties, revising it, and then reintroducing it using continuous quality improvement with standardized metrics throughout the state within 24 months.

The underlying rationale is that we will continue to face ongoing pandemics and endemics. Pandemics worsen socioeconomic health disparities. Thus, interest groups that represent disadvantaged populations should be looking for comprehensive yet realistic solutions that will significantly benefit their constituencies. Pandemics, and COVID in particular, also represent a significant drain on our overall economy (trillions in economic cost![6]), and thus should be of vital interest to the commercial sector. If commercial interests work together with advocacy groups representing the disadvantaged, then these two groups can make this proposal reality and, in turn, encourage healthcare organizations to facilitate greater linkages between PH and PCC.

Public Health Challenges in the United States: The Massachusetts Healthcare Landscape

The United States, like the rest of the world, preferentially invests in the acute healthcare system rather than public health. Of the $3 trillion in health spending in this country, public health receives at most 3%.[7] This figure does not reflect the wide variation in state and local investments in public health; where you live determines the level of public health protection you receive.

As another example of disparity, MassHealth, the health insurance program for low-income people, provides coverage for more than 1.8 million people—over a quarter of the state's residents. MassHealth is an important contributor to the state's high insured rate—currently, more than 97%. (For comparison, the uninsured rate in Texas is 19%; in the United States overall it is 9%.[8])

Who delivers traditional public health services today in Massachusetts? Its 351 cities and towns are independently organized for the delivery of local public health services and operate autonomously from the Massachusetts Department of Public Health. Massachusetts local boards of health, or local health departments (LHDs), are charged with a complex set of responsibilities, including enforcement of state sanitary, environmental, housing, and health codes. Within a county, one town might have a mask mandate and the next one might not; one town might have professionally trained public health staff, while the next town might rely on volunteer staff.

To begin to address inadequacies in our public health system, the Massachusetts legislature signed the SAPHE 1.0 (State Action for Public Health Excellence) into law in 2020. In this chapter, I propose a new bill, which we will call Community Health Resilience Plan, or CHRP. It builds on what has been accomplished (SAPHE 1.0) and what passed the Massachusetts House of Representatives and

Senate but did not come into law because the governor returned the bill for further consideration (SAPHE 2.0).[9] CHRP is much more ambitious than SAPHE 2.0. See Appendix 1 for further description of both bills.

The Critical Role of Community Health Workers (CHWs) in a Coordinated PH-PCC System

In a *community-centered* health and social care ecosystem as defined in the proposal, the CHW will implement both neighborhood and family-centered care. A nationally recognized definition adopted by the American Public Health Association (APHA), CHW section, describes the CHW as a:

> Frontline public health worker who is a trusted member of and/or has an unusually close understanding of the community served. This trusting relationship enables the worker to serve as a liaison/link/intermediary between health/social services and the community to facilitate access to services and improve the quality and cultural competence of service delivery. A community health worker also builds individual and community capacity by increasing health knowledge and self-sufficiency through a range of activities such as outreach, community education, informal counseling, social support, and advocacy.[10]

CHWs are extensively trained in their field.[11] Practically speaking, CHWs constitute the ideal link between PH and PCC and, in fact, would serve as the focal point of the healthcare and social work professional team to fulfill several specific Joint Committee recommendations. The titles of these Joint Committee recommendations directly relevant to CHWs are: "Create a mechanism to report at-home and rapid testing results to local board of public health and the Department of Public Health"; "Invest and Prepare for Contact Tracing" and "Fund contact tracing efforts by investing in local public health and supplemental funding during disease outbreaks"; and "Improve data gathering and release by the Commonwealth to make it more transparent, readily accessible, detailed and timely." CHWs in both PH and PCC that communicate and coordinate with each other are the ideal human interface for implementing each of these recommendations.

Another Joint Committee recommendation involves CHWs but merits additional comment and, in some ways, goes to the heart of the challenge that the United States faces in rebuilding our public health system and effectively addressing this and future pandemics. In "Establish a temporary COVID-19 Recovery Corps," the Joint Committee highlights how such a Corps would "engage volunteers in the ongoing need for response and recovery assistance in the Commonwealth. Throughout the pandemic volunteers played a crucial role in our response and recovery and organized volunteerism can continue to be an important part of the ongoing response to this and future crises."

Researchers have amply documented the relationship between health and civic engagement. The latter is an important social determinant of health and, importantly, can impact the outcomes of the political determinants of health. The National Academy of Sciences (NAS) in June 2022 published a report entitled "Civic Engagement and Civic Structure to Enhance Health Equity."[12] According to this NAS report:

> Civic engagement, like affordable housing, a living wage, and a good education, is a social driver of health status, affecting the health of both engaged individuals and society. "In other words, ... the health of members of a democratic society and the health of the democracy are intertwined." Good outcomes for democracy and for health equity require:
>
> ■ Authentic community organizing by local people
> ■ Civic engagement that brings together and lifts up diverse voices which are crucial for a healthy democracy
> ■ Taking community needs into account
> ■ Research, such as community-based participatory research and participant-driven interviews that treat participants with dignity and respect (e.g., explaining to community members how data will be used)

Simply put, CHWs working together with COVID-19 Recovery Corps would provide the person power and local credibility to connect social and political determinants of health with improved outcomes, especially during a pandemic. CHWs represent the point person for maximizing the efficacy of this Joint Committee's recommendation. CHWs are the key to a community-focused population-based health system that links PH and PCC. In turn, such an effectively implemented population-based health system can be a critical element in not only dealing well with this and future pandemics but also, in fact, rebuilding trust in American institutions.

Community Health Resilience Plan (CHRP): Coordinating Public Health and Patient-Centric Care Systems; The Next Step in Pandemic Preparedness

A dramatically improved public health system could decrease the fractionation of current public health resources and maximize communication between traditional government-provided/funded public health services and PCC organizations. CHRP, which builds on the Joint Committee report of the Massachusetts legislature and SAPHE 1 and SAPHE 2, aims to significantly enhance the public health system by inextricably coordinating LHDs with the PCC health systems in Massachusetts. CHRP accomplishes this integration by

■ distributing CHWs throughout both LHDs and the PCC system, making CHWs the linchpin of this coordinated dual system;

■ encouraging quality improvement through financial and administrative incentives for LHDs and PCC to work collaboratively. Together, they can continuously improve public health quality outcomes that are adjusted for socioeconomic disparities.

Both legislation and regulation are required to implement CHRP. Legislation must be passed to provide the overall framework of a coordinated PH and PCC system, including

■ the CHW linchpin;
■ the establishment of a special assistant to the governor for COVID-19 vaccine administration;
■ the specification, via a senior executive-level position, of the relation between the Department of Public Health and MassHealth;
■ funding for a strengthened PH infrastructure (Recommendations pertaining to funding are specified in the Joint Committee Report.);
■ funding for improved indoor air quality in schools and public spaces also requires legislation and should follow the specific recommendations identified in the Joint Committee Report.

In addition, critical elements of CHRP need to be addressed via regulation. It will be critical to specify how to embed CHWs as the center of the spokes of the public health "wheel." The most recent Massachusetts ACO waiver extension request to the federal government states that ACOs will: "Streamline care coordination to ensure members have a single accountable point of contact."[13] CHWs should be the single accountable point of contact. Regulation, in particular, can encourage communication between LHDs and PCC via a CHW on what constitutes "high and rising-risk members." Contact-tracing regulations can highlight the best-practice patterns in light of what we have learned from initial efforts, such as the contact-tracing contract that the state gave to Partners in Health at the start of the pandemic.[14]

CHWs can also provide the critical link between the community, primary care, and the schools. Schoolchildren are among those who have suffered the most during this pandemic, especially from an emotional and social perspective. During the pandemic, education inequality has widened.[15] CHWs should be engaged with, for example, school counselors to best coordinate family-centered public health, emotional, and physical care, especially as it pertains to children under stress.[16]

Regulations will be needed to specify CHW-based outcomes and process metrics to be tracked for the entire state, with a particular focus on areas with significant socioeconomic disparities. See Appendix 3 for a suggested set of metrics that improve quality outcomes, measure the impact of PH and PCC coordination, and specify the financial incentives to improve outcomes of socioeconomic disparities. These metrics are all validated. In addition, the current payment system must be adjusted, with a particular focus on payment adjustment based on the burden of illness of the population (risk adjustment) and how to incorporate CHWs into the payment system.

Conclusion

In summary, this proposal provides a politically challenging but much-needed approach to addressing our pandemic public health needs by

a. encouraging coordination between public health and patient-centric health systems;
b. using validated quality metrics with accompanying financial metrics and CHWs to guide the implementation of this coordination;
c. addressing the needs of the entire population, with a special focus on those most at risk;
d. implementing as soon as practicable a small-scale test of this approach so that necessary details for its feasibility, budgetary implications, effectiveness, and sustainability can be appraised. Small-scale interventions (in several counties) could occur within 6 months and full-scale implementation within 24 months.

Passing CHRP legislation depends on engaging interest groups outside healthcare, including the commercial sector and groups advocating on behalf of those who have suffered the most during the pandemic.

Notes

1 Commonwealth Fund. (2022) Meeting America's Public Health Challenge. Available at: https://www.commonwealthfund.org/publications/fund-reports/2022/jun/meeting-americas-public-health-challenge. Accessed: August 31, 2022.
2 Rabin, RC. (2022) US Life Expectancy Falls Again in Historic Setback. *New York Times*. Available at: https://www.nytimes.com/2022/08/31/health/life-expectancy-covid-pandemic.html. Accessed: August 31, 2022.
3 Commwealth Fund Op cit.
4 Report of the Joint Committee on Covid-19 and Emergency Preparedness and Management (2022) *Massachusetts State Legislature*. Available at: https://www.politico.com/f/?id=00000181-ad90-d667-abfb-efbd009f0000. Accessed: November 23, 2022.
5 Goldfield, NI., Crittenden, R., Fox, D., McDonough, J. et al (2020) COVID-19 Crisis Creates Opportunities for Community-Centered Population Health: Community Health Workers at the Center. *J Ambul Care Manage*. 43: 3: 184–90.
6 Centers for Disease Control and Prevention (2016) *Health United States, 2016*. Available at: https://www.cdc.gov/nchs/data/hus/hus16.pdf#094. Accessed: November 23, 2022.

7 Shalal, A. (2022) IMF sees cost of COVID pandemic rising beyond $12.5 trillion estimate. *Reuters*. Available at: https://www.reuters.com/business/imf-sees-cost-covid-pandemic-rising-beyond-125-trillion-estimate-2022-01-20/. Accessed: November 23, 2022.

8 Conway, D. and Mykyta, M. (2022) Decline in Share of People Without Health Insurance Driven by Increase in Public Coverage in 36 States. *United States Census Bureau*. Available at: https://www.census.gov/library/stories/2022/09/uninsured-rate-declined-in-28-states.html. Accessed: November 23, 2022.

9 Shoenberg, S. (2022) Lawmakers, advocates hit Baker's opt-in approach to public health. *Commonwealth*. Available at: https://commonwealthmagazine.org/politics/lawmakers-advocates-hit-bakers-opt-in-approach-to-public-health/?fbclid=IwA R3H_-VRP_Oi14R1Dya4SS5Wnoj04TUHC6nM9GuKjxrb3jH7IKoJDPIdePw. Accessed: November 23, 2022.

10 American Public Heealth Association, Community Health Worker Section (2022) *Community Health Workers American Public Health Association*. Available at: https://www.apha.org/apha-communities/member-sections/community-health-workers. Accessed: November 23, 2022.

11 See https://nachw.org/membership/chw-networks-and-certification-programs/

12 Ayers, J., Dawes, D., Ramakrishnan, K. (2021) Civic Engagement and Civic Infrastructure to Advance Health Equity: A Workshop. *National Academies, Science, Engineering, Medicine*. Available at: https://www.nationalacademies.org/event/06-14-2021/civic-engagement-and-civic-infrastructure-to-advance-health-equity-a-workshop. Accessed: November 23, 2022.

13 Massachusetts 1115 Waiver Extension Proposal (2021) *Mass Health*. Available at: https://www.mass.gov/doc/1115-waiver-extension-request-summary/download. Accessed: November 23, 2022.

14 Partners in Health (2020) Partners in Health Helping State Trace Contacts of COVID-19 Patients in Landmark Agreement with MA Gov's Office *Partners in Health*. Available at: https://www.pih.org/ma-response. Accessed: November 23, 2022.

15 Samuels, CA. and Prothero, A. (2020) Could the 'Pandemic Pod' Be a Lifeline for Parents or a Threat to Equity? *Education Week*. Available at: https://www.edweek.org/leadership/could-the-pandemic-pod-be-a-lifeline-for-parents-or-a-threat-to-equity/2020/07. Accessed: November 23, 2022.

16 Gysbers, NC. (2022) Embrace the past, welcome the future: A brief history of school counseling. *American School Counselors Association*. Available at: https://www.schoolcounselor.org/getmedia/52aaab9f-39ae-4fd0-8387-1d9c10b9ccb8/History-of-School-Counseling.pdf. Accessed: November 23, 2022.

Appendix 1: Summary of SAPHE 1 and SAPHE 2 (the latter passed the Massachusetts House of Representatives and Senate in 2022, but the governor returned it to the legislature for further consideration)

SAPHE 1.0.

The Massachusetts legislature signed SAPHE 1.0 into law in 2020. The act provides resources to elevate performance standards to improve the municipal and regional public health system. In addition, it increases cross-jurisdictional sharing of public health services to strengthen the service delivery capabilities of the municipal and regional public health system. It improves planning and system accountability of the municipal and regional public health system, and it establishes workforce standards, including, but not limited to, education and training standards for municipal and regional public health officials and staff. Under SAPHE 1.0, the above are all recommendations and are subject to appropriations.

SAPHE 2.0

SAPHE 2 did not become law in the session that finished in July 2022. It proposes to:

- Ensure minimum public health standards for every community.
- Increase capacity and effectiveness by encouraging municipalities to share services.
- Create a uniform data collection and reporting system.
- Establish a sustainable state funding mechanism to support local boards of health and health departments.

Appendix 2: Summary of the Report of the Joint Committee on Covid-19 and Emergency Preparedness and Management: Findings and Recommendations of the Committee. January 2021–June 2022

Scope of the Committee: The Committee on COVID-19 and Emergency Preparedness and Management serves as an oversight and advisory committee to monitor and investigate issues related to coronavirus disease (COVID-19) emergency response and recovery.

Purpose of the Report: While this report does not make recommendations on all areas that are affected by the COVID-19 pandemic, the Committee has endeavored to highlight key areas focused on emergency preparedness and management.

Recommendation: Statewide Response Must Be Transparent, Predictable, and Well-Communicated

The Committee recommends that the statewide response to COVID-19 be communicated thoroughly and with significant advance notice of any changes. Where appropriate, the state must consider and integrate input from responding local and regional officials into its response plans.

The Committee heard consistently about sudden and dramatic shifts in the state's response, particularly around COVID-19 testing and the vaccine rollout. For example, some local and regional boards of public health and HMCC [Health and Medical

Coordinating Coalitions] stakeholders prepared to administer and manage vaccine clinics, with some stakeholders conducting local vaccine drills, before the Commonwealth suddenly shifted its early strategy to focus on high throughput mass vaccination sites.

Recommendation: Plans for Vaccines Should Be Suited to Communities, Particularly Communities of Color and Other High-Risk Populations

The Committee recommends that emergency response planning prioritize those who are hardest hit to promote racial equity and cultural competency. Building trust among high-risk communities requires bringing people into the planning process and the implementation of response actions. Adhering to existing local action plans will help the state reach these populations.

While mass vaccination sites may have been efficient at delivering large quantities of vaccinations, the Commonwealth's initial, almost singular, focus on these vaccine super-sites raised substantial and persistent equity concerns. In all, the state launched eight mass vaccination sites, located at Gillette Stadium in Foxborough, Fenway Park/the Hynes Convention Center in Boston, the Reggie Lewis Center in Boston, the Natick Mall, a Doubletree Hotel in Danvers, the Eastfield Mall in Springfield, and the former Circuit City in Dartmouth. Some of these sites were poorly served by public transportation, and only accessible via car or ridesharing.

Recommendation: Strengthen Local and Regional Public Health Infrastructure

The Committee recommends strengthening local and regional public health infrastructure so local officials can lead and plan for local emergency response. This will require sufficient funding streams and expanding regional initiatives.

However, there are stark differences and long-standing inequities between and within public health departments in the state's 351 cities and towns. The Commonwealth is one of the few states that does not dedicate annual baseline or formulaic funding to local public health departments. As a result, municipalities in the Commonwealth have widely varying abilities to provide public health protections to residents. While some cities and towns have well-funded, professionally-staffed local public health departments, some local boards of health are staffed solely by volunteers, and others have only a single part-time staff member. This is always dangerous for public health, and during the pandemic the consequences were severe.

Recommendation: Fortify Supply Chains and Stockpiles

The Committee recommends that the Commonwealth have a well-maintained stockpile of personal protective equipment (PPE) and additional medical and non-medical supplies that can be immediately accessed and distributed when needed. The

Commonwealth should also take efforts now to increase its capacity to manufacture key supplies in Massachusetts in order to fortify its supply chains.

Recommendation: Create a Mechanism to Report At-Home and Rapid Testing Results to Local Boards of Public Health and the Department of Public Health

The Committee recommends the creation of a mechanism to report at-home and rapid testing results. Once implemented, DPH should publish the relevant data on how many positive rapid tests have been reported daily.

At the start of the pandemic testing was sparse, reflecting the limited available supplies and high demand. As the pandemic progressed, supplies of tests have generally improved. Now, at-home, self-administered, rapid COVID-19 antigen tests have been authorized for use by the FDA and can be purchased online or over the counter at pharmacies. These tests are covered by health insurance, providing up to 8 tests per person per month, at no cost to the consumer.

Recommendation: Prepare and Plan for Testing Needs, Including Local Production of Testing Materials

The Committee recommends that the Commonwealth prepare a scalable plan to increase testing and production of testing materials locally during emergencies. The Commonwealth should be prepared to be self-sufficient in its ability to provide testing for its residents during a pandemic.

Efforts to provide Commonwealth residents with COVID-19 testing resources faced many challenges in the early days of the pandemic, and some of those challenges persisted throughout, or resurfaced through multiple spikes. Some of these testing challenges were unique to COVID-19, some of those challenges were outside of the state's control, and some could have been avoided with better preparation and by following previously developed plans.

Recommendation: Invest and Prepare for Contact Tracing

The Committee recommends that the state invests in developing a branch of the MAVEN software or its equivalent specifically for contact tracing that contact tracers who are not from local health departments can access directly.

Because the state was unprepared to conduct contact tracing, the system that was developed was inefficient, ineffective, and expensive. Laboratories would upload COVID-19 test results into the state's Massachusetts Virtual Epidemiologic Network (MAVEN) system where local boards of health, local health departments, or their representatives at regional health collaboratives could access the information on positive COVID-19 test results. Local boards of health could then conduct contact tracing on a positive case within their jurisdiction or could assign a case, multiple cases, or all cases to the CTC.

These difficulties in part stemmed due to the initial lack of representation of local public health in the process. Public health nurses and other local and regional board of health staff could have brought their expertise to the software design and workflow protocols.

Recommendation: Fund Contact Tracing Efforts by Investing in Local Public Health, with Supplemental Funding during Disease Outbreaks

The Committee recommends that the Commonwealth prepare and fund local health officials to lead contact tracing in future pandemics.

The Committee recommends that the Commonwealth prepare local health jurisdictions to lead contact tracing in future pandemics (emphasis added). Having both local public health jurisdictions and the CTC conduct contact tracing meant that two entities were responsible for performing the same task, which is inefficient. Local health jurisdictions experience cross-jurisdictional problems when conducting contact tracing, such as when a resident lives in one town but works in another. Regional health collaboratives are the solution, but they require flexible funding as recommended by this report.

The Committee recommends that local health jurisdictions should also be funded to deliver baseline public health protections. Local health departments and regional health collaboratives should be the Commonwealth's first choice for conducting contact tracing, and any emergency funding should support their work.

Recommendation: Continue and Expand State Supported Wastewater Monitoring and Epidemiology

The Committee recommends that the Commonwealth use wastewater surveillance as an essential tool for detecting and tracking the presence of COVID-19 and other diseases over time. This surveillance should be used as a mechanism to warn of re-emergences or outbreaks of disease and trigger the deployment of countermeasures to reduce transmission. The Commonwealth should initially expand additional wastewater monitoring, focused on adding more within municipalities, institutions of higher education, office campuses, congregate care settings, and prisons.

Recommendation: Improve Data Gathering and Release by the Commonwealth to Make It More Transparent, Readily Accessible, Detailed, and Timely

The Committee recommends that when making pandemic data public, DPH should work to include cross-tabulations detailing infections, hospitalizations, and deaths by racial and ethnic background, and by age. To track surges, the data should be as granular as possible, mindful of the complexities in reporting for small populations.

Recommendation: Restructure and Update the Commonwealth's Incident Management Structure to Better Align with Well-Established Standardized Incident Organizational Structures

Recommendation: Utilize Anchor Dates and Trigger Thresholds for Emergency Planning, Response, and Recovery

The Committee recommends identifying key indicators that provide early signals about virus transmission rather than relying on lagging indicators such as hospitalizations or mortality rates to trigger response actions.

The implementation of anchor dates, key data indicators, and trigger thresholds will enable better collaboration and increase trust in the government response. Projecting dates or publicizing thresholds for action helps the public know the purpose of and what to expect, as well as any collective pandemic management goals.

Recommendation: Establish a Temporary COVID-19 Recovery Corps

The Committee recommends establishing a temporary COVID-19 Recovery Corps to engage volunteers in the ongoing need for response and recovery assistance in the Commonwealth.

Throughout the pandemic volunteers played a crucial role in our response and recovery and organized volunteerism can continue to be an important part of the ongoing response to this and future crises. The Medical Reserve Corps, which includes both clinical and non-clinical volunteers, along with student volunteers in the Academic Public Health Corps played important roles. In addition, the Massachusetts Service Alliance (MSA) was a consistent supporter of volunteerism throughout the pandemic.

The MSA is a private, non-profit organization that works to expand volunteerism and service in Massachusetts by providing individuals and organizations with funding, training, and support to enable them to strengthen our communities. The MSA also operates the Commonwealth Corps program, a service program founded by Governor Patrick in 2007, that focuses on cultivating, training, and placing service members and nurturing volunteerism across the Commonwealth.

MSA's network of service members assisted with the distribution of face masks, hand sanitizer, and other safety supplies to residents in Worcester. MSA service members also distributed hand warmers, a particular help to people experiencing housing insecurity or homelessness during the pandemic. Additionally, service members assisted with health education and youth education programs, adapting lessons to be conducted completely outside or shifting to remote online learning. The MSA also assisted organizations in increasing the capacity for volunteers, administering over $200,000 worth of COVID-19 resilience grants to 56 non-profit organizations. These grants targeted organizations that needed additional financial support for volunteer capacity, supplies, or projects that were impacted by COVID-19.

The Committee recommends that a COVID-19 Recovery Corps be established to further aid the recovery process, given the quantity and quality of work done by the MSA and Commonwealth Corps before and during the pandemic. If established, service members could be placed with health-focused organizations, including municipal public health departments, community health centers in high-risk communities, and service organizations providing food and supply distribution. As the recovery progresses, service members could help connect residents with job training, adult education, work readiness, and employment opportunities.

Creating a COVID-19 Recovery Corps will cultivate a class of service members with the skills and commitment needed to remedy the deep scars this pandemic has left on the Commonwealth.

Recommendation: Improve Indoor Air Quality in Schools and Other Public Settings

The Committee recommends that the Commonwealth establish a plan and funding mechanism to improve indoor air quality in schools and other public buildings.

Air quality is important for population health. Prolonged exposure to polluted air can cause respiratory disease. Those with pre-existing respiratory conditions were more likely to become severely ill from COVID-19. In addition, adequate ventilation and filtration in indoor settings can help reduce transmission of COVID-19 and other airborne respiratory viruses. However many school buildings in the Commonwealth are old, have poor ventilation, or lack right-sized filtration devices. The Commonwealth also does not have comprehensive data on the air quality of our K-12 classrooms, where students and teachers alike spend at least eight hours per day.

Recommendation: Designate a "Special Assistant to the Governor for COVID-19 Vaccine Administration" for All Efforts Related to Vaccinations

The Committee recommends that a special assistant to the Governor be created to serve as the senior level position in the administration for the purposes of reinvigorating the efforts to close existing vaccination gaps, planning for future surges, and setting and meeting immediate and long term goals for COVID-19 vaccination rates in the Commonwealth.

Many of these recommendations are included in omnibus legislation approved by the Committee, H. 4714, *An Act for a Better Prepared Massachusetts*. As of June 23, 2022, the legislation was also approved by the Health Care Financing Committee and is pending before the Senate Committee on Ways and Means.

While the Committee has presented a number of recommendations to improve our future preparedness and emergency response capacity and capabilities, these observations are by no means exhaustive of all possible improvements. Similarly, the successes and challenges that have been described above represent only a piece of the overall response to the pandemic. A statewide after-action-report will be needed to properly outline the Commonwealth's response in the past two years with the level of detail that it deserves, including a substantive analysis of the entirety of our pandemic response, especially as we transition into a new phase(s) of pandemic management. This kind of after-action analysis could be accomplished as part of a comprehensive commission charged with a complete review of what transpired during the pandemic.

Despite these challenges, there is reason for optimism. Our understanding of how the virus behaves and what we can do to protect individuals and communities and minimize its spread has improved. The COVID-19 vaccines have proven to be effective at limiting transmission, hospitalizations, and death. Researchers and scientists have published studies that detail the effectiveness of the pharmaceutical and non-pharmaceutical tools we have available to protect ourselves via collective and coordinated action if another surge arises.

Early in the pandemic, the state government acted with diligence to make substantive changes—from a public health order to stay home, to strong eviction protections, and more. In so doing, the state has proven it can lead adaptively. Dedicated officials at all levels clearly demonstrated that they can be trusted during a pandemic to get the job done. Legislation and funding have been passed to bolster local public health infrastructure so that we enter the next pandemic with stronger tools to fight back. The reflections in this Committee report and the efforts of so many continue to point the way forward toward what is needed now and the work to prepare for the next contagion, the next pandemic, the next disaster. These recommendations include components that require unwavering commitment in order to achieve the intended reforms. The Committee recommends that the state begin this work without delay.

Appendix 3: A Suggested "Flight Instrument Panel," or Dashboard of Quality and Financial Metrics—*System-Wide, Public and Patient Care–Centric Health Systems; Patient-Reported Outcome Information*

General Approach: Bull, C., Teede, H., Watson, D., Callander, EJ. (2022) Selecting and Implementing Patient-Reported Outcome and Experience Measures to Assess

Health System Performance. *JAMA Health Forum*. 3:4 e220326. doi:10.1001/jamahealthforum.2022.0326

What Matters Index: Wasson, JH., Ho, L., Soloway, L, Moore, LG. (2018) Validation of the What Matters Index: A brief, patient-reported index that guides care for chronic conditions and can substitute for computer-generated risk models. *PLoS One*. 13:2: e0192475. Doi: 10.1371/journal.pone.0192475. PMID: 29470544; PMCID: PMC5823367.

Patient Activation/Empowerment Measure: Hibbard, JH., Stockard, J., Mahoney, ER., Tusler, M. (2004) Development of the Patient Activation Measure (PAM): conceptualizing and measuring activation in patients and consumers. *Health Serv Res*. 39: pp: 1005-26. doi: 10.1111/j.1475-6773.2004.00269.x. PMID: 15230939; PMCID: PMC1361049.

Health Confidence: Wasson, J. and Coleman, EA. (2014) Health confidence: an essential measure for patient engagement and better practice. *Fam Pract Manag*. 21:5 pp: 8-12. PMID: 25251348.

Claims Data

Background Information: Greene, J., Hibbard, JH., Sacks, R., Overton, V., et al (2015) When patient activation levels change, health outcomes and costs change, too. *Health Aff* (Millwood). 34:3 pp:431-7. Doi: 10.1377/hlthaff.2014.0452. PMID: 25732493.

Risk-Adjusted ER rate, divided into the following categories: Potentially Preventable Conditions, including Ambulatory Care Sensitive Conditions, COVID-related, Mental Health/Substance Abuse

Risk-Adjusted Hospitalization rate, divided into the following categories: Potentially Preventable Conditions, including Ambulatory Care Sensitive Conditions, COVID-related, Mental Health/Substance Abuse

   Immunization Status
   Timeliness of Prenatal and Postpartum Care

Chapter 9

Reform of Our National and International Organizations

Leadership, Trust, Power—and Money

In 2017, before the COVID pandemic, the World Bank concluded:

> Multiple pandemics, numerous outbreaks, thousands of lives lost, and billions of dollars of national income wiped out—all since the turn of this century, in barely 17 years—and yet the world's investments in pandemic preparedness and response remain woefully inadequate.[1]

And then the COVID pandemic hit. According to the Lancet Commission on Lessons for the Future from the COVID-19 Pandemic:

> The multiple failures of international cooperation include (1) the lack of timely notification of the initial outbreak of COVID-19; (2) costly delays in acknowledging the crucial airborne exposure pathway of SARS-CoV-2, the virus that causes COVID-19, and in implementing appropriate measures at national and global levels to slow the spread of the virus; (3) the lack of coordination among countries regarding suppression strategies; (4) the failure of governments to examine evidence and adopt best practices for controlling the pandemic and managing economic and social spillovers from other countries; (5) the shortfall of

DOI: 10.4324/9781003426257-11

global funding for low-income and middle-income countries (LMICs), as classified by the World Bank; (6) the failure to ensure adequate global supplies and equitable distribution of key commodities—including protective gear, diagnostics, medicines, medical devices, and vaccines—especially for LMICs; (7) the lack of timely, accurate, and systematic data on infections, deaths, viral variants, health system responses, and indirect health consequences; (8) the poor enforcement of appropriate levels of biosafety regulations in the lead-up to the pandemic, raising the possibility of a laboratory-related outbreak; (9) the failure to combat systematic disinformation; and (10) the lack of global and national safety nets to protect populations experiencing vulnerability.[2]

A recent article in *Newsweek* recently highlighted that

The old saying, never let a crisis go to waste, has never been so relevant. COVID-19 is certainly a crisis of historic proportions. Its dangers to health and prosperity are graphically demonstrated by the number of deaths, currently heading to 4 million, and the lost output, projected to reach 22 trillion. But the dangers are not limited to the present crisis. Today's global pandemic was predictable and predicted. Eleven separate reports[3] proposed important changes to the global approach to health security that would have mitigated or even snuffed out this crisis at an earlier stage. And today there is a real threat that as vaccines beat variants in the richer parts of the world, the crisis does go to waste.[4]

At a global level, the *Newsweek* article succinctly gets it right:

■ Pandemic preparedness must be considered a global public good.
■ All countries should collectively finance pandemic preparedness and response as global public goods with strategic value, not as aid.

Over the next five years, significant short-term improvements might take place in American national public health organizations such as the Centers for Disease Control and Prevention (CDC). Little will occur at the international level until and unless China and the United States can effectively collaborate. Even in this case, on the current difficult relationship between the United States and China, I maintain—as I have throughout this book—that health professionals can make a significant impact.

This chapter will focus on opportunities for organizational improvement at the national and international levels. It is an arena where health professionals could make an even greater difference than they already do. In 1980, physicians Bernard Lown and Yevgeny Chazov founded International Physicians for the Prevention of

Nuclear War (IPPNW), an organization that received the Nobel Peace Prize for its efforts. Using this model, we look for another pair or, better yet, a group of health professionals from different continents to come forward and address this and future pandemics. A new group of health professionals pursuing effective pandemic responses could represent the next generation of health-based peacebuilding. Such a group of health professionals would constitute leadership in its best form. In the meantime, leaders can concentrate on making necessary changes in national and international health organizations. That is the focus of this chapter. In particular, this chapter will center on needed reforms at the federal level, with a separate section on the CDC and international engagement/agencies, with a particular emphasis on the World Health Organization (WHO).

The Federal Level

Background

In the United States and its territories, public health officials from 59 state and territorial health departments conduct a variety of public health functions.[5] These functions include disease detection, vaccine administration, and emergency preparedness and response. In addition, approximately three thousand county, city, and tribal health departments; about two hundred thousand public and private clinical laboratories; and multiple federal agencies also conduct these functions.

Because of the many entities involved, the identification and management of a public health emergency call for effective communication and collaboration across all levels of government and the public health community. Efficient information sharing among these entities is essential to prepare for, respond to, and manage a public health emergency.

In 2009, 43% of Americans had a positive view of the nation's public health system—not exactly a ringing endorsement. During the pandemic, this figure fell to 34%.[6] This means that a frightening number of Americans lack trust in our country's ability to deal with the pandemic. This concerns both trust in the science of public health and the ability to deliver interventions. The federal government is involved in both. With health professions playing the key role, the federal government can lead the way to increase trust by engaging in effective communication with both public health professionals and the public at large. Specifically, developing trust in science involves, in addition to leadership, a multipronged approach that begins with national leadership appreciating the critical importance of the public's belief in science. It is remarkable that, according to Roger Pielke, the United States:

> "is almost alone worldwide in its lack of a high-level expert advisory body on COVID-19, and this matters for policy, politics, and trust."
> Trust has many dimensions, he explained, which can include trust in

experts and institutions, but trust between institutions is also important. He posited that the lack of such an advisory body is a core failing of intelligence in the pandemic response.[7]

The specifics of increasing trust are key. What can largely happen only at a federal level? At this level, we need leadership and money on the following issues and for the following federal organization:

■ Health and National Security
■ Stockpiling essential supplies
■ Crisis Standards of Care
■ Data
■ Protection of public health professionals
■ Food and Drug Administration (FDA)
■ Centers for Disease Control and Prevention (CDC)

Health and National Security

These three words, "health" and "national security," do not typically go together in the United States. But a sustained effort to link health with national security at both a national and international level is essential. That calls for structuring organizational relationships between national security and public health agencies at a federal level. If this had been in place in 2019 it is very likely we would have been better prepared to face the COVID pandemic. It's even possible that we would not be continuing to argue about the origins of the COVID virus.

And, as discussed by Scott Gottlieb,[8] federal interest in coupling health and national security waxes and wanes with the visibility of the health issue—Clinton with AIDS, Bush with bioterrorism, Obama with SARS. It is one thing for the general public to completely ignore safe public health practices, such as the appropriate use of masks during COVID. However, at a national political level, leadership that remains constantly aware of pandemics in general, and the connection between health and national security specifically, together with the appropriate resources to remain prepared and act instantly, makes a critical difference in outcomes.

The following paradox illuminates the importance of connecting health and security in the United States. As will be discussed below, it is important that individual countries strengthen the World Health Organization's ability to facilitate cooperation between countries in all aspects of pandemic preparedness. We face the challenge, though, that future pandemics will likely see a repeat of what happened at the start of COVID—the shutting down of countries, leading to crippling economic consequences. Knowing this, countries may well curb the communication of outbreaks of potentially emerging pandemics. Thus, it is likely that even if WHO reform because of COVID leads to increased cooperation between countries "on paper," these lofty words will be no substitute for a closer integration between health and national security at a national level in the United States. Such closer integration could "strongly encourage" countries to increase cooperation.

Stockpiling Essential Supplies

I constantly remind myself, as reported elsewhere in this book, of what the hospital to which I admit patients, Baystate Medical Center in Springfield, Massachusetts, went through, as reported in the *New York Times Magazine*, to try and obtain personal protective equipment (PPE). Yes, hospitals everywhere learned to not depend on the federal government. But the fact that the federal government was missing in action was the key ingredient in the disastrous US COVID response, with its tragic consequences.

At a minimum, it is imperative that we either establish an adequate stockpile of predicted necessary pandemic supplies or put in place legislative and/or regulatory tripwires that force the federal government to declare a national emergency when a pandemic occurs. Such a declaration allows the federal government to require companies to produce essential supplies—in this case, for example, PPE.[9] But this is not enough; part of pandemic preparedness is making sure in advance of a pandemic that an appropriate stockpile of necessary supplies, such as PPE, is on hand, which did not occur consistently in the Trump administration.[10] The situation has improved after Biden became president.[11]

Crisis Standards of Care

Crisis standards of care (CSCs) make it possible to make a "substantial change in usual healthcare operations ... made necessary by a pervasive (e.g., pandemic influenza) or catastrophic (e.g., earthquake, hurricane) disaster."[12] Developed by the Institute of Medicine as a concept in 2009, the federal government has a unique role in laying the groundwork for the effective deployment of CSCs. Unusually, some cities can act without the engagement of the federal government, as in the case of El Paso:

> El Paso, Texas ... used its unity to meet the needs of the population, even without political support at the state level. *The state did not have a CSC plan* [emphasis added] ... the significant surging of patients in El Paso during the first wave of the pandemic resulted in all hospitals being confronted with the need to conduct very aggressive resource-sparing strategies. Among those strategies was the use of an alternate care site, but there were concerns about the need for a common message to patients and the community about what the facility would be. ... The community did have strong political leadership and support at the local level from the mayor and the county judge executive, who supported hospitals collectively taking advantage of alternate care sites with common messaging and discharge criteria.[13]

Yet this situation is unusual; at a national level, effective CSC implementation did not occur. There has been little federal leadership on the many ingredients that go into appropriate CSCs including providing systemic approaches to the many health workforce shortages and together with scientific and non-technical aspects of CSCs. Importantly, at a recent National Academies meeting on this topic, several people spoke to the need for a closer relationship between acute health and public health leaders.[14] This need echoes aspects of what I discussed in the last chapter. It is likely that these bonds can best truly occur at a state level.

Data

Ensuring actionable, reliable, and timely data is largely a federal responsibility. Sadly, we have a long way to go even as of this writing in December 2022. According to a Government Accounting Office (GAO) report published in *June 2022*, two years after the start of the COVID pandemic:

> In January 2021, we reported on the need for more complete and con-sistent COVID-19 data to inform health care indicators. We noted that the lack of complete and consistent data limited the ability to monitor trends in the pandemic and assess the impact of public health actions to prevent and mitigate the spread of COVID-19. Addition-ally, we noted that incomplete and inconsistent data had limited the ability to prioritize the allocation of health resources in specific geographic areas or among certain populations most affected by the pandemic.
>
> As of March 2022, HHS [Health and Human Services, the main Federal health agency] had not fully implemented most of the statu-tory requirements related to supporting the establishment of systems of public health communications and surveillance. Further, HHS had not implemented any of the … requirements related to moderniz-ing public health situational awareness and biosurveillance. Conse-quently, more than 15 years after the law initially mandated it, the federal government does not yet have an interoperable network of sys-tems for near real-time public health situational awareness. Had the network been available, it could have been used to provide vital infor-mation to public health officials to better manage a timely COVID-19 response.[15]

The GAO identified a major problem in coordinating the many streams of (often inconsistently collected) data gathered at a federal level. The GAO has laid out a clear path for improvement. It is the federal government that is ultimately responsible. See below under "The Federal Level: Centers for Disease Control and Prevention (CDC)" for actions that the CDC should take.

Protection of Public Healthcare Professionals

Making every effort to elevate the status of public health professionals would send a strong signal of a federal-level commitment to address this and future pandemics. Without our front-line public health professionals, who must not feel under regular threat of physical, emotional, or social media attacks, we will never be able to deal effectively with pandemics. Accordingly:

> HHS should charge an independent group, such as the National Academies of Sciences, Engineering, and Medicine, with developing a model law to provide protections for federal, state, local, tribal, and territorial public health leaders in case of inappropriate interference with core public health functions.[16]

Legislation alone will not make the difference. When political officials at a federal level disparage and discredit our public health professionals, it causes immense harm to efforts to deal with public health issues. Conversely, when they express approval of public health professionals and offer helpful suggestions for areas of improvement as needed, that facilitates their work. But without legislation protecting public health professionals and without top-level federal commitment, we will simply be unable to cope with pandemics at all. It would make a difference if health professionals and, specifically, healthcare organizations, were to take a much more visible role in elevating the issue of protecting public health professionals.

Food and Drug Administration

The Food and Drug Administration (FDA) heroically, but with serious blemishes, attempted to resist the politicization of the agency under Trump.[17] Much has been written on the politicization of the entire federal health bureaucracy under Trump's administration. While challenges and efforts to politically influence decisions will always be an issue, the Biden administration has at least begun to tone down the politicization, though much progress remains to be made.[18] This is the key issue that many federal agencies, in particular, the CDC and the FDA, will always face. Other areas tied to the pandemic that call for attention are:

■ Laboratory diagnostic tests. The current approach of the FDA has created confusion and needs a legislative fix. Scott Gottlieb and Mark McClellan have specified a solution and legislation is ready as of the fall 2022.[19]
■ Vaccine and drug approval process. In response to overt pressure from the Trump administration, FDA staff very early set clear and high markers for vaccine approval.[20] In light of the controversy involving Aduhelm (an FDA-approved medication for Alzheimer's disease), questions have been raised about how to best improve the drug[21] and vaccine[22] development process.

Centers for Disease Control and Prevention (CDC)

What does the CDC do? Its website describes its mission as follows:

> CDC works 24/7 to protect America from health, safety, and security threats, both foreign and in the U.S. Whether diseases start at home or abroad, are chronic or acute, curable or preventable, human error or deliberate attack, CDC fights disease and supports communities and citizens to do the same. CDC increases the health security of our nation. As the nation's health protection agency, CDC saves lives and protects people from health threats. To accomplish our mission, CDC conducts critical science and provides health information that protects our nation against expensive and dangerous health threats and responds when these arise.[23]

There are two crucial omissions in this virtually impossible-to-achieve mission statement. To begin with, the CDC should focus on gathering the most accurate scientific information available. Then another branch of the CDC or, more likely, another federal agency, should focus on providing health information to the public. It is critical for the CDC to communicate with Americans more quickly—even when it doesn't know everything.

The CDC website contains an astonishing set of facts pertaining to the gathering of data:

How does CDC get its data? *CDC does not have direct authority to require data reporting [emphasis added throughout]*. Understanding the data CDC receives means understanding a few key factors involved in what we get and how we get it:

The data used by public health comes from a wide variety of places within our local communities: hospitals, laboratories, doctors' offices—anywhere that a person receives health care. Increasingly, public health is also tapping into new sources of data, such as wastewater and environmental data, that provide even more insights into what's happening with diseases.

■ CDC receives data from 50 states and 3000+ local jurisdictions and territories. *Each jurisdiction creates its own data-sharing agreements with CDC and with each other. For the most part, it is up to each city, county, and state to decide what information is collected, as well as how and when it can be shared with CDC. These decisions can vary widely, leading to big differences in the data CDC receives.*

■ Data comes to CDC in a variety of formats. As we modernize public health data, more and more information is being shared through automated, electronic data exchange. *However, some data are still sent via excel spreadsheets, fax machines, or even by phone or by hand.*

■ It can take different amounts of time for data to reach CDC. *Because each state has its own systems and capabilities, and also because the data first travels a path from the local to state levels before coming to CDC, the speed and timing of the data will vary.* CDC and our partners are working to create modern, interoperable systems that will allow us to share more real-time data at every level of public health and with the public.[24]

While the CDC is making efforts to improve its data collection efforts,[25] it still has a long way to go.[26]

Another challenge pertains to the public release of data. Rochelle Walensky, the current director, best expresses the overall communication conundrum: "In a pandemic, you don't have time to wait. You have to take action to help people," said Walenksy, who has faced her own communications problems during the crisis. "We haven't been able to be as nimble as we've needed to be."[27]

Walensky said she is trying to steer the agency toward the "sweet spot" between its old way of publishing its findings, which can take weeks or months, and ensuring that the science going out to the public is safe and reliable.[28]

As one CDC briefing document stated, the CDC should be producing "data for action" rather than "data for publication."[29] This challenge is more difficult to address, as it involves the interpretation of data and importantly reflects the political polarization in this country. When parts of the country will not "take action" on the basis of "data for action," the CDC could separately, publicly, and in a relentless fashion highlight states and localities implementing best practice patterns in the hope that "laggards" will consider it in their interest to ramp up their efforts. Demonstrating the positive health impact of this approach could lead to not only better data but more funding.

Lastly, adequate funding is a critical part of the functioning of any organization. For example, the CDC operates the Quarantine Station Program that:

works 24/7 to safeguard America from public health threats, both foreign and domestic. We are scientists, doctors, nurses, veterinarians, data experts, educators, communicators, and emergency responders. Our public health officers help protect more than 360 million travelers who arrive at US ports of entry by land, air, and sea—nearly 1 million per day.[30]

Yet, as the National Academy of Medicine clearly demonstrated in a report published in 2022:

The current level of funding and personnel for the Quarantine Station Program of the DGMQ is inadequate and is preventing the organization from effectively and efficiently carrying out its many responsibilities and activities. The continuous challenge of emergencies and pandemics over the last decade have stretched the DGMQ's capacity and ability to respond to global disease threats. The committee's assessment of the agency's organizational capacity finds that it is designed to operate in a past era—before the last decade's unprecedented and profound health events. ... Even after the COVID-19 pandemic has subsided, it is highly unlikely that the organization will ever return to "normal."[31]

Simply put, our pandemic prevention and readiness activities are woefully underfunded. Will we respond as a country and set aside the necessary funds? Will we address any number of other challenges that the CDC should have met, such as the ready availability of reliable COVID tests?[32] I am doubtful, but it will help to highlight the need continuously and publicly.

World Health Organization

The COVID pandemic daily put the World Health Organization (WHO) in the news. The mission of the WHO, according to its website, is simple and yet impossible to attain:

> Founded in 1948, WHO is the United Nations agency that connects nations, partners and people to promote health, keep the world safe and serve the vulnerable, so everyone, everywhere can attain the highest level of health.[33]

The WHO has the following enormous challenge: the extent to which it can meet its mission depends on the willingness and ability of member countries to participate. Let's start with the positive, showing how one country demonstrated an effective governmental response to the COVID pandemic. Qatar strongly responded with governmental engagement in a setting of universal coverage (a full description of Qatar's engagement appears in the reference).[34] The WHO provided necessary assistance so Qatar could achieve its remarkable success.

Clearly, many countries, with the United States among the worst, did not pursue Qatar's approach. The Lancet Commission on Lessons for the Future from the COVID-19 Pandemic, referenced at the beginning of this chapter, offered these general recommendations:

> We call for a dual track to prevent future emerging infectious diseases. To prevent natural spillovers, governments should coordinate on the global surveillance and regulation of domestic animal and wild animal trade and take stronger measures against dangerous practices.
>
> To prevent research-related spillovers, WHO should be given new oversight authority regarding the biosafety, biosecurity and bio-risk management of national and international research programmes that are engaged in the collection, testing, and genetic manipulation of potentially dangerous pathogens.[35]

How does the WHO prevent the spread of pandemics such as COVID? From the WHO website:

> Articles 21(a) and 22 of the WHO Constitution assign the World Health Assembly (WHA) the authority to adopt regulations "designed to prevent the international spread of disease." These regulations, known as the International Health Regulations (IHR), were first adopted in 1969 and have been amended three times, most recently in 2005 after the outbreak of severe acute respiratory syndrome in 2003. ...Nonetheless, these measures failed to ensure a sufficiently robust global response to the emergence of SARS-CoV-2.[36]

I agree with the Lancet Commission's conclusion that

> The WHO—acting under the IHR (2005)—repeatedly erred on the side of reserve rather than boldness. ...Although over-reaction can be politically embarrassing, the COVID-19 pandemic has shown that centralised under-reaction can be devastating.[37]

Going forward, in addition to the need for more funds, I would highlight two critical recommendations that many commissions, including the Lancet Commission, have put forward:

■ The importance of the speed with which the vaccines were developed cannot be overemphasized. Yet this miracle of modern science was available to very few countries. The WHO could help lower-income countries gain rapid access to vaccines. At least in part, the WHO could accomplish this through the development of low-income-country vaccine capacity. But this will not be enough. Right now vaccine development is in the hands of pharmaceutical companies that are understandably not interested in relinquishing patents even after earning billions for shareholders and individual developers.[38] A major donor to the WHO, the Gates Foundation, is very strongly in favor of maintaining intellectual property exactly as is, meaning that patents are not waived, nor are low-income countries allowed to develop vaccine development capacity.[39] The resolution of this conundrum will require effective implementation of the next recommendation.
■ Dealing with pandemics that involve health and security calls for the involvement of the heads of state. There has been no shortage of reports advocating for new political mechanisms that bring heads of state together.[40] The National Academy of Medicine, for example, recommended

> the establishment of a global health threats council composed of heads of state and government to ensure ongoing high-level political leadership and awareness around pandemic preparedness and

response. Such leadership has been lacking in the current crisis. Future crises, recognizing that another pathogen with pandemic potential could emerge at any moment, should not repeat the experience of a worldwide scramble for such global public goods as personal protective equipment and other supplies.[41]

The Lancet Commission's recommendation on this point is very attractive:

A WHO Global Health Board composed of the six WHO regions, represented by heads of state on a rotating basis, and selected by the governments of each region.[42]

Lastly, while none of the many reports I've read have highlighted this recommendation, I strongly believe, as emphasized throughout this book, that political leadership is critical and that health professionals can make a difference. Important to this effort is the reform of the WHO at the highest levels. Despite problems during this pandemic documented by many commissions, including the Lancet Commission, and other reports,[43] the current WHO director, Dr. Tedros Adhanom Ghebreyesus, recently won reappointment to another five-year term.[44] In return for adequate funding from member countries, WHO reform should include transitioning to new leadership.

Conclusions

This chapter has highlighted how every level of government, starting at a local level and extending to the national and international levels, has critical roles to play if we are to deal well with this and future pandemics. The challenges that we face go beyond what this chapter has put forward. Leadership is key and drives all the issues discussed here. But there is one aspect of leadership I would like to bring up that I have not yet emphasized. Effective leadership starts with an inquisitive mind, one that is not bound only to the political needs of the moment. An article in the *Times Literary Supplement* written by Paul Collier published shortly after the start of the pandemic summarizes the type of leadership that works during a pandemic—starting at the preparedness phase but extending to all aspects of dealing with a pandemic. Such leaders

start out by specifying the concept of radical uncertainty which orients our thought to two fundamental questions: "how to face identifying known unknowns" and "how to face unknown unknowns." Collier continues: "The answers to the former are to build resilience while encouraging rival teams of experts. The answers to the latter are to learn from others while investing in finding out new information. Resilience is all about assigning responsibilities to the multiplicity of entities best equipped to understand how to build the capacity to withstand shocks. ... Facing many unknowns, the primary use of models should be to highlight those among the known unknowns that critically affect policy choices. These then become the ones most urgent to resolve whether by learning from others or collecting data. The value of using rival teams is that this method flushes out these known unknowns while discouraging exaggerated claims to knowledge."[45]

Leadership, and specifically health professional leadership, taking such an approach engages with all points of view as described above and inculcates humility in all. And, importantly, health professional leadership taking this approach can more effectively empower politicians to make tough, possibly unpopular, decisions. These decisions will understandably keep national interests at the forefront. For the United States—and the rest of the world—it can only be hoped that coupling health and national security together with achieving international cooperation can actually materialize and lead to better outcomes for this and future pandemics.

Notes

1 International Working Group on Financing Preparedness. (2017) From panic and neglect to investing in health security: Financing pandemic preparedness at a national level. *World Bank.* Available at: https://documents1.worldbank.org/curated/en/979591495652724770/pdf/115271-REVISED-FINAL-IWG-Report-3-5-18.pdf. Accessed: December 4, 2022.

2 The Lancet Covid-19 Commission. (2022) The Lancet Commission on lessons for the future from the Covid-19 pandemic. *The Lancet.* Available at: https://www.thelancet.com/commissions/covid19. Accessed: December 4, 2022.

3 The Independent Panel for Pandemic Preparedness and Response. (2021) Building on the past. *The Independent Panel.* Available at: https://theindependentpanel.org/wp-content/uploads/2021/05/Background-paper-1-Building-on-the-past-.pdf. Accessed: December 4, 2022.

4 Milliband, D., O'Neill, J., and Rottingen, JA. (2022) Never Let a Crisis Go to Waste: Preventing the Next Pandemic. *Newsweek.* Available at: https://www.newsweek.com/never-let-crisis-go-waste-preventing-next-pandemic-opinion-1605717. Accessed: December 4, 2022.

5 For more background see: https://health.gov/news/202009/association-state-and-territorial-health-officials-helping-public-health-agencies-improve-health-nationwide. Accessed: December 4, 2022.

6 Pielke, R. (2021) Science advice and trust in the U.S. during the pandemic. *National Academies of Science, Engineering and Medicine.* Available at: https://www.nationalacademies.org/event/07-27-2021/docs/DF652102EC097359A73C0FFEBC66999C617C9202DF73. Accessed: December 4, 2022.

7 Robert Wood Johnson Foundation/ Harvard TH Chan School of Public Health. (2021) *The public's perspective on the United States public health system.* RWJ/ Harvard TH Chan School of Public Health. Available at: https://cdn1.sph.harvard.edu/wp-content/uploads/sites/94/2021/05/RWJF-Harvard-Report_FINAL-051321.pdf. Accessed: December 4, 2022.

8 Gottlieb, S. (2021) *Uncontrolled Spread: How Covid-19 crushed us and how can defeat the next pandemic.* New York: Harper Collins. See especially Chapter 18: A new doctrine for national security.

9 Federal Emergency Management Agency [FEMA]. (2021) Applying the Defense Production Act. *FEMA*. Available at: https://www.fema.gov/press-release/20210420/applying-defense-production-act. Accessed: December 4, 2022.

10 Ward, A. (2020) Trump's excuses for not using the Defense Production Act are wrong – and dangerous. *Vox*. Available at: https://www.vox.com/2020/3/23/21191003/coronavirus-trump-defense-production-act-venezuela. Accessed: December 4, 2022.

11 Krackov, D., Blanchard, C., Sklamberg, H., Blackwood, K. et al. (2021) Expanded use of the Defense Production Act and focus on building the domestic supply chain. *Arnold Porter*. Available at: https://www.arnoldporter.com/en/perspectives/advisories/2021/01/expanded-use-of-the-dpa. Accessed: December 4, 2022.

12 National Academies of Sciences, Engineering, and Medicine. 2022. *Evolving crisis standards of care and ongoing lessons from COVID-19: Proceedings of a Workshop Series*. Washington, DC: The National Academies Press. Available at: https://doi.org/10.17226/26573. Accessed: October 10, 2022.

13 Ibid. 10, 24.

14 Ibid. 74.

15 Government Accounting Office. (2022) Pandemic lessons highlight need for public health situational awareness network. *Government Accounting Office*. Available at: https://www.gao.gov/products/gao-22-104600. Accessed: December 4, 2022.

16 The Commonwealth Fund Commission on a National Public Health System. (2022) Meeting America's public health challenge. *Commonwealth Fund*. Available at: https://www.commonwealthfund.org/sites/default/files/2022-06/TCF-002%20National%20Public%20Heath%20System%20Report-r4-final.pdf. Accessed: December 9, 2022.

17 Facher, L. (2020) Trump has launched an all-out attack on the FDA, Will its integrity survive. *Stat News*. Available at: https://www.statnews.com/2020/08/27/trump-has-launched-an-all-out-attack-on-the-fda-will-its-scientific-integrity-survive/. Accessed: December 9, 2022.

18 Howard, S. (2022) CDC, FDA, NIH workers did not report incidents of political interference, 'fearing retaliation' government watchdog says. *CNN Health*. Available at: https://www.cnn.com/2022/04/21/health/political-interference-gao-report/index.html. Accessed: December 9, 2022.

19 Gottlieb, S. and McClellan, MB. (2022) Reforms Needed to Modernize the US Food and Drug Administration's Oversight of Dietary Supplements, Cosmetics, and Diagnostic Tests. *JAMA Health Forum*. 3:10. Available at: https://jamanetwork.com/journals/jama-health-forum/fullarticle/2797520. Accessed: December 5, 2022.

20 Gottlieb, S. Uncontrolled Spread op cit. 299.

21 Barrueeta, A., Dupont, S., Joyce, K., and Ross, M. (2022) Restoring provider confidence in FDA-approved drugs. *Health Affairs*. Available at: https://www.healthaffairs.org/do/10.1377/forefront.20220623.43556/. Accessed: December 9, 2022.

22 Suwondo, P., Westmoreland, T., and Forman, H. (2020) Ten urgent reforms to protect the CDC and FDA from harmful political interference. *Health Affairs*. Available at: https://www.healthaffairs.org/do/10.1377/forefront.20201120.456386/. Accessed: December 9, 2022.

23 CDC. (2022) Mission role and pledge. *Centers for Disease Control*. Available at: https://www.cdc.gov/about/organization/mission.htm. Accessed: November 30, 2022.

24 CDC. (2022) Where does our data come from? *Centers for Disease Control*. Available at: https://www.cdc.gov/surveillance/projects/dmi-initiative/where_does_our_data_come_from.html. Accessed: December 10, 2022.

25 CDC. (2022) What is the data modernization initiative. *Centers for Disease Control.* Available at: https://www.cdc.gov/surveillance/projects/dmi-initiative/index.html. Accessed: December 4, 2022.

26 Mandavilli, A. (2022) The CDC isn't publishing large portions of the Covid data it collects. *New York Times.* Available at: https://www.nytimes.com/2022/02/20/health/covid-cdc-data.html. Accessed: December 10, 2022.

27 Mahr, K. and Banco, E. (2022) No quick fixes: Walensky's push for change at CDC meets reality. *Politico.* Available at: https://www.politico.com/news/2022/10/21/rochelle-walensky-change-cdc-00062874. Accessed: November 24, 2022.

28 Mahr, K. (2022) CDC Director orders agency overhaul, admits flawed COVID-19 response. *Politico.* Available at: https://www.politico.com/news/2022/08/17/cdc-agency-overhaul-covid-19-response-00052384. Accessed: November 24, 2022.

29 Pezenik, S. and Hazlett, C. (2022) Review finds CDC mishandled Covid-19 pandemic response. *ABC News.* Available at: https://abcnews.go.com/Politics/cdc-covid-guidance-confusing-overwhelming-organization-overhaul/story?id=88502792. Accessed: December 4, 2022.

30 CDC. (2021) Quarantine and border health services. *Centers for Disease Control.* Available at: https://www.cdc.gov/ncezid/dgmq/focus-areas/quarantine.html. Accessed: December 4, 2022.

31 National Academies of Sciences, Engineering, and Medicine. (2022). *Improving the CDC Quarantine Station Network's Response to Emerging Threats.* Washington, DC: The National Academies Press. Available at: https://doi.org/10.17226/26599. Available at: https://nap.nationalacademies.org/download/26599. Accessed: December 10, 2022.

32 Gottlieb, S. (2022) *Uncontrolled Spread* op cit. see especially. 270–4.

33 WHO. (2022) Who we are. *World Health Organization.* Available at: https://www.who.int/about. Accessed: December 4, 2022.

34 National Academies of Sciences, Engineering, and Medicine. (2022) *Toward a Post-Pandemic World: Lessons from COVID-19 for Now and the Future: Proceedings of a Workshop.* Washington, DC: The National Academies Press. Available at: http://nap.nationalacademies.org/26556. Accessed: December 4, 2022.

1. Lessons Learned in Qatar as Presented by H. E. Hanan Al Kuwari A pandemic like COVID-19 needs strong government response. Goals for Qatar were to prioritize human life over economic effects. A national COVID-19 committee with diverse membership was formed that engaged the public throughout its efforts, which was vital to its approach.

2. Response to the crisis needs to be scientific, data-driven, prudent, and trans- parent. Though little was known at the beginning, all available information was shared. Public communications clarified that decisions were made based on information known at the time, but that new information was still being as- sessed. The national COVID-19 committee created an approach to share all the government data with academia so anyone could conduct research.

3. "Universal health coverage (UHC) and whole-of-government approach are necessary to tackle the social determinants of health," she said. Everyone was treated for COVID-19 with the same standard of care. Hotel isolation facilities were free and available to everyone, as well as shared housing and ensuring quick distribution of free phones or internet access where needed.

4. "A strong integrated health system can save lives and make a difference, but only if it is well prepared, she said." In addition to UHC, the health system in Qatar

is based on principles of accountable care. Primary care centers are responsible for the population, and all hospitals and centers are accredited and connected by one electronic medical record. The government invested heavily in infrastructure, workforce development, and quality of care over the last 10 years, with more recent investments in preparedness and resilience. The investment in a culture of safety ensured prioritization of staff safety.

5. "During a health crisis, it is important to adapt health system governance that is integrated, inclusive, agile, and has clear lines of responsibility," she concluded. The national health system built upon community-based care with online consultations, emergency home visits, and supplies delivered directly to the patient's home.

35 The Lancet Covid-19 Commission. (2022) *The Lancet*. Available at: https://www.thelancet.com/commissions/covid19. Accessed: December 4, 2022.

36 World Health Organization. (2022) Available at: https://www.who.int/news/item/01-12-2021-world-health-assembly-agrees-to-launch-process-to-develop-historic-global-accord-on-pandemic-prevention-preparedness-and-response.

37 The Lancet Covid-19 Commission. (2022) *The Lancet*. Available at: https://www.thelancet.com/commissions/covid19. Accessed: December 4, 2022.

38 Ibid.

39 Cao, S. (2021) Bill Gates' comments on Covid-19 vaccine patent draws outrage. *The Observer*. Available at: https://observer.com/2021/04/bill-gates-oppose-lifting-covid-vaccine-patent-interview/. Accessed: December 4, 2022. The Gates Foundation later reversed course. Cheney, C. (2021) Gates Foundation reverses course on Covid-19 vaccine patents. Available at: https://www.devex.com/news/gates-foundation-reverses-course-on-covid-19-vaccine-patents-99810. Accessed: December 4, 2022.

40 See for example. The Independent Panel. (2021) Building on the past. The Independent Panel for Pandemic Preparedness and Response. Available at: https://theindependentpanel.org/wp-content/uploads/2021/05/Background-paper-1-Building-on-the-past-.pdf. Accessed: December 4, 2022.

41 National Academies of Science, Engineering and Medicine. (2022) *Toward a Post-Pandemic World*. op cit. Available at: http://nap.nationalacademies.org/26556. Accessed: December 4, 2022.

42 The Lancet Covid-19 Commission. (2022) The Lancet Commission on lessons for the future from the Covid-19 pandemic. *The Lancet*. Available at: https://www.thelancet.com/commissions/covid19. Accessed: December 4, 2022.

43 Dentico, D. and Fletcher, ER. (2020) World Health Organization's censorship of Italy's pandemic response sets dangerous precedent – critics say. *Health Policy Watch*. Available at: https://healthpolicy-watch.news/the-world-health-organizations-censorship-of-report-on-italys-pandemic-response-sets-dangerous-conflicts-of-interest-precedent/. Accessed: December 4, 2022.

44 Maxmen, A. (2022) WHO chief Tedros looks guaranteed for re-election amid Covid pandemic. *Nature*. Available at: https://www.nature.com/articles/d41586-022-00019-4. Accessed: December 4, 2022.

45 Collier, P. (2020) The problem of modelling: Public policy and the Coronavirus. *Time Literary Supplement*. Available at: https://www.the-tls.co.uk/articles/problem-modelling-public-policy-coronavirus-paul-collier/. Accessed: December 4, 2022.

Chapter 10

What Can Health Professionals Do to Better Address This and Future Pandemics?

Introduction

How can health professionals best engage with senior-level politicians, especially those for whom electoral success is predicated on opposition to scientific approaches to control of this (and future) pandemics? How can health professionals best engage with those most affected by the pandemic—low-income people, people of color, and Republicans? What can professional associations representing health professionals and licensure boards and individual health professionals do to improve their impact on this and future pandemics?

In Chapter 8, I wrote about a state-level approach to effectively address this and future pandemics. But how can health professionals help pass this legislation or similar efforts? In this chapter I make suggestions that individual health profession-als and health professional organizations can consider to mitigate needless suffering when dealing with a pandemic. I do this at both the micro (starting with myself) and macro (professional organization) levels. Until now, I've had limited success engaging with professional organizations. My conclusion is that to have a successful engagement with a professional association such as the one I belong to, American Medical Association (AMA), I need to tie my interest in fruitful engagement in this pandemic to the economic self-interest of its members.

DOI: 10.4324/9781003426257-12

In addition, in this chapter, I will make references to and synthesize some of many reports that international and US organizations have produced over the past two years. I am partial to the work of the American National Academy of Medicine. Their publications and publications of other organizations, such as the *Lancet*,[1] provide excellent ideas on how we can move forward. Unfortunately, few of the major recommendations pertaining to either the availability of additional streams of money or the fundamental restructuring of our public health system (as discussed in Chapter 8) are likely to be implemented—at least not on a national level. Lastly, I offer recommendations, such as what I advocate in Chapter 8, that most other publications have neither highlighted nor even mentioned.

What I've Tried to Do and How I Might Adjust My Actions Going Forward

As a health professional dealing with this pandemic, I have acted in three concentric circles—my family/friends/colleagues; as an individual physician; and as a physician who has tried to be involved organizationally in my professional associations. I've involved myself organizationally in two ways: I started the organization Ask Nurses and Doctors (AND) and I tried to engage with the AMA, the main organization representing physicians in the United States. I rejoined the AMA in an effort to encourage the group to become more active in addressing the COVID pandemic in ways that to date it hasn't. I believe that I have failed, thus far, in my efforts with the AMA, but I feel I have no choice but to keep trying, whether with the AMA and/or other organizations. My efforts via AND to organize health professionals in support of Congressional candidates, as I detail in my COVID Notes (Chapter 3), have been modestly successful.

Many states in the summer of 2022 began to diminish or eliminate COVID mitigation measures (such as mask requirements) as the pandemic evolved. (Some states, such as Texas and Florida, had almost none to begin with.) In response, the National Academy of Medicine published a report that provided an excellent research summary stating that:

> Individuals must assess their level of risk and risk tolerance amid different mitigation measures, regulations, and metrics across states and localities. The public is also exposed to misinformation and disinformation through social and mainstream media—all occurring within a politically polarized environment.[2]

In many ways, their guidance (summarized below) is exactly how I, for the past two years, have tried to behave with my family/friends/colleagues and as an individual physician with my patients.

■ **Build trust and credibility:** Transparency is essential to building trust in public health officials, evidence, and recommendations. It requires candor about the limits to existing knowledge and the likelihood that it will change as the pandemic continues to evolve.

■ **Foster autonomy and empowerment:** Public health officials must recognize and respect individuals' autonomy in making decisions for themselves and their families. Empowering that autonomy means making the information people need to exercise it authoritative, comprehensible, and accessible.

■ **Honor people's emotions and personal stories:** Public health officials must acknowledge the deep emotions and practical challenges that can accompany the decisions individuals are now asked to make. They can demonstrate their concern by hearing personal stories and translating scientific information into terms relevant to individual decisions.

■ **Encourage public engagement:** Individuals will be and will feel less alone if they make these decisions as part of a community. Public health officials can foster public engagement by partnering with trusted community organizations that support two-way communications, helping to convey health information and hear individuals' needs.

The first three apply to my behavior with family/friends/colleagues and patients. The last, encouraging public engagement, I have done via my work at Ask Nurses and Doctors. In this work, I've engaged with health professionals living in states where competitive electoral races occurred in the 2022 cycle. I was particularly focused in this cycle on Pennsylvania and Florida and worked with local health professionals to produce letters to the editor (LTEs), op-eds, and videos. I mostly communicated my recommendations about COVID mitigation through the COVID diary, "COVID-19 Notes," sent approximately every two weeks to 1000 colleagues and friends.

While I have no choice but to respect my patients' decision to reject taking the COVID vaccine, I continue to bring up the subject while trying different approaches. One of the more interesting episodes I report on in my diary concerns one of my impoverished patients who was an adamant vaccine refuser. I asked him what he thought the best way was to predict those who don't get the vaccine. He tried a few guesses; I was sure he wouldn't know the answer, which is being a Republican. And I, in turn, wasn't expecting his response: "I am a Republican."

My message, framed in a virtually infinite number of ways, is the same for everyone—at least thus far, and who can predict the future? Going forward on a personal level, I don't see much of a future that doesn't involve masks and/or vaccines (at least from time to time); that doesn't involve greater caring about how I engage in large crowds— especially indoor large crowds where neither vaccines nor masks are mandated. I am used to wearing the N-95 mask, even though it is uncomfortable. The masks will get better.[3] But for now and the foreseeable future, I wear the mask and I encourage all my family, friends, and patients to don a mask when in crowds and/or indoors with a large group of people. In addition, we all need to be "fully" vaccinated—whatever the CDC recommends. I wouldn't be surprised if my clinical practice requires a mask for some time to come.

Engaging with Politicians and Medical Societies

I resigned in 2016 from my research work of thirty years and started Ask Nurses and Doctors (AND) in 2018. I had always hoped that my research on how to better connect health care payment to improved quality would impact health policy; I also hoped that enhancing the connection between payment and quality would tie into health reform. But after the presidential election of 2016, I knew that I had to try something that might have a more direct impact.

My idea was not to run for office but to encourage local health professionals to get politically involved in their electoral district or state. I never will run for office; where I live in western Massachusetts, we have great incumbents and a ready pipeline of excellent candidates. At the same time, health professionals have a long tradition of political involvement, including electoral office, throughout the world.[4] In the United States, there are both Republican and Democratic physicians in Congress.

I wasn't sure how to become more politically involved. I spent much of 2017 trying to formulate what eventually would become AND. After I founded AND in the spring of 2018, I went up and down the northeastern seaboard looking for a competitive Congressional race with a candidate or incumbent, I could support. Ideally, I would then find at least one health professional whom I knew who resided in the district or state that I wanted to work in. I found all these ingredients in the second district in Maine, where Jared Golden, a Democrat, was trying to unseat Bruce Poliquin, essentially a pre-Trump Trumpite. I knew one health professional residing in Maine-2 from my research days. I met with Jared in the summer. How did AND do? Working under the direction of Jared's campaign, we recruited and organized 130 health care professionals to write op-eds, LTEs, and coordinate with Jared's campaign on press conferences. We met once a week to decide how we would deploy health professionals in the coming week.

The outcome: Jared won on ranked-choice voting. AND made a measurable difference in the election outcome. Representative Golden recognized this when he came with me and my Congressman, Jim McGovern, for a meeting with the Democratic Congressional Campaign Committee (DCCC) in February 2019. They helped AND obtained a contract to continue the efforts that we began and expand from there. We continued to provide this service through the 2020 cycle. We worked on behalf of a significant number of candidates/incumbents: most of them won.

After the 2020 election cycle, the DCCC completely changed its staff, and they let all existing consultants go, including AND. In the 2022 cycle the focus of AND went in two directions. As discussed below, I personally tried to become organizationally involved in my health professional societies, specifically, the American Medical Association and the Massachusetts Medical Society. In addition, AND concentrated on elections in Florida and Pennsylvania. Working with local health professionals, we published a good number of op-eds and LTEs,[5] and we tried to become engaged with state medical societies.

Though I am pleased with our political engagement, what were the results of our efforts to work with medical organizations? Here, by way of example, is a response AND received from a senior executive at a state medical society after we sent an email asking if we could work together. AND hoped to engage with the physician members of the medical society first on COVID issues (such as vaccines) and subsequently, in a nonpartisan manner, on election issues. Her negative response:

> Right now, the number 1 issue for physicians in our state is the recent change by the state supreme court in the venue rule (*an issue pertaining to malpractice—my note*). Our members, no matter the work setting, are concerned about medical malpractice cases being dragged to find a friendly court.

Medical organizations are reputed to focus primarily on economic and/or licensure issues, including malpractice. This is borne out in the research literature, which examined AMA campaign contributions and determined that economic issues of benefit to AMA members drove campaign contributions even if, as discussed in an article published in 1988, pro-tobacco candidates were given AMA support![6]

It is true that the AMA has gone on record supporting good public health practices such as COVID vaccinations. But the reality I found in discussions with senior AMA officials is sadly different. That is, aside from public pronouncements and a web page, the efforts that the AMA and state medical societies have made on behalf of public health, such as best COVID practices, pales in comparison with the efforts that these organizations have made for its members' economic interests.

A prime example is seen in these excerpts from the AMA web page (as of November 2022) entitled "COVID-19: AMA's Recent and Ongoing Advocacy efforts."[7] The first sections of the document have headings such as "Financial Relief (for physicians)." The first item is

> Due to organized medicine advocacy, Health Resources and Services Administration has provided an extenuating circumstances exception for physicians who missed the reporting period for the Provider Relief Fund. AMA provides a new workflow resource which outlines the steps necessary for submitting a "Request to Report Late."

The next heading is "Telehealth," and the first item under this section is:

> Sought and secured broad telehealth coverage expansion and improved payments at the federal and state levels to increase access to care and provide patients with a safer way to receive care.

The following section dealt with personal protective equipment and how the AMA was able to secure more PPE for physicians. After that came the section "Urging the Surgeon General to take action against COVID-19 misinformation."

In the end, I was unable to convince the senior leadership at the AMA that I engaged with to become more engaged in the COVID-19 pandemic. I am sure that this doesn't surprise anyone engaged in health care politics at either a state or national level. Whether it is payment for physicians that uses a methodology called the resource-based relative value scale (RBRVS) or health policy issues pertaining to equity, the AMA senior leadership examines the issue via the lens of "what's in it for our members from an economic point of view."

What Are My Concrete Recommendations for Organized Medicine?

It would make an enormous difference if the AMA (and I use them only as an example; my recommendations apply to any health professional organization) became much more public in its fight against COVID, especially against misinformation. Simply put, the AMA and other professional organizations need to stand up for science. It should be emphasized that there are many aspects to this fight that will benefit physicians, including compensation, via, for example, telehealth. It is in the AMA's self-interest to pursue a strategy of standing up for science, as this will lead to better control of the pandemic, which, in turn, will positively affect such issues as physician burnout.

As spelled out below, the AMA could forcefully stand up for science in a variety of ways, but this cannot happen until the senior leadership makes this fight an existential priority. To do so, the AMA could hire an individual reporting directly to their president who would be responsible for both internal and external efforts in this fight. The following are just examples of the type of activities that the person reporting to the AMA president could undertake, here divided into two broad categories:

a. Internal:

- Coordinate with state medical societies on COVID activities and vaccine misinformation, especially in those states where the political leaders (and even the public health leaders, such as in Florida) are against science and good COVID practices.
- Work with all interested parties to legally enable state medical licensure boards to be much more aggressive in disciplining physicians who purvey COVID and vaccine misinformation.
- Develop resources that physicians (and other health professionals) who continue to work on the front lines could utilize to avoid burnout; much more than is currently on offer is needed.[8]

b. External:

■ Privately meet with the US surgeon general and health professional leaders in the federal government to see how the AMA could engage with all aspects of public efforts to fight against COVID misinformation and assist with vaccine boosters. Currently, when the federal government is trying to push a COVID vaccine booster campaign, it advertises its partnering with participating pharmacies. The AMA, which has not been visible in this life-saving effort, should be prominently mentioned in the government's social media campaign.[9]

■ Organize regular AMA participation on all social media and talk shows (especially conservative ones) on all aspects of COVID and vaccine misinformation. A small example: for all states, especially those with the lowest vaccination rates, the AMA could partner with Democratic and Republican physicians extolling the virtues of science and, specifically, vaccination. It is particularly important for Republican physicians to be engaged, as tragically, Republicans, having a greater proportion of people who reject vaccination, are afflicted with a much higher mortality risk than Democrats.[10]

■ The AMA could step up to be at the forefront of the fight against misinformation. Right now, the AMA is doing little in an arena where the purveyors of misinformation, such as Robert F. Kennedy Jr.[11] and America's Frontline Doctors,[12] have millions of dollars backing the misinformation machine. In contrast, the organizations involved in the fight against misinformation, sadly, have minimal resources at their disposal.[13] Clearly, there is space for a major effort by the AMA and many other health professional organizations.

■ Given the existing political polarization at the federal level, more activity could pivot to the state level. Health professionals under the aegis of state medical societies could be engaged in two types of activities. For one, I will try to work with the Massachusetts Medical Society to encourage passage of legislation such as that described in Chapter 8. Second, the MMS should coordinate with managed care organizations to encourage beneficial practices such as the widespread use of COVID vaccines.

Where will the money come from for these efforts? I believe that donations from its members could be a prime source (I would certainly donate). And surely many foundations would agree to match funds raised. The AMA could undertake these internal and external steps on its own, or preferably with other organizations, especially health care professional organizations representing other physician specialties, nurses, pharmacists, and other health care professionals.

But what if the AMA decides, as is highly likely, against this path? Should we just give up? The problem is that, even though it is much weaker than in its heyday fifty years ago,[14] the AMA is "the main game in town." Thus, in addition to trying to influence it from within, as I will continue doing, it is important that concerned people engage with other organizations that could in turn encourage the AMA to pursue the options discussed above. For example, at an individual level, the US surgeon general, the director of the US Department of Health and Human Services, and other senior-level federal government officials could privately approach the AMA. As many of my recommendations involve engaging with social media broadly defined, media foundations such as the Pulitzer Center could, in turn, approach the AMA for partnership opportunities. The Pulitzer Center already has a tradition of partnership with many organizations.[15] I have reached out to some of these foundations.

What about the state medical boards (responsible for physician licensure) and the umbrella national organization, the Federation of State Medical Boards (FSMB)? Have they fulfilled their duty to protect the public from physicians peddling misinformation? I agree with those who argue that:

> State medical boards must immediately act to revoke the medical licenses of doctors who use their professional status to deliberately mislead patients for reasons of politics or profit. Thus far, regulatory bodies have largely failed in this duty.[16]

Most recently, on September 30, 2022, California governor Gavin Newsom signed legislation that would allow the state medical board to discipline physicians and surgeons who spread misinformation about COVID-19 during patient care. Misinformation is defined in the legislation as "false information that is contradicted by contemporary scientific consensus contrary to the standard of care."[17] The key words added are "during patient care." Thus, physicians who peddle in COVID misinformation outside of direct patient care, such as social media, will not suffer any consequences.[18]

I believe that the medical profession should have one standard for practice and that it should guide our behavior as individual health professionals and as members of organizations—and that is to uphold faith in science as our standard. I understand that medicine has art and science built into it. But the reality is that COVID vaccines work and hydroxychloroquine does not. Physicians should not be allowed to glibly mouth lies about COVID and vaccines. Yet, while it is easy to insist that physicians should not lie, practically speaking, when does attempting to stop the spread of scientific misinformation impinge on free speech? In a recent article, law professor Carl Coleman stated:

- In most cases, imposing disciplinary penalties on physicians for speech that takes place outside a physician–patient relationship would have dangerous policy implications and would almost certainly be unconstitutional.
- Drawing on examples from the regulation of the legal profession, it argues that disciplinary actions would be appropriate under one set of circumstances:

if a board can establish that a physician has disseminated information that she knows to be false or with reckless disregard as to whether it is true—i.e., with the "actual malice" standard applied to defamation cases brought by public officials and public figures.[19]

In this respect, a carrot-and-stick approach would work best for both the FASB and physician organizations such as the AMA. We should have been employing carrots all along, even before the start of the pandemic, in order to strengthen the high trust that already exists between the public and the medical professions. Certainly, the public expects licensure boards to discipline physicians who peddle misinformation.[20] If the public sees organized medicine disciplining physicians espousing patently false information to their patients, they will have even greater trust in the medical profession. In addition, if the AMA follows through on some of the above recommendations, it will further strengthen trust.

But we could go much further. The FSMB in particular, but also the AMA and other physician organizations, could also strengthen ties with politicians for the explicit purpose of fighting for vaccines and against misinformation. If we are ever to address this and future pandemics, they must go beyond pushing for legislation pertaining to malpractice and payment, as discussed above, and emphasize to politicians the importance of following science. Knowing that actively practicing physicians do not have the time, both the FSMB and organizations such as the AMA could, for example, coordinate the efforts of thousands of retired physicians to regularly meet with politicians on best scientific practices pertaining to COVID and other public health threats.

From a stick perspective, for example, both the FSMB and the AMA missed an opportunity to publicly oppose the successful effort in 2021 of Tennessee Republicans to browbeat the Tennessee state Board of Medical Examiners into rolling back regulations against physicians purveying misinformation.[21] The FSMB could work with legislators at both the state and national level to push for maximum adherence to scientific standards when dealing with COVID practices without stepping on free speech rights. Thus far, I've seen little evidence, even considering the concerns expressed in the Coleman article quoted above, that any systematic actions against physician misinformation have been taken by the FSMB and/or any physician licensing body.

Short of the very challenging option of revoking a physician's medical license for COVID lies, health professional societies have other options that they can pursue. According to Carl Coleman:

> For example, private hospitals and other health care organizations could revoke physicians' privileges[22] or terminate their employment for spreading false or misleading information about medical matters. Medical specialty boards (which, unlike licensing boards, are nongovernmental entities) could treat disseminating medical falsehoods as grounds for revoking certifications.[23]

Conclusion

As of now, neither the AMA nor any other health professional organizations have seen it in their self-interest to forcefully fight publicly and aggressively to protect the public against COVID-19 and future pandemics. If enough health professionals put pressure on AMA leaders to convince them that it is, in fact, in their self-interest to protect the public in ways they have not done to date, that could change the AMA's mindset. At the same time, health professionals could pressure outside organizations, such as the federal government, to provide the necessary encouragement. Will health professional organizations make this essential change? Will health professional organizations become more aggressive if for no other reason than to confront health professional burnout? As pandemics are here to stay, I have to believe that they will have no choice, precisely because it will be in their self-interest to step up and take actions on behalf of the public in much more visible ways than they have in the past.

Notes

1 Sachs, J., Abdool Karim, SS., Aknin, L., et al. (2022) The Lancet Commission on lessons for the future from the Covid-19 pandemic. *The Lancet*. Available at: https://www.thelancet.com/journals/lancet/article/PIIS0140-6736(22)01585-9/fulltext. Accessed: November 23, 2022.

2 National Academies of Sciences, Engineering, and Medicine (2022) *Supporting Individual Risk Assessment During COVID-19*. Washington, DC: The National Academies Press. Available at: https://nap.nationalacademies.org/catalog/26629/supporting-individual-risk-assessment-during-covid-19. Accessed: December 4, 2022.

3 Stern, J. The masks we'll wear in the next pandemic (2022). *The Atlantic*. Available at: https://www.theatlantic.com/science/archive/2022/10/pandemic-n95-mask-protection-shortcomings-indoor-air-quality/671723/?utm_campaign=KHN%3A%20First%20Edition&utm_medium=email&_hsmi=229702065&_hsenc=p2ANqtz-kMt0mKOf9py5VKGYFAQWncpp3-RQ_oLctJ2TCpd3PSKvq0CGNr7hi-Puo8PBegneo-IqlLefRXysFfCWxe24dUYa9zQ&utm_content=229702065&utm_source=hs_email. Accessed November 23, 2022.

4 Goldfield, N. (2021) *Peace-building through women's health*. New York: Routledge. See chapter 15.

5 Goldfield, N., Kaminski, M., and Lerner, J. (2022) Voting for the common health of PA *Tribune Live*. Available at: https://triblive.com/opinion/dr-norbert-goldfield-dr-mitch-kaminski-and-jeffrey-c-lerner-voting-for-the-common-health-of-pa/. Accessed: November 23, 2022.

6 Sharfstein J. (1998) 1996 congressional campaign priorities of the AMA: tackling tobacco or limiting malpractice awards? *Am J Public Health*. 88: 8: 1233–36. 10.2105/ajph.88.8.1233. PMID: 9702157; PMCID: PMC1508293. Available at: Accessed: October 10, 2022.

7 American Medical Association (2022) Covid 19 – AMA's recent and ongoing advocacy efforts. *American Medical Association*. Available at: https://www.ama-assn.org/delivering-care/public-health/covid-19-amas-recent-and-ongoing-advocacy-efforts. Accessed: October 10, 2022.

8 Berg, S. (2022) With physician burnout soaring, 28 health organizations step up. *American Medical Association*. Available at: https://www.ama-assn.org/practice-management/physician-health/physician-burnout-soaring-28-health-care-organizations-step. Accessed: November 23, 2022.

9 Weiland, N. (2022) As White House presses for booster shots, Americans are slow to get them. *New York Times*. Available at: https://www.nytimes.com/2022/10/15/us/politics/covid-booster-shots.html. Accessed: November 23, 2022.

10 Wallace, J., Goldsmith-Pinkam, P., Schwartz JL. (2022) Excess death rates for Republicans and Democrats during the Covid-19 pandemic. *National Bureau of Economic Research*. Available at: https://www.nber.org/papers/w30512. Accessed: November 23, 2022.

11 Kennedy, RF. Jr. (2021) *The Real Anthony Fauci*. New York, NY: Skyhorse Publishing.

12 See https://americasfrontlinedoctors.org

13 Krisberg, K (2022) Health misinformation a "threat to public health". *The Nation's Health*. Available at: https://www.thenationshealth.org/content/52/1/1.1. Accessed: November 23, 2022.

14 Collier R. (2011) American Medical Association membership woes continue. *CMAJ*. 183: 11: E713–14. 10.1503/cmaj.109-3943. Epub 2011 Jul 11. PMID: 21746826; PMCID: PMC3153537.

15 See https://pulitzercenter.org

16 Sawyer, N., Bloomgarden, E., Cooper, N., Nicols, T. et al. (2021) State medical boards should punish doctors who spread false information about Covid and vaccines. *Washington Post*. Available at: https://www.washingtonpost.com/opinions/2021/09/21/state-medical-boards-should-punish-doctors-who-spread-false-information-about-covid-vaccines/. Accessed: November 23, 2022.

17 Radcliffe, S. (2022) Did California just ban medical misinformation? What we know. *Healthline* Available at: https://www.healthline.com/health-news/did-california-just-ban-medical-misinformation-what-we-know. Accessed: November 23, 2022.

18 Purtill, C. (2022) Doctors feel that California law aimed at Covid-19 misinformation could do more harm than good. *Los Angeles Times*. Available at: https://www.latimes.com/science/story/2022-10-06/spreading-lies-about-covid-19-could-get-doctors-disciplined-in-california. Accessed: November 23, 2022.

19 Coleman, C. (2021) Physicians who disseminate medical misinformation: Testing the constitutional limits on professional disciplinary action. *Seton Hall Public Law Research Paper*. Available at: https://papers.ssrn.com/sol3/papers.cfm?abstract_id=3925250. Accessed: October 16, 2022.

20 Der Beeamont Foundation (2022) Disinformation doctors licensed to mislead. *De Beaumont Foundation*. Available at: https://debeaumont.org/news/2021/disinformation-doctors-poll/. Accessed: November 23, 2022.

21 Meyer, H. (2021) Medical board stops warning docs against giving false COVID information. *Medscape*. Available at: https://www.medscape.com/viewarticle/964451. Accessed: October 16, 2022.

22 Salcedo, A. (2021) Hospital revokes Houston doctor's privileges for 'spreading serious misinformation' about Covid on Twitter. *Washington Post*. Available at: https://www.washingtonpost.com/nation/2021/11/15/houston-doctor-suspended-hospital-misinformation-covid/. Accessed: December 28, 2022.

23 Coleman, C. (2022) License revocation as a response to physician misinformation: Proceed with caution. *Health Affairs Forefront*. Available at: https://www.healthaffairs.org/do/10.1377/forefront.20211227.966736/. Accessed: December 28, 2022.

Chapter 11

Health Professionals Can Have an Even Greater Impact on This and Future Pandemics

Final Arguments and a Call to Action

October 29, 2022. As I begin to pull together my concluding comments, I am in Italy, my birthplace, on my first vacation of the year. The weather today in Venice is picture-perfect – sunny and in the seventies; it is the warmest October on record. Of the literally tens of thousands of people who have "flooded in" to see the beauty of this city, my wife and I are among the few wearing masks. (I've never seen Venice so crowded, and local Venetians agree with this impression.) We were on boats traveling between the Venetian islands packed in like sardines, a super spreader event, and yet again, unfortunately, virtually no one except for ourselves was wearing masks. Today there are several thousand people hospitalized with COVID-19 in Italy; a week ago, there were more than a hundred at Baystate Medical Center, the hospital in Springfield, Massachusetts, to which I admit patients, among the more than 25,000 people hospitalized in the United States.

Although Ali S. Khan, dean of the College of Public Health at the University of Nebraska Medical Center, in late 2022 stated in a recent National Academy of Medicine (NAM) report "We have witnessed the greatest political and public health

DOI: 10.4324/9781003426257-13

failure in our nation's history,"[1] the world's population is by and large behaving as if COVID never happened.

COVID and Other Pandemics Are Here to Stay: What Actions Health Professionals Can Undertake

In this last chapter, I will first briefly restate the impact of COVID on American society. I will do this with respect to both the pandemic itself and how our response to the pandemic reflects the overall societal forces at play. I will then highlight one particularly important NAM report released in 2022, *Emerging Stronger from COVID-19*, which attempts to glean lessons learned and to specify paths forward. I will detail the key points from the report while pointing to areas that could have been usefully brought up.

I will then discuss the three areas health professionals could focus on that would, if well implemented, make a significant impact on the course of this and future pandemics. These are: increasing vaccination rates, decreasing misinformation, and implementing, at least at a state level, community-oriented linkages between public health and acute health. I will specify the avenues available to address these three areas, including an approach that some will consider controversial. As one who considers being a health professional core to my identity, I will also outline what I hope to do in the coming years in this lifelong struggle. It is a struggle that I am committed to participating in for as long as I am able, physically and emotionally. While I am not optimistic about the overall chance of success, I strongly believe that the only way to arrive at a better American pandemic response and, consequently, a healthier American population is to have more health professionals take leadership roles in COVID and pandemic politics. This engagement has to occur at the level of individuals, through our own organizations that we create, through our health professional societies, and finally through political/electoral involvement. Considering that pandemic politics is intimately tied into overall societal forces at play in the United States, this conclusion is a call for much greater health professional political engagement. Our very country is at stake.

Our Challenge – My Challenge

Speaking at the Conservative Political Action Conference in Orlando in February 2022, Florida Governor Ron DeSantis boasted that "had Florida not led the way, this country would look like Canada or Australia."[2] With Florida among the states leading the "American way," population death rates in the country soared to ten times the rate in Australia. While, as a health professional, it is painful for me to write this tragic fact, we must ask ourselves what to do about this sad state of affairs.

The Impact of COVID on Society: A Summary

As of May 31, 2022, there were 6.9 million reported deaths and 17.2 million estimated deaths from COVID-19, as detailed by the Institute for Health Metrics and Evaluation.[3] Tragically, more than *one hundred thousand* health care workers have died of COVID.[4] And there have been more than 600 million cases worldwide – almost certainly an undercount.[5] According to the Lancet COVID-19 Commission published in September 2022 on the lessons for the future from the COVID-19 pandemic:

> There are five basic pillars of a successful fight against emerging infectious diseases. The first is prevention: to stop an outbreak before it occurs by taking effective measures to prevent the emergence of a new and dangerous pathogen. The second is containment: to eliminate the transmission of disease from infected individuals to susceptible individuals after a disease has emerged. The third is health services: to save the lives of people with the disease and ensure the continuity of other health services, including those for mental health. The fourth is equity: to ensure that economic and social burdens are shared among the population and that the most vulnerable groups and individuals are protected. The fifth is global innovation and diffusion: to develop, produce, and distribute new therapeutics and vaccines in an equitable and efficient manner.
>
> To accomplish these five pillars requires an ethical framework of prosociality – the orientation of individuals and government regulations to the needs of society as a whole, rather than to narrow individual interests. In the fourteenth century, authorities in Venice battled plague outbreaks by requiring ships to remain at anchor for forty days before landing (the word "quarantine" derives from the Italian *quarantagiorni*, or forty days), as an early and incipient form of prosocial regulation. Prosociality nowadays includes voluntary behaviors by individuals, such as the proper use of face masks, in addition to government regulations, such as the enforcement of workplace safety standards, to prevent the transmission of disease. [6]

According to Ed Young, a journalist for the *Atlantic* magazine who chronicled every misstep we made during this pandemic, "Every adult in the U.S. has been eligible for vaccines since mid-April [2021]; in that time, more Americans have died of COVID-19 per capita than people in Germany, Canada, Rwanda, Vietnam, or more than 130 other countries did *in the pre-vaccine era*."[7] Chapter 1 of this book brings up the debate between highlighting the social economic disparities in health (Rudolf Virchow) and blaming the poor for their "condition" (Edwin Chadwick).[8] As Chapter 1 states and Ed Young emphasizes, the poor have suffered disproportionately. And, as Ed Young again reports infectious diseases can spread beyond the poor:

> Even though 62 percent of Americans believe that pandemic-related restrictions were worth the cost, Republican legislators in 26 states have passed laws that curtail the possibility of quarantines and mask mandates. But inequity reduction is not a side quest of pandemic preparedness. It is arguably the central pillar – if not for moral reasons, then for basic epidemiological ones. *Infectious diseases can spread*, from the vulnerable to the privileged. "*Our* inequality makes *me* vulnerable," Mary Bassett, who studies health equity at Harvard, told me. "And that's not a necessary feature of our lives. It can be changed."[9]

As discussed in Chapters 9 and 10, the medical profession, and health professionals in general, has largely stood by as health professionals continue to spread misinformation.[10] Politicians in states with low vaccination rates are dismantling[11] public health services and discouraging[12] vaccines. And again, organized medicine in those states and at a national level has done virtually nothing to impact the political process other than to make public pronouncements. Health professionals spreading misinformation are influencing patients of mine who believe that COVID is a government conspiracy. The impact: Alabama, which has one of the country's lowest COVID vaccination rates, recorded more deaths in 2020 than births – a first in state history.[13]

At the same time, some Republicans haven't stopped at decrying efforts to increase vaccination rates; some are also threatening people with harm at the individual level.[14] The result: people living in counties that went 60 percent or higher for Trump in November 2020 had 2.7 times the death rates of those that went for Biden.[15] Senator Ron Johnson from Minnesota stated that gargling mouthwash kills COVID and received virtually no forceful pushback from health professional organizations.[16] We are more than three years into this pandemic and a recent assessment indicated that we are not ready for the next one.[17]

The National Academy of Medicine Report, Emerging Stronger from COVID-19: Priorities for Health System Transformation

At almost six hundred pages, the NAM report is by far the most comprehensive assessment produced in the United States of our unsung heroes, successes, failures, and recommendations for the future. I will quote directly from the report, as the passages give a sense of the tone of this important contribution to our national scientific conversation about this country's response to the pandemic. See Appendix 2 for more detailed quotes from the book.

I will then focus my assessment on the opportunities for improvement in this NAM report, particularly as they pertain to recommendations concerning health professionals and public health. It is important to acknowledge the following absolutely remarkable success that the NAM spotlighted:

> Despite the many challenges, there were remarkable successes. Less than 11 months after SARS-CoV-2 was first discovered, at least two vaccines were developed, tested, and found to be more than 90 percent effective in pivotal trials.[18]

At the same time, on an individual health professional level, the NAM pointed to the tremendous personal sacrifices that health professionals assumed in caring for COVID patients. Many paid with their own lives:

> Throughout the pandemic, health care and public health workers across the country met the needs of their communities and called attention to the importance of preparedness, often suffering great personal costs to respond to the crisis.[19]

Starting with the public health sector, the NAM recommends focusing on:

1. Transforming public health funding;
2. Affirming the mandate for public health;
3. Promoting structural alignment across the public health sector;
4. Investing in leadership and workforce development;
5. Modernizing data and IT capabilities; and
6. Supporting partnerships and community engagement.[20]

With respect to community engagement, the NAM recommends that we:

■ Establish and maintain regional and/or state-level backbone entities that can be leveraged during crises for shared action
■ Cultivate relationships with nontraditional partners including employers, the business sector, and technology
■ Identify a new backbone national entity that can support collaboration to achieve unified policy recommendations from all the core components of the public health sector
■ Enhance trust and credibility through improved risk communication with public health authorities.[21]

The NAM appropriately emphasizes the importance of supply chain (a network of individuals and companies who are involved in creating a product and delivering it to the consumer[22]) redundancy:

> Ensure federal policies encourage manufacturers and laboratories to invest in and maintain sufficient redundancy at all levels of the supply chain across geographies and distribution channels.[23]

Despite the in-depth analyses and recommendations on where we should go from here, there are three significant areas that the NAM report could have explored in much more depth, adding greater specificity together with concrete recommendations:

- The important role of health care professionals in addressing the pandemic
- The impact of the pandemic on political polarization in the United States
- Greater linkages and/or communication between public health and acute health systems

On the very first page of the NAM report, the authors of Chapter 1, entitled "Patients, Families and Communities COVID-19 Impact Assessment: Lessons Learned and Compelling Needs," ambitiously assert: "community-driven solutions are necessary, as communities are in a unique position to drive priorities and actions tailored to their needs that address many of the determinants of health."

In general terms, the NAM states:

> A life stage, population-centered approach may have mitigated these disparate outcomes by engaging wraparound, holistic strategies to prevent chronic disease, maintain mobility, and provide home- and community-based care in lieu of institutional care.... Meaningful change will require all individuals to be able to recognize their own interests, perspectives, and culture at the center of their experiences throughout the health system and across the continuum of care. These foundational principles are the basis for transformative action:
>
> 1. Centering health system actions and accountability on *individuals, families, and communities;*
> 2. Committing to the pursuit of *equity* as core to health system performance;
> 3. Securing the *public health infrastructure* for twenty-first century population health challenges;
> 4. Building a robust and integrated digital health and *data sharing infrastructure;*
> 5. Integrating *telehealth* into payment and delivery systems;
> 6. Investing in *workforce* capacity and readiness;

7. Streamlining *innovation pathways* for biomedical science;
8. Strengthening stewardship of the health product *supply chain*;
9. Restructuring health care payments to focus on *outcomes and population health*; and
10. Fostering *communication and collaboration* across sectors and stakeholders.[24]

The NAM report gets us tantalizing closer to what needs to happen if we are to effectively deal with this and future pandemics:

Centering Health System Actions and Accountability on Individuals, Families, and Communities

- Understand and prioritize the health and health care goals that matter most to individuals, families, and communities.
- Ensure access to the health services that individuals, families, and communities need, when and where they need them.
- Provide active individual, family, and community roles in co-designing health, health care, and research initiatives.
- Orient data and accountability systems to the most important needs and goals of individuals, families, and communities.[25]

Restructuring Health Care Payments to Focus on Outcomes and Population Health

- Identify and translate to sustainable practices those pandemic-era reimbursement flexibilities most effective in accelerating care improvements.
- Identify the services and approaches that successfully use nontraditional fee-for–service models in improving the effectiveness, efficiency, and equitability of care.
- Accelerate design and emphasize implementation of alternative payment models oriented to broad movement from fee-for-service payment models to risk-adjusted prospective payment incentives.
- Design and foster locally based partnership strategies to marshal community resources so as to improve progress in public health, the social determinants of health, and health equity.[26]

Yet the above is as specific as the recommendations get. Nowhere does one find the specificity that the NAM could have presented in laying out the different options pertaining to tying individuals, families, and communities together – the key to eventually addressing this or any other pandemic. Unlike my proposals in Chapter 8 and other chapters in this book, the NAM did not provide any paths forward on how to actually link public health and acute health systems. In fact, while there are statements recommending connecting public and acute health systems, nowhere are there any concrete recommendations either on how to achieve this and/or the absolute necessity of making these linkages happen if we are to ever to successfully address this or future pandemics.

And what about the role of health professions and their engagement? The NAM report highlights the many statements emanating from numerous professional societies:

> Statements from numerous professional societies affirmed the health consequences of structural racism and the necessity of embedding a focus on equity into clinical education and practice, and the Rainbow PUSH Coalition and National Medical Association collaborated to develop the COVID-19 Public Health Manifesto (AAN, 2020; AMA, 2020e; ANA, 2020b).[27]

> The "Principles of Trustworthiness," developed by the Association of American Medical Colleges, has the potential to serve as a useful tool in this regard (AAMC, 2022).[28]

The NAM report stops at these statements. There is nothing, for example, on the role of health professionals in propagating misinformation, because, as discussed in other chapters, health professional societies have done little either politically or in any other way to try to impact the epidemic other than to issue statements. The lack of concrete recommendations for what health professional societies could consider doing in the future with respect to misinformation, vaccination, or anything else for that matter, other than public pronouncements, represents an unfortunate missed opportunity.

Next Steps Forward: A Summing Up, Together with One Additional Tool to Be Considered in These Pandemic Times

Health professionals should focus on the following outcomes if we are to effectively deal with this and future pandemics:

■ Increased acceptance of vaccination
■ Decreased misinformation
■ Greater community health linkages between acute and public health systems.

There are three broad options on how to achieve these three outcomes:

■ Engagement from outside the health professional organizations
■ Engagement from within health professional organizations
■ Engagement in the political process and pressure groups.

Throughout this book, I've specified actions we could take to accomplish these three outcomes. Professional associations such as the American Medical Association and American Nurses Association, among many others, at a state level, could use an aggressive social media strategy to both promote vaccinations and fight against misinformation. If the state association is too politically weak as might be the case in Florida, with Joseph Ladapo, an anti-vaxxer, in place as surgeon general, the AMA at a national level could be engaged in a social media strategy focused on Florida and privately work with local health professionals and politicians to accomplish these three outcomes.

In addition, at a state level, licensure boards could play a major role in the fight against misinformation and outright lies. Both professional and licensure boards at a national level could push the legal envelope to try and hold health professionals accountable, as far as is feasible, for their public pronouncements on vaccines and pandemic facts. Surely, licensure boards can be much more aggressive in disciplining health professionals who do not adhere to science while taking into consideration the constitutionally based right to free speech. That may mean having national professional associations such as the AMA clarify the constitutional boundaries of free speech as they take up the political and legal fight to defend science and enable society to effectively address pandemics.

I realize that the vaccination and misinformation issues are larger than health care; the pandemic has contributed to the unleashing of forces ranging from anti-Semitism[29] to anti-Asian attacks[30] to political violence directed at senior leaders of our government.[31] The pandemic is certainly not the only cause of these unleashed forces. The anti-vax political[32] and religious leaders[33] have proved a major obstacle to dealing with the COVID pandemic effectively, and they will undoubtedly hamper efforts in future pandemics. Lamentably, many of these leaders around the world, including from Israel,[34] compare coronavirus restrictions to Nazi anti-Jewish laws; in the United States, Fauci has been compared to the concentration camp doctor Josef Mengele.[35] Tragically, increased anti-Asian sentiment in the United States has escalated to killings of Asian Americans.[36]

We read about frequent deaths among the anti-vax political and religious leaders; the evangelist Marcus Lamb died of COVID-19 after his network discouraged vaccines, but some Christian evangelists don't want to talk about it.[37] Many corporations are not helping.[38]

Tragically, as discussed in previous chapters, these political and religious leaders have been aided and abetted by health professionals. I am a health professional – that is my identity and the identity of hundreds of thousands of others committed to a healthier society. I and we as health professionals have the possibility and responsibility to act and be open to new ways of creating awareness and action in response to the pandemics that are here to stay. Right now, we as health professionals have the potential to impact the political process and health professional organizations as described above. By fighting against COVID misinformation, in favor of vaccinations, and advocating for linkages between public and acute health, we will do our part to address the broader societal forces in play.

A Strong Tool for a Tragic Time: The Pros and Cons of Civil Disobedience

> I would remind you that extremism in the defense of liberty is no vice. And let me remind you also that moderation in pursuit of justice is no virtue.[39]

This was written not by a defender of government health care insurance for all and/or an effective pandemic response but by Harry Jaffa, a mid-twentieth-century philosopher, in defense of a Barry Goldwater presidency. In quoting these words, however, I conclude this book with a defense of civil disobedience.

What if working with the political process and health professional organizations doesn't bring about a more forceful and concrete response to the pandemic, which continues to result in unnecessary hospitalizations and deaths? What other tools can health professionals consider to pressure the United States to take a more effective approach to a pandemic that has caused so much suffering and the dramatic loss of life expectancy?

At the start of the pandemic, and after seeing the appalling reaction of the last administration, I hoped to see health professionals take a more forceful stand. For example, back in the summer of 2020, I advocated that Anthony Fauci and Devorah Birx should have resigned instead of clinging to a fig leaf of power. Birx has estimated that hundreds of thousands of individuals unnecessarily died in 2020 alone.[40] Had Fauci and Birx operated from the outside, working with and leading thousands of health professionals, they might have had a greater impact.

What if health professionals both in and out of government service had not only resigned but also considered acts of civil disobedience to push the US government into a more forceful response to the pandemic? Could they have garnered support from Fauci and Birx in 2020? How many more lives could have been saved if Fauci and Birx, supported by health professionals committing acts of civil disobedience, had acted to change US government pandemic policies, as ACT-Up in particular managed to do during the AIDS epidemic?[41] Could actions of civil disobedience have resulted in essential public health measures and contact tracing, as Republican health officials Mark McClellan and Scott Gottlieb advocated, as discussed in other chapters of this book, back in March 2020?

Clearly, a struggle involving health professionals committing acts of civil disobedience back in 2020 is simply impossible to imagine, and not just because of the national and worldwide COVID shutdown at that point in time. And even though Fauci communicated with ACT-UP leadership in the 1980s, it is unlikely that he and Birx would have been supportive of civil disobedience. We simply don't know what could have been. At a time when hospitalizations and deaths from COVID remind us that the pandemic is still very active, the question is how can we bring civil disobedience into play when most people have returned to "lives as usual." Since virtually all experts state that we are not coping effectively with the pandemic today, civil disobedience should be considered. If we as health professionals lead the way, we can finally effectively deal with this and future pandemics. Appendix 1 at the end of this chapter provides a suggested approach on how to explore the pros and cons of civil disobedience for health professionals who, like myself, are interested in pursuing, and will not give up, the three key areas of increasing vaccination, combating misinformation, and advocating for community linkages between acute and public health.

Imagine the power and impact on public opinion if health professionals – both Republicans and Democrats – committed acts of civil disobedience simply because they care for the entire population.

Concluding Comments

From a lead 2020 editorial of the *Irish Times* from Dublin: "The world has loved, hated and envied the US. Now, for the first time, we pity it."[42] Yes, "pity" is the right word.

And looking to the future, I agree with the following sentiment by J. Demsas with respect to COVID and future pandemics:

> Growing up, I remember hearing a common refrain from environmentalists: We would take action on climate change only when the water hit our ankles. Once the crisis presented less as a hypothetical and more as an immediate danger, the public would pay serious attention and invest in countering it. Today, I'm not even sure that's true.[43]

With respect to public health, Rachel Kohrs said it best in January 2023: "Will America's public health reckoning ever come?"[44] Or knowing what we know today, I am not sure that the public will pay greater attention if COVID comes roaring back, or a new pandemic emerges and kills and hospitalizes even more than the almost 40,000 patients (as of January 2023) hospitalized or dying every week in the United States. Both in terms of its impact on the health of Americans and a dramatic downturn in economic performance,[45] the COVID pandemic has been disastrous. The United States, rated first among industrialized countries in the ability to respond to disasters, squandered this status with a performance that was the worst of any industrialized country.[46]

Or to put it differently, an expert at a 2022 NAM conference plaintively asked: "How do we engage our society when there is active disinformation and opposition to scientifically based practices in both traditional media and social media, as well as leadership?"[47] My response, in part, is that health professionals have not effectively stepped up and assumed our fiduciary responsibility. We have not succeeded at peace through health. The pandemic has exacerbated an already polarized US population to such an extent that the country at a minimum is in danger of sliding into "populism, cronyism and corruption."[48] The conservative historian Robert Kagan believes that the constitutional crisis has arrived.[49]

While Reagan's presidency offered political challenges in its effort to stamp a conservative but not authoritarian vision onto the United States, the reality is that the Trump administration constituted a clear and present danger.[50] It is remarkable and a sign of the times that we are faced with the possible return of Trump. And, if not Trump, there are other would-be authoritarians, such as Governor's Ron DeSantis and Greg Abbott, waiting in the wings.[51]

The specter of climate change and pandemics is ever present. A remarkable article connecting climate change with COVID concluded: "reduced human activity resulting from COVID-19 restrictions contributed to a brighter, earlier, and greener 2020 spring season in China." I was born in Italy. During the height of the pandemic, unusual fish and birds returned to the canals of Venice after an absence of many years.[52]

Can we similarly imagine the eventual end to this pandemic and develop effective responses for inevitable future pandemics?[53] Mark and Paul Engler, among others, recently detailed ways of addressing our political divide.[54] This is our long-term challenge. While health professionals to date have not played a significant role in healing our political divide, an increasing number of health professionals are running for electoral office, and even more are engaged politically. Such efforts would be enormously magnified if health professional organizations took a more proactive role in addressing COVID misinformation, the need for vaccinations, and advocate for better coordination between our acute and public health systems.

Trust in authorities is key to effectively dealing with pandemics in the United States[55] or abroad[56]. Health professionals can play a key role in increasing trust. A bipartisan comprehensive public health response undertaken by Republican and Democratic health professionals would go a long way to further this effort. While action appears unlikely at a national level, health professionals across the board can make a difference at a minimum at a state level, as outlined in Chapter 8. As recently quoted by the writer and surgeon Atul Gawande, C. Everett Koop, surgeon general under Ronald Reagan, once said, "Health care is vital to all of us some of the time, but public health is vital to all of us all of the time."[57] Many of us became health professionals aspiring to better serve the society we live in. We know the power that effective public health can have on the entire population. Even if the challenges are daunting, health professionals, armed with the specific actions recommended in this book, can help increase trust in our government's ability to deal with pandemics and, by extension, other forces polarizing American society.

Pandemics are here to stay. The price of failure is severe. Without public trust, American fragility and the resultant polarization in American society will only increase. The lack of effective and coordinated public health at the time of a pandemic undermines public trust. Health professionals may be the key to reestablishing trust and reversing American fragility. Health professionals can be a force for the public good.

Notes

1 National Academies of Sciences, Engineering, and Medicine. (2022) *Future planning for the public health emergency preparedness enterprise: Lessons learned from the COVID-19 pandemic: Proceedings of a workshop.* Washington, DC: The National Academies Press. Available at: https://doi.org/10.17226/26805. Accessed: December 28, 2022.

2 Available at: https://www.youtube.com/watch?v=QI9couOvu2Q. Accessed: November 23, 2022.

3 See Institute for Health Metrics and Evaluation. Available at: https://covid19.healthdata.org/global?view=cumulative-deaths&tab=trend. Accessed: November 23, 2022.

4 World Health Organization. (2021) Health and care worker deaths during Covid-10. *World Health Organization.* Available at: https://www.who.int/news/item/20-10-2021-health-and-care-worker-deaths-during-covid-19. Accessed: November 23, 2022.

5 For an up to date summary of Covid deaths Worldometer. Available at: https://www.worldometers.info/coronavirus/coronavirus-death-toll/. Accessed: November 23, 2022.

6 Sachs, J., Abdool Karim, SS., Aknin, L. et al. (2022) The Lancet Commission on lessons for the future from the Covid-19 pandemic. *The Lancet.* Available at: https://www.thelancet.com/journals/lancet/article/PIIS0140-6736(22)01585-9/fulltext. Accessed: November 23, 2022.

7 Young, E. (2022) We're already barrelling towards the next pandemic. *The Atlantic.* Available at: https://www.theatlantic.com/health/archive/2021/09/america-prepared-next-pandemic/620238/. Accessed: October 3, 2022.

8 As discussed in Snowden, F. (2020). *Epidemics and society: From the Black Death to the present* New Haven: Yale University Press, pp. 184–85.

9 Young op. cit.

10 Edwards, J. (2021) Georgia's medical board mum as doctors spread Covid-19 misinformation. *The Atlanta Journal-Constitution.* Available at: https://www.ajc.com/news/coronavirus/georgias-medical-board-mum-as-doctors-spread-covid-19-misinformation/CRWP7IZFBBEBPFSAVIW7AGD7CM/?utm_source=Iterable&utm_medium=email&utm_campaign=campaign_3110932. Accessed: December 26, 2022.

11 Weber, L. and Barry-Joseph, AM. (2021) Over half of states have rolled back public health powers in pandemic. *Kaiser Health News.* Available at: https://khn.org/news/article/over-half-of-states-have-rolled-back-public-health-powers-in-pandemic/?utm_campaign=KHN%3A%20First%20Edition&utm_medium=email&_hsmi=159714944&_hsenc=p2ANqtz-_BLjbTwjJZKUFzbMdGYpvxSeELQ9m LoRScd_ZxnPmU42DTQhW7LSYWannAv6wS-UFLOHyk67JorpfrBYNo3N_WujhZGGQ&utm_content=159714944&utm_source=hs_email. Accessed: December 26, 2022.

12 Caputo, M. and Fineout, G. (2021) DeSantis flirts with the anti-vaccine crowd. *Politico.* Available at: https://www.politico.com/states/florida/story/2021/09/15/desantis-flirts-with-the-anti-vaccine-crowd-1391038. Accessed: December 26, 2022.
    And most recently Morgan, I. (2022) Governor DeSantis, Surgeon General Ladapo go after Covid vaccines; request state-wide grand jury. *Florida Phoenix.* Available at: https://floridaphoenix.com/2022/12/13/gov-desantis-surgeon-general-ladapo-go-after-covid-vaccines-requests-statewide-grand-jury/. Accessed: December 26, 2022.

13 Archibald, R. (2021) Alabama saw more deaths in 2020 than any year in history. *Alabama*. Available at: https://www.al.com/news/2021/09/alabama-saw-more-deaths-in-2020-than-any-year-in-history.html?utm_source=newsletter&utm_medium=email&utm_campaign=newsletter_axiosam&stream=top. Accessed: December 26, 2022.

14 Mello, MM., Greene, J., and Scharfstein, J. (2020) Attacks on public health officials during Covid-19. *JAMA*. Available at: https://jamanetwork.com/journals/jama/fullarticle/2769291. Accessed: November 23, 2022.

15 Abutaleb, Y., Parker, A., Dawsey J., and Tucker, P. (2020) The inside story of how Trummp's denial, mismanagement and magical thinking led to the pandemic's dark winter. *Washington Post*. Available at: https://www.washingtonpost.com/graphics/2020/politics/trump-covid-pandemic-dark-winter/?itid=hp-top-table-main. Accessed: November 23, 2022.

16 Jeong, A. (2021) A GOP Senator suggested gargling mouthwash to kill the coronavirus. Doctors and Listerine are skeptical. *Washington Post*. Available at: https://www.washingtonpost.com/health/2021/12/09/ron-johnson-mouthwash-covid/. Accessed: November 23, 2022.

17 Demsas, J. (2022) The U.S. has no plans to prevent the next pandemic. *The Atlantic Magazine*. Available at: https://www.theatlantic.com/newsletters/archive/2022/07/monkeypox-covid19-us-next-pandemic/670946/. Accessed: November 23, 2022.

18 Anise, A., Adams, L., Ahmed, M., and Bailey, A. eds. (2020) *Emerging Stronger from COVID-19: Priorities for Health System Transformation*. Washington, DC: National Academies Press. p. 395. Available at: https://nap.nationalacademies.org/catalog/26657/emerging-stronger-from-covid-19-priorities-for-health-system-transformation. Accessed: November 23, 2022.

19 Ibid. p. 478.

20 Ibid. p. 257.

21 Ibid. p 275.

22 Hayes, A. (2022) The supply chain. *Investopedia*. Available at: https://www.investopedia.com/terms/s/supplychain.asp. Accessed: November 23, 2022.

23 Anise, A. (op cit). p. 373.

24 Ibid. p 494.

25 Ibid. p. 507.

26 Ibid. p. 519.

27 Ibid. p. 490

28 Ibid. p. 89.

29 Milbank, D. (2022) American Jews start to think the unthinkable. *Washington Post*. Available at: https://www.washingtonpost.com/opinions/2022/10/28/american-jews-exile-fears/. Accessed: November 23, 2022.

30 Associated Press. (2021) More than 9,000 Anti-Asian incidents have been reported since the pandemic began National Public Radio. Available at: https://www.npr.org/2021/08/12/1027236499/anti-asian-hate-crimes-assaults-pandemic-incidents-aapi; Accessed: January 16, 2023.

31 Parker, A., Allam, H., and Sotomayor, M. (2022) Attack on Pelosi's husband follows year's of demonizing her. *Washington Post*. Available at: https://www.washingtonpost.com/politics/2022/10/29/paul-pelosi-attack-republicans-target/. Accessed: November 23, 2022.

32 Millbank, D. (2021) Sarah Palin's anti-vax talk show Republicans have become a death cult. *Washington Post*. Available at: https://www.washingtonpost.com/

opinions/2021/12/20/sarah-palin-anti-vax-tpusa-tconference/. Accessed: December 26, 2022.

33 Gerson, M. (2022) Trump should fill Christians with rage. How come he doesn't? *Washington Post.* Available at: https://www.washingtonpost.com/opinions/2022/09/01/michael-gerson-evangelical-christian-maga-democracy/. Accessed: November 23, 2022.

34 Shpigel, N. (2021) Netanyahu party lawmaker likens Covid restrictions to 'concentration camps'. *Haaretz.* Available at: https://www.haaretz.com/israel-news/2021-12-26/ty-article/.premium/likud-lawmaker-calls-covid-restrictions-to-concentration-camps/0000017f-dbff-d856-a37f-ffffb3450000. Accessed: December 26, 2022.

35 Grynbaum, MM. (2021) Fox New's host's incendiary Fauci comments follow a network pattern. *New York Times.* Available at: https://www.nytimes.com/2021/12/23/business/media/fox-anthony-fauci-jesse-watters.html. Accessed: December 26, 2022.

36 Findling, M., Blendon, R., Benson, J., and Koh, H. (2022) COVID-19 has driven racism and violence against Asian Americans: Perspectives from 12 national polls. *Health Affairs Forefront.* Available at: https://www.healthaffairs.org/do/10.1377/forefront.20220411.655787/. Accessed: January 16, 2023.

37 Boorstein, M. (2020) Marcus Lamb died of Covid-19 after his network discouraged vaccines. But some Christian leaders don't want to talk about it. *Washington Post.* Available at: https://www.washingtonpost.com/religion/2021/12/03/marcus-lamb-daystar-vaccine-televangelist-graham/. Accessed: December 26, 2022.

38 Kimball, S. (2021) Business groups ask White House to delay Biden Covid vaccine mandate until after the holidays. *CNBC.* Available at: https://www.cnbc.com/2021/10/25/businesses-ask-white-house-to-delay-biden-covid-vaccine-mandate-until-after-holidays.html. Accessed: December 26, 2022.

39 Berkowitz, P. (2021) Harry Jaffa's love-hate relationship with moderation. *Free Beacon.* Available at: https://freebeacon.com/culture/harry-jaffas-love-hate-relationship-with-moderation/. Accessed: November 23, 2022.

40 Wang, A. (2021) Birx tells CNN most Covid deaths "could have been mitigated "after the first 100,000. *Washington Post.* Available at: https://www.washingtonpost.com/politics/2021/03/27/birx-tells-cnn-most-us-covid-deaths-could-have-been-mitigated-after-first-100000/. Accessed: November 23, 2022.

41 Aizenman, N. (2019) How to demand a medical breakthrough: Lessons from the AIDS fight. *National Public Radio.* Available at: https://www.npr.org/sections/health-shots/2019/02/09/689924838/how-to-demand-a-medical-breakthrough-lessons-from-the-aids-fight. Accessed: December 26, 2022. And see Act Up Historical Archive. Available at: https://actupny.org. Accessed: December 26, 2022.

42 O'Toole, F. (2021) Donald Trump has destroyed the country he promised to make great again. *The Irish Times.* Available at: https://www.irishtimes.com/opinion/fintan-o-toole-donald-trump-has-destroyed-the-country-he-promised-to-make-great-again-1.4235928. Accessed November 10, 2022.

43 Demsas, J. (2022) The U.S. has no plan to prevent the next pandemic. *The Atlantic.* Available at: https://www.theatlantic.com/newsletters/archive/2022/07/monkeypox-covid19-us-next-pandemic/670946/. Accessed: January 11, 2023.

44 Kohrs, R. (2023) Will America's public health reckoning ever come? *Stat.* Available at: https://www.statnews.com/2023/01/11/will-americas-public-health-reckoning-ever-come/?utm_source=STAT+Newsletters&utm_campaign=54c4f3805c-MR_

COPY_01&utm_medium=email&utm_term=0_8cab1d7961-54c4f3805c-152403458. Accessed: January 14, 2023.

45 Collier, P. (2021) Locked and loaded Times Literary Supplement. Available at: https://www.the-tls.co.uk/articles/shutdown-adam-tooze-book-review-covid-paul-collier/. Accessed: December 26, 2022.

46 GHS Index. How the United States squandered its capacities to respond to the pandemic. *GHS Index.* Available at: https://www.ghsindex.org/news/how-the-united-states-squandered-its-capacities-to-respond-to-the-pandemic/. Accessed November 10, 2022.

47 National Academies of Sciences, Engineering, and Medicine. (2022) *Future planning for the public health emergency preparedness enterprise: Lessons learned from the COVID-19 pandemic: Proceedings of a workshop.* Op cit. p 13. Available at: https://doi.org/10.17226/26805. Accessed: December 28, 2022.

48 Hill, F. (2021) The Kremlin's strange victory. *Foreign Affairs.* Available at: https://www.foreignaffairs.com/articles/united-states/2021-09-27/kremlins-strange-victory?utm_campaign=Brookings%20Brief&utm_medium=email&utm_content=164798306&utm_source=hs_email. Accessed: December 26, 2022.

49 Kagan, R. (2021) Our constitutional crisis is already here. *Washington Post.* Available at: https://www.washingtonpost.com/opinions/2021/09/23/robert-kagan-constitutional-crisis/. Accessed: December 26, 2022.

50 Kanno-Youngs, Z., and Shear MD. (2022) Biden warns that American values and under assault by Trump-led extremism. *New York Times.* Available at: https://www.nytimes.com/2022/09/01/us/politics/biden-speech-trump-maga.html. Accessed: November 23, 2022.

51 Biden, J. (2022) Full transcript of President Biden's Speech in Philadelphia. *New York Times.* Available at: https://www.nytimes.com/2022/09/01/us/politics/biden-speech-transcript.html?action=click&module=Well&pgtype=Homepage&section=US%20Politics. Accessed: November 23, 2022.

52 Brunton, J. (2020) Nature is taking back Venice. *The Guardian.* Available at: https://www.theguardian.com/environment/2020/mar/20/nature-is-taking-back-venice-wildlife-returns-to-tourist-free-city. Accessed: November 23, 2022. And Su, F., Fu, D., Yan, F., Xiao, H. et al. Rapid greening response to China's spring vegetation to Covid-19 restrictions: Implications for climate change. *Science.* Available at: https://www.science.org/doi/10.1126/sciadv.abe8044?_ga=2.82591638.1255382000.1629735222-862897998.1619546695. Accessed: December 26, 2022.

53 Carroll, A. (2021) When can we declare the pandemic over? *New York Times.* Available at: https://www.nytimes.com/2021/04/27/opinion/covid-lockdown-end.html?action=click&module=Opinion&pgtype=Homepage. Accessed: December 26, 2022.

54 Engler, M. and Engler, P. (2021) Can social movements realign America's political parties to win big change? *Democracy Uprising.* Available at: https://democracyuprising.com/2021/03/25/can-social-movements-realign-americas-political-parties-to-win-big-change/. Accessed: December 26, 2022.

55 De Marco, H. (2021) Vaccine promoters struggle to get people boosted in California's fields. *Kaiser Health News.* Available at: https://khn.org/news/article/vaccine-promoters-struggle-to-get-people-boosted-in-californias-fields/?utm_campaign=KHN%3A%20First%20Edition&utm_medium=email&_hsmi=197756001&_hsenc=p2ANqtz-_8NFoioARtg51YPx6G8eNp0FM31hVpUY0lXGNVA0zZNyN6Lc2TVrk_kvkMIcbLKOmQQxQG8wGbhpeMPxomVjQC

uAATPA&utm_content=197756001&utm_source=hs_email. Accessed: December 26, 2022.

56 Chu, L. (2021) Vaccine politics follows political choice in the U.S. Why doesn't it in Germany. *Christian Science Monitor.* Available at: https://www.csmonitor.com/Daily/2021/20211209?cmpid=ema:ddp:20211209:1137066:read&sfmc_sub=61636896&id=1137066#1137066. Accessed: December 26, 2022.

57 Gawande, A. (2020) We can solve the Coronavirus mess now – if we want to. *New Yorker.* Available at: https://www.newyorker.com/science/medical-dispatch/we-can-solve-the-coronavirus-test-mess-now-if-we-want-to?utm_source=nl&utm_brand=tny&utm_mailing=TNY_Daily_090220&utm_campaign=aud-dev&utm_medium=email&bxid=5bea06da24c17c6adf125b09&cndid=50856718&hasha=5c81c9183ba5aa9fd682e58291889859&hashb=cebff94d072ef16164c89170fc47fd36337bb64d&hashc=8c6ed225fce9f934f5b1b6d643f99d2a761bd86aefbc7f884c1cbe64c9dce77f&esrc=bounceX&utm_term=TNY_Daily. Accessed: December 26, 2022.

58 Committee of Interns and Residents, SEIU Healthcare. (2022) Our History. Committee of Interns and Residents. Available at: https://www.cirseiu.org/our-history-2/. Accessed: November 23, 2022.

59 Harmon, RG. (1978) Intern and resident organizations in the United States: 1934–1977. *Milbank Mem Fund Q Health Soc.* 56: 4: 500–30. PMID: 366458. Available at: https://www.jstor.org/stable/3349574. Accessed: November 23, 2022.

60 Bogage, J. and Mark., J. (2023) New York nurses end strike after reaching tentative deals with hospitals. *Washington Post.* Available at: https://www.washingtonpost.com/business/2023/01/12/new-york-nurses-strike-deals-hospitals-tentative/. Accessed: January 16, 2023.

61 Sunrise Movement. (2017) Young people sit in at offices of House Republicans to demand they vote against tax breaks for 1% and fossil fuel billionaires. *Sunrise Movement.* Available at: https://www.sunrisemovement.org/movement-updates/young-people-sit-in-at-offices-of-house-republicans-to-demand-they-vote-against-tax-breaks-for-1-de654ea3462f/. Accessed: November 23, 2022.

62 Anise, A. op. cit. p. 510.

63 Ibid. p. 198.

64 Ibid. p. 220.

65 Ibid. p. 339.

66 Ibid. p. 360.

Appendix 1: A Suggested Approach to Civil Disobedience with the Goal of Increasing Vaccinations and Decreasing Pandemic Misinformation

In the United States, health care professionals have historically participated in large demonstrations and engaged in acts of civil disobedience. In the 1970s, large groups of New York City–based interns and residents, myself included, went on strike to improve not only their own pay and working conditions but also access to care for the poor.[58] In 1989, unionized interns and residents at Boston City Hospital held a three-day "heal-in" to improve care conditions for patients and work requirements for staff, filling up the hospital and resulting in the closure of the emergency department.[59] During the COVID pandemic, health professionals, especially nurses, have gone on strike.[60]

Ensuring that acts of civil disobedience will be successful and their goals – of increasing vaccination and decreasing misinformation – are not misinterpreted calls for carefully thinking through tactics and strategies. Two types of general actions fall under the rubric of civil disobedience, both of which should, ideally be publicly announced in advance to have maximum impact:

■ actions that explicitly violate a state or federal law
■ actions that violate administrative procedures of an organization (that is, monkey-wrenching or gumming up the system).

When considering civil disobedience, the following preliminary organizational steps should be implemented:

■ Create a nationwide umbrella organization of groups and individuals that would be interested in being kept abreast of strategic thinking and ongoing events
■ Assemble a group of three to five individuals in each state willing to serve as leaders/committee leaders of the umbrella organization
■ Assemble a group of at a minimum of three to five individuals willing to lead "teach-ins" or information exchanges with groups around the country
■ Create a national steering committee to direct and present "thought" and "practical" papers.

"Thought" and "practical" papers together with "Teach-ins" would pose the following types of questions and issues:

■ What is the metaphor or theme we will base any action on to increase vaccination and decrease pandemic misinformation? Can we frame the theme around justice and, yes, freedom? A curriculum surrounding issues pertaining to increasing vaccination, fighting against misinformation, and community linkages between public and acute health has yet to be conceived. Such a curriculum should address all controversies, be seen as complete and unbiased, and be tailored to audiences including health professional students, professionals in practice, retired health professionals, and, in particular, the broader public.
■ Decide what kind of specific political program is needed for implementation. Specify legislation addressing vaccination, misinformation, and community public/acute health linkages.

Prior to undertaking any civil disobedience actions, the following external outreach should occur:

- Identify and have meetings with sympathetic members of Congress and other organizations or individuals engaged in health care politics. Send letters to the editor and to members of Congress advocating specific vaccine and misinformation policies.
- Reconvene and decide, based on the results of these meetings, whether further actions, including civil disobedience, merit attention.
- Assess whether to work in those states with the greatest needs – lowest vaccination rates, high misinformation, and completely inadequate public health – or those states where we might have the broadest public support.
- Debate what type of follow-through is necessary: rolling action or political follow-up or both?
- Assess whether it is sufficient to just rely on health professionals. What about other groups that have a vested interest, such as senior citizens and/or groups assisting the underserved?
- Of critical importance, assess the specific legal implications for any action we might undertake.

Civil disobedience calls for two types of people: those who are willing to commit acts of civil disobedience and supporters. The latter group is just as important as the former and critical to the success of the effort. Supporters can fill the following roles:

- Communications with the public
- Legal advocacy
- Negotiations with political representatives
- Negotiations with grassroots organizations and other entities that might be supportive in a variety of ways.

After thinking through goals, strategies, and tactics, what types of actions should be considered? Demonstrations and sit-ins could take place at the following types of organizations: licensure boards, offices of professional organizations such as the AMA and ANA, managed care organizations, and hospital systems. Each of these organizations has a part to play in fighting to increase vaccinations and decrease misinformation. Health professionals and their supporters should also consider sit-ins in the offices of members of Congress, a tactic deployed by the Sunrise Movement in pursuit of environmental reform.[61]

What is the minimum number of individuals needed? Effectively implemented, 50 committed individuals nationwide could catalyze the process to systematically deal with low vaccination rates and pandemic misinformation.

In considering civil disobedience as a tool to effectively address this and future pandemics, I believe that the public, in the aggregate, would be supportive.

Appendix 2: Additional Details from the NAM Report, *Emerging Stronger from COVID-19: Priorities for Health System Transformation*

With respect to "enhancing stewardship of the health product supply chain":

■ Restructure, strengthen, and maintain the designations, tracking protocols, and decision rules needed to ensure the availability and distribution of health products for which unanticipated demand surges are most critical.
■ Identify product categories most likely to require future iterations of improvements, and establish cooperative agreements with companies who are best positioned to undertake product development.
■ Assess and streamline regulatory processes as needed for cross-sector and cross-national partnerships to replenish stockpile shortages and encourage innovations that promote supply chain resilience.
■ Foster the development of international protocols and agreements to enhance the prospects for success in global responses in supply shortage circumstances.[62]

In bold, the authors of the NAM report state:

As the U.S. looks to the future, it will need to embrace the importance of data architecture for any coordinated national or international response to health crises and find effective ways to define such an architecture and then create the infrastructure to put it into action. This need includes attention to every aspect of health care, including:

■ supply chains, such as "Adopting internet-of-things (IoT) connectivity and digitization that will allow hospitals to better track products throughout the supply chain"
■ digital therapeutics, such as mental health services (discussed at length in chapter)
■ digital architecture to help understand this new virus via "real world data," or RWD
■ Cybersecurity as it pertains to, for example, health care organizations.[63]

The NAM report also has a chapter on data architecture (referring to both available data elements and digital interoperability, meaning communication between different computer systems). Regulations facilitating communication between data systems must balance the need for privacy with the need for individuals to communicate their information with and between organizations. The NAM report looks to the future and provides the following recommendations on digital capacity and architecture, each of which is critical:

1. options and strategies for computing architecture, data architecture, and data interoperability;
2. elements of a national public health crisis pre-warning system;
3. these issues and options around a national "data trust" for public health;
4. how to operationalize and advance telemedicine and virtual care;
5. approaches to incentivize digital medicine solutions;
6. strategies for using digital capacity to create new evidence and appropriately update clinical care while ensuring data quality and protection; and
7. system-wide cybersecurity.[64]

With respect to product testing and diagnostics capacity, including the diagnostics supply chain:

> There is acknowledgement that involving private-sector laboratories earlier would have allowed for a more rapid scale-up of testing capacity. If labs had begun receiving information earlier, when other countries were facing the crisis, they could have helped earlier. Once private labs were allowed to provide testing under emergency-use conditions, the U.S.'s ability to test for the virus dramatically expanded. The authors of this manuscript believe that engaging both public and private labs early in the national response to COVID-19 would have helped scale up testing supplies and infrastructure more quickly.[65]

Notwithstanding the dramatic developments in vaccines and all health products relevant for COVID-19 prevention and treatment, numerous opportunities remain related to better understanding of the COVID virus:

■ Fundamental human biology – e.g., in the case of pandemic preparedness, better understanding of the innate immune response to infections and how it differentiates "friend vs. foe"
■ Therapeutic modality research – e.g., the use of RNA therapeutics for rapid response to pandemic threats either as antiviral or as vaccine

- Human toxicology science
- Manufacturing science – especially of new therapeutic modalities
- Clinical trial design – e.g., modifications to design that allow for non-placebo-controlled trials in conjunction with the use of data science to generate better controls and identify other ways to assess comparator arms.[66]

Index

Abbott, Greg 6, 70, 236
ACA *see* Affordable Care Act
Academic Public Health Corps 193
accountable care organizations (ACOs) 174,
    182, 186
ACOs *see* accountable care organizations
ACT-Up 234
Adams, Jerome 45
Affordable Care Act (ACA) 7, 47, 51, 79–80,
    160, 167, 171, 173, 176, 182
AHIP *see* America's Health Insurance Plans
Alabama 70, 228
American Board of Internal Medicine
    (ABIM) 131
American Medical Association (AMA) 66, 79,
    125–126, 130, 213, 216–222, 233
American Nurse 80
American Nurses Association 233
American Public Health Association (APHA)
    165, 184
America's Frontline Doctors 134, 219
America's Health Insurance Plans (AHIP) 173
anti-Asian attacks 233
anti-Semitism 233
Ask Nurses and Doctors (AND) 39–41, 43,
    55–59, 61–62, 69–70, 77, 79–82, 84, 86–87,
    89–90, 214–217
Association of American Medical Colleges
    (AAMC) 232
Atlanta Journal-Constitution 59
Atlas, Scott 55
Australia 60, 126, 181, 226–227

Barr, Bill 46
Baystate Medical Center 3, 58, 71, 201, 225
Berger, Peter 12
Biden, Joe 56–59, 65–66, 68–69, 72–76,
    83–84, 89–90, 134, 201, 203, 228

Birx, Deborah 45, 234
Blacks/Black Americans 5, 48, 49, 50, 51, 79,
    85, 147
Blacks 50, 79, 147
British Medical Journal 82
Burston, Ahriel 153

California 86, 128, 134, 143, 175, 220
Canada 226, 228
CCA *see* Commonwealth Health Insurance
    Connector Authority
CDC *see* Centers for Disease Control and
    Prevention
CDSMP *see* Chronic Disease Self-Management
    Program
Center for Countering Digital Hate
    (CCDH) 133
Centers for Disease Control and Prevention
    (CDC) 55, 198, 204–206
Chazov, Yevgeny 22, 198
China 64, 78, 142, 198, 236
Christensen, Cathryn 29
Christian evangelists 74, 233
Christian Science Monitor (CSM) 149
Chronic Disease Self-Management Program
    (CDSMP) 25
CHR *see* Community Health Representative
    Program
CHRP *see* Community Health Resilience Plan
CHWs *see* Community Health Workers
civil disobedience 67, 234–235, 241–244
Cliniquita, La 151
Coleman, Carl 132, 220–221
Collier, Paul 46, 208
Collins, Francis 73–74
Commonwealth Corps 193–194
Commonwealth Health Insurance Connector
    Authority (CCA) 164, 176

community health centers 172
Community Health Representative (CHR)
Program 52
Community Health Resilience Plan (CHRP)
165–166, 171–174, 176–178, 181–183, 185
Community Health Workers (CHWs) 63,
161–163, 165, 174, 181–182, 184
conflict 6–7, 11–12, 22–29, 125; impact of
14–15; Israeli-Palestinian 14, 18, 25; political
20; protracted 25; societal culture of 12–13
consumer groups 172
contact tracers (CTCs) 164, 177
contact tracing 45–47, 50, 54–55, 57, 67, 163,
191–192, 234
COVID-19 Recovery Corps 185, 193–194
Crespin, Emperatriz 28–29
crisis standards of care (CSCs) 201–202
CSCs *see* crisis standards of care
CSM *see* Christian Science Monitor
CTCs *see* contact tracers
curriculum development 37

Das, Veena 13
data 143–146, 202; environmental 204;
interpretation of 205; preliminary 45;
wastewater 204
Democratic Party 5, 127
Democrats 46, 48, 55, 83, 85, 87, 89,
125–127, 219
DeSantis, Ron 6, 8, 70, 89, 226–227, 89
Detroit Public Health Department 77–78

Economist 11, 40
Edwards, Anbrasi 29
El Salvador 20
Emergency Preparedness and Management 182
emergency response systems (EMS) 161, 164
emergency use authorization (EUA) 54
employers 172
EMS *see* emergency response systems
epidemics 4–5, 161–162, 232

Facebook 67, 70, 152
FASB 132, 221
Fauci, Anthony 42, 45, 49, 66, 73–74, 83, 127,
129, 233–234
FDA *see* Food and Drug Administration
federal government 4, 44, 55, 58, 65, 69, 77,
88, 127, 176, 186, 199, 201–202, 219–220,
222; Congress 173; executive branch 172;
judiciary 173
Federation of State Medical Boards (FSMB)
126, 131, 220–221

Fineberg, Harvey, *New England Journal of
Medicine* 42
Florida 7–8, 44, 57–58, 67–68, 70, 78, 86–87,
89, 136, 171, 214–216, 226, 233
Florida Department of Health Medical Quality
Assurance Program 132
Florida Department of Health Services 134
Florida Medical Licensure Board 89, 136
Food and Drug Administration (FDA) 67,
129–130, 191, 200, 203
FSMB *see* Federation of State Medical Boards
Fukuyama, Francis, *Trust: The Social Virtues and
the Creation of Prosperity* 175

Galtung, Johan 13–14
Garber, Randi 18, 36–37
Gates Foundation 207
Gawande, Atul 236
Geneva Conventions 15, 22
Germany 44–45, 170, 173, 175, 228
Gessen, Masha 177
Gohmert, Louie 6, 133
Gold, Simone 6, 126, 133–134
Gorbachev, Mikhail 20
Gottlieb, Scott 44, 164, 167, 200, 203, 234
Government Accounting Office (GAO) 73, 76,
80, 86, 143, 202
Grant, James 20
"Green Pass" 70–71
Grounder, Celine 88
gun violence 145

Hahn, Stephen 55
Hammad, Jeyda 25
HATD *see* Healing Across the Divides
Hawaii 67
Healing Across the Divides (HATD) 23, 26
health: care 7, 22, 127; community-centered
160, 182, 184; diplomacy 16, 19–20;
impact of conflict on 14–15; insurance
50–51, 57, 74, 83, 177; interventions 16;
peace to 17, 26–29; peace to public 26–29;
professionals (*see* health professionals);
public (*see* public health); and well-being
14, 27, 144
Health and Human Services (HHS) 202, 203
Health and Medical Coordinating Coalitions
(HMCC) 189–190
Health and National Security 200–201
Health Care Financing Committee 195
health insurers 173
HHS *see* Health and Human Services
Hispanics/Latinos 51, 64, 79, 83, 144–145

homelessness 146, 193
Hong Kong 40, 78
hospital associations 174
hydroxychloroquine 125, 128–130, 220

IHR *see* International Health Regulations
Inflation Reduction Act (IRA) 84
International Campaign to Ban Landmines 16
International Committee of the Red Cross
    (ICRC) 16, 21
International Health Regulations (IHR) 207
International Physicians for the Prevention of
    Nuclear War (IPPNW) 16, 19–22, 198–199
IRA *see* Inflation Reduction Act
Irish Times 47, 235
isolation 40, 60, 80, 142, 146, 160, 162–164
Italy 40, 41, 48, 70–71, 225, 236
Ivermectin 17, 72, 78, 132, 135

Jacksonville Union 52
Jaffa, Harry 234
Jensen, Scott 85
Johnson, Ron 228
Jones, Camara 163
Journal of the American Medical Association
    (*JAMA*) 75

Kawachi, Ichiro 150
Kemp, Brian 68
Kim, Jim Yong 160
Klaas, Brian, *Corruptible: Who Gets Power and
    How It Changes Us* 126
Kleinman, Arthur 13
knowledge: bureaucratic use of 13;
    communication of 16, 21–23; cross-cultural
    36; intimate 22, 167; and skills 36, 38;
    technical 175
Kohrs, Rachel 235
Koop, Everett 236

Labor Unions 174
Ladapo, Joseph 7, 86, 89, 132, 136, 233
Lamb, Marcus 74, 233
Lancet 82, 214
The Lancet COVID-19 Commission 227
LaTulippe, Steven 132
leadership 56–57, 74, 88, 172, 175–176,
    199–200, 235; active 7, 162; American 154;
    charismatic 13; effective 208; governmental
    177; health professional 209; medical 55;
    national 199; political 45, 170, 208; roles
    161; senior 218; state 171, 177
legitimacy 126

LMICs *see* low-income and middle-income
    countries
local health departments (LHDs) 183
Louisiana 67–68
low-income and middle-income countries
    (LMICs) 198
Lown, Bernard 22, 198
Luckmann, Thomas 12

Maddocks, Ian 19–20
managed care organizations (MCOs) 173
Mann-Shalvi, Hanni 35
Massachusetts, State of 89, 131, 161–162, 167,
    174–175, 177
Massachusetts Community Tracing
    Collaborative 164
Massachusetts Department of Public Health
    (DPH) 162, 164
Massachusetts Joint Committee on COVID-19
    182, 189–195
Massachusetts Medical Society 216
Massachusetts Service Alliance (MSA) 193–194
Massachusetts Virtual Epidemiologic Network
    (MAVEN) 191
MassHealth 183, 186
McClellan, Mark 44, 203, 234
McConnell, Mitch 66
MCOs *see* managed care organizations
Médecins sans Frontières/Doctors without
    Borders 16, 22
medical debt 83
Medical Reserve Corps 193
Mengele, Josef 74, 233
mental health and substance abuse (MHSA)
    142–143; family, community, and societal
    responses 149–150; and inevitable human
    response of resilience 147–148; integrated
    primary and 147; racism and the 147; social
    factors 146–147; systemic changes to health
    system 148–149
MHSA *see* mental health and substance abuse
Mississippi 67
Mollica, Richard 146, 151

Nathan, Marty Dr 153
National Academy of Medicine (NAM) 205,
    207, 214, 225–226, 228–232, 245
National Academy of Sciences (NAS) 185
National Center for Health Statistics 63
National Education Association 174
National Institute of Allergy and Infectious
    Diseases 49
National Institutes of Health (NIH) 129

Native Americans 51, 85
Newsom, Gavin 220
New York 171
New York Times 3, 15, 41, 46, 48, 58, 76,
    78, 201
NIH *see* National Institutes of Health
Nobel Peace Prize 16, 20, 199
nonpharmaceutical interventions (NPIs) 161
NPIs *see* nonpharmaceutical interventions

Obama, Barack 41, 182, 200
Occupied Palestinian Territory (OPT) 23
Osterholm, Michael 59
Ottawa Charter for Health Promotion 14

Pan, Richard 86
Pan American Health Organization (PAHO)
    16, 20
Partners in Health (PIH) 160–161, 164, 167,
    176, 186
patient care-centric systems (PCC) 182–186
Paxlovid 76, 81, 85–86, 88–89
peace 26; and health 13–14, 17–18; negative 13;
    positive 13; work 38
peace through health (PtH) 6, 8, 11–12, 16,
    235; articles and/or monographs 18–19;
    communication of knowledge; health
    professional practice across the divides
    21–22; definition 15–17; evocation and
    extension of altruism 22; health diplomacy:
    mediation and conflict transformation;
    construction of goals in common;
    superordinate goals 19–20; limiting the
    destructiveness of war 20–21; peace to
    health, or peace to public health and public
    trust 26–29; personalizing the enemy 23;
    social healing strengthening resilience;
    increasing trust 24–26; sociological
    underpinnings of 12–14; solidarity and
    support; noncooperation and dissent 23–24
Pennsylvania 82, 86, 215–216
People's Action 66
personal protective equipment (PPE)/mask
    wearing 57, 63, 65, 190, 201, 218
Pfizer vaccine 67–68
PH *see* public health
Physicians for Human Rights-Israel
    (PHR-Israel) 22–24
Physicians for Human Rights-USA
    (PHR-USA) 23
post-traumatic stress disorder (PTSD) 15
PPE *see* personal protective equipment
PtH *see* peace through health

public health 17, 56–57, 77, 136, 182–186,
    204, 217; crises 49, 147, 160, 176; emergency
    199; infrastructure 68, 190, 195, 230;
    interventions 54, 150; officials 79, 83–84,
    215; professionals 40, 199, 203; sector
    229; system 7, 17, 56, 78, 127, 176–177,
    181–185, 189, 199, 214, 236; workers
    164–165
public healthcare professionals 203; *see also*
    public health

Qatar 88, 206

Raoult, Didier 128, 129
Reagan, Ronald 134, 236
Rebuild Consortium 26–28
recovery 151
Red Crescent 22
regulation 174, 182, 206–207, 220–221,
    245; biosafety 198; contact-tracing 186;
    government 227
Republican Party 5, 14, 126–127
Republicans 4–5, 40, 55, 65, 72, 80, 83, 85, 87,
    89, 125–127, 131, 213, 219, 228
resilience 25–26, 151
resource-based relative value scale (RBRVS) 218
Rigano, Gregory 128–129
Rodriguez-García, Rosalía, *How Can Health
    Serve as a Bridge to Peace?* 18
Rush, Benjamin 134

State Action for Public Health Excellence 1.0
    (SAPHE 1.0) 183, 184, 188,189
State Action for Public Health Excellence 2.0
    (SAPHE 2.0) 183, 184, 189
school 55, 84, 186; buildings 194; children 36;
    closing 58; closures 144, 163; loss of 146;
    medical 37; opening 62, 127; shootings 145
Schumacher, Carol 85, 150
Scott, Dylan 57, 69
SEIU *see* Service Employees International Union
Service Employees International Union
    (SEIU) 174
short of breath (SOB) 50–51
social capital 28, 150–153
social care ecosystem 160, 182, 184
social distancing 40, 50–51, 54, 57–58, 63,
    162–163, 176
socio-economic disparities 5–6, 25, 78, 149,
    153, 186, 228
Soviet Union 20, 64
Stages of Change Model 24
State of Massachusetts 131, 161–162

Steinberg, Darrell 143
Stockpiling Essential Supplies 201
suicide 49, 63, 143–147, 149
Sunrise Movement 243
Supreme Court 24, 51, 75, 83, 173, 177, 217
Sweden 79

Taylor-Robinson, Simon 20
telehealth 148–149, 217
Tennessee 67, 80, 221
testing 54, 162
Texas 214
Times Literary Supplement 46, 208
Tribe, Rachel 25
Trump, Donald 4–6, 39, 41–42, 44–45, 47,
    55, 57–58, 72–73, 78–79, 80, 127–130,
    177–178, 201, 228, 236
trust 24–26; and credibility 214–215, 229;
    importance of 175–176; interpersonal 150;
    public 17, 26–29

UNICEF *see* United Nations Children's Fund
United Auto Workers 174
United Kingdom 170
United Nations Children's Fund (UNICEF) 20
U.S. attorneys 46
USA Today 47

US Department of Health and Human
    Services 220
US Public Health Service 167
U.S. Senator 65

Vermont 58
violence 26; cultural 13; direct 13–14; domestic
    27, 142; gun 145; police 49, 147; political
    13–14, 233; structural 13–14

Walensky, Rochelle 87, 205
Washington Post 47, 49, 52, 77, 128
Washington, State of 161, 163–164, 167,
    175, 177
White House Council of Economic Advisers 47
white supremacy 127
WHO *see* World Health Organization
World Bank 160, 197–198
World Health Assembly (WHA) 207
World Health Organization (WHO) 22, 25, 64,
    149, 162, 206–208
World War II 25–26, 40
Wuhan 61, 142

Young, Ed 227–228

Zwirner, David 48

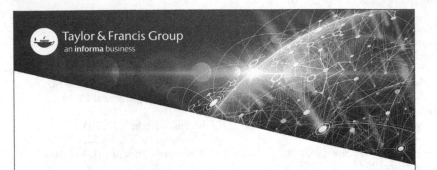

Printed in the United States
by Baker & Taylor Publisher Services